ROSS & WILSON

Anatomy and Physiology

Colouring and Workbook

6th Edition

ROSS & WILSON

6th Edition

Anatomy and Physiology

Colouring and Workbook

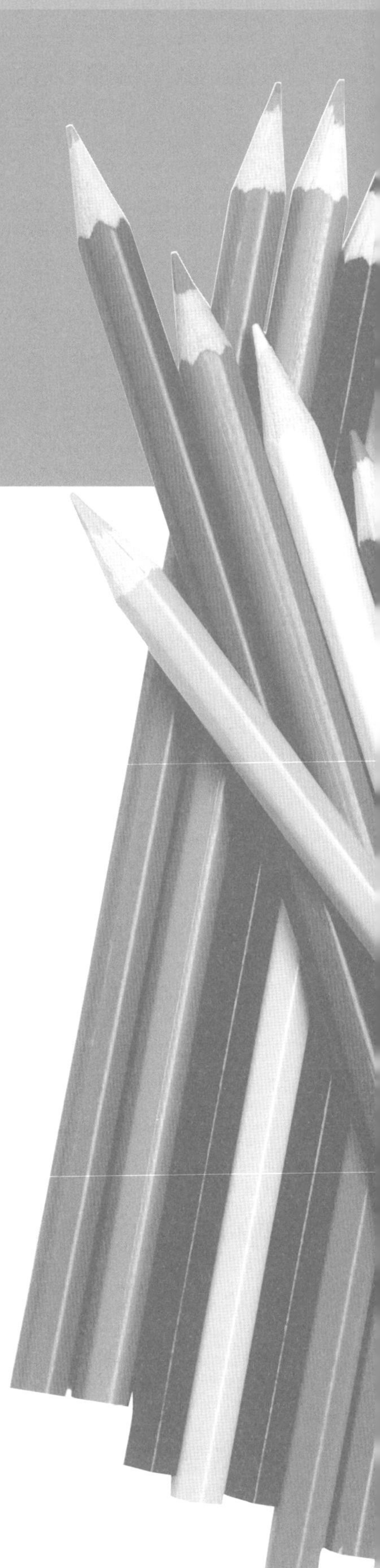

Anne Waugh BSc (Hons) MSc CertEd SRN RNT PFHEA
Former Senior Teaching Fellow and Senior Lecturer,
School of Health and Social Care, Edinburgh Napier University,
Edinburgh, UK

Allison Grant BSc PhD FHEA
Lecturer, School of Health and Life Sciences, Glasgow
Caledonian University, Glasgow, UK

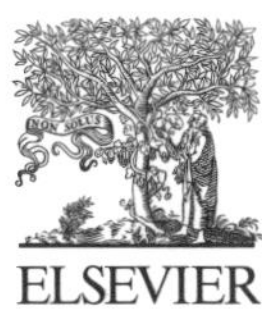

ELSEVIER

First edition 2004
Second edition 2006
Third edition 2010
Fourth edition 2014
Fifth edition 2019

Notices

Practitioners and researchers must always rely on their own experience and knowledge in evaluating and using any information, methods, compounds or experiments described herein. Because of rapid advances in the medical sciences, in particular, independent verification of diagnoses and drug dosages should be made. To the fullest extent of the law, no responsibility is assumed by Elsevier, authors, editors or contributors for any injury and/or damage to persons or property as a matter of products liability, negligence or otherwise, or from any use or operation of any methods, products, instructions, or ideas contained in the material herein.

ISBN: 978-0-323-87240-9

Content Strategist: Poppy Garraway/Robert Edwards
Senior Content Development Specialist: Elizabeth McCormac
Senior Project Manager: Anne Collett
Senior Book Designer: Margaret Reid

Printed in the UK

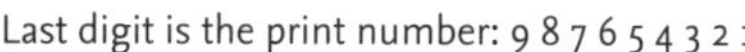
Last digit is the print number: 9 8 7 6 5 4 3 2 1

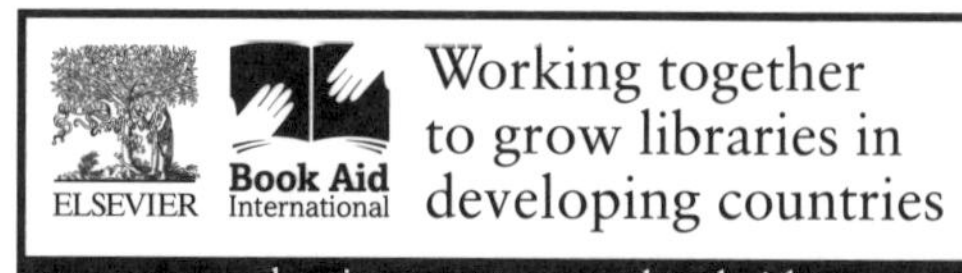

Contents

Preface

Ross & Wilson has been a core text for students of anatomy and physiology for almost sixty years. Although this companion text has been extensively revised to match the 14th edition of the main text, providing a range of revision activities to facilitate and consolidate your learning, it can also be used to support any general anatomy and physiology course. Readers who own the new 14th edition of *Ross & Wilson* will also find many more online activities to support their studies.

The systems approach used in the main text forms the framework for the exercises, many of which are based on clear illustrations of body structure and functions. A variety of activity styles is used to maintain interest and provide choice, recognising that students study, learn and revise in different ways. The section on 'How to use this book', p. ix, explains how the icons and exercises are used in the text.

We hope that you will find this book a stimulating and useful companion to your anatomy and physiology studies, particularly when you need to test your learning or are preparing for assessments. We are always delighted to receive feedback, especially from students, so please continue to send your comments to us via the publishers.

We are very grateful for the support we have received from the project team at Elsevier, particularly Poppy Garraway, Betsy McCormac and Anne Collett.

We would also like to thank our families, Andy, Seona and Struan, for their love and support.

Anne Waugh
Allison Grant
October 2022

How to use this book

ICONS AND EXERCISES

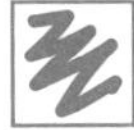 **Colouring:** identify and colour structures on diagrams.

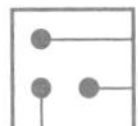 **Labelling:** identify and label structures on diagrams.

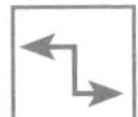 **Matching:** match statements with reasons; structures with functions; key choices with blanks in a paragraph; and organs on diagrams.

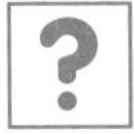 **Multiple-choice questions (MCQs):** identify the correct option from a list of four. Where there is more than one correct option, this is indicated in the question.

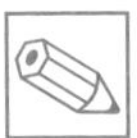 **Completion:** identify the missing words to complete paragraphs.

 **Definitions:** explain the meaning of a common anatomical or physiological term.

 **Pot luck:** a variety of other exercises is also used to facilitate learning. Simple guidance about completion is provided.

 **Applying what you know:** indicates revision exercises to apply what you have learned.

Combinations of these activities are also used to provide variety in the text.

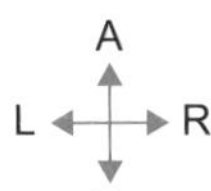

A/P: anterior/posterior
S/I: superior/inferior
L/R: left/right
L/M: lateral/medial
P/D: proximal/distal

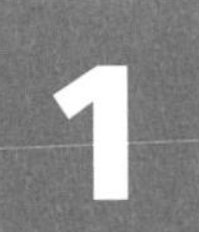

1 Anatomy and organisation of the body

The human body is complex, like a highly technical and sophisticated machine. Although it operates as a single entity, it is made up of several parts that work interdependently. This chapter will help you learn about the major systems and control mechanisms that maintain integrated body functioning. The last sections consider the organisation of the body, including anatomical terminology, the skeleton and body cavities.

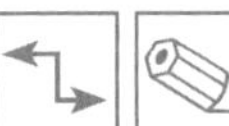

MATCHING AND COMPLETION

1. Match the key choices below with the labels on Figure 1.1.

Key choices:
System level
Cellular level
Organ level
The human being
Chemical level
Tissue level

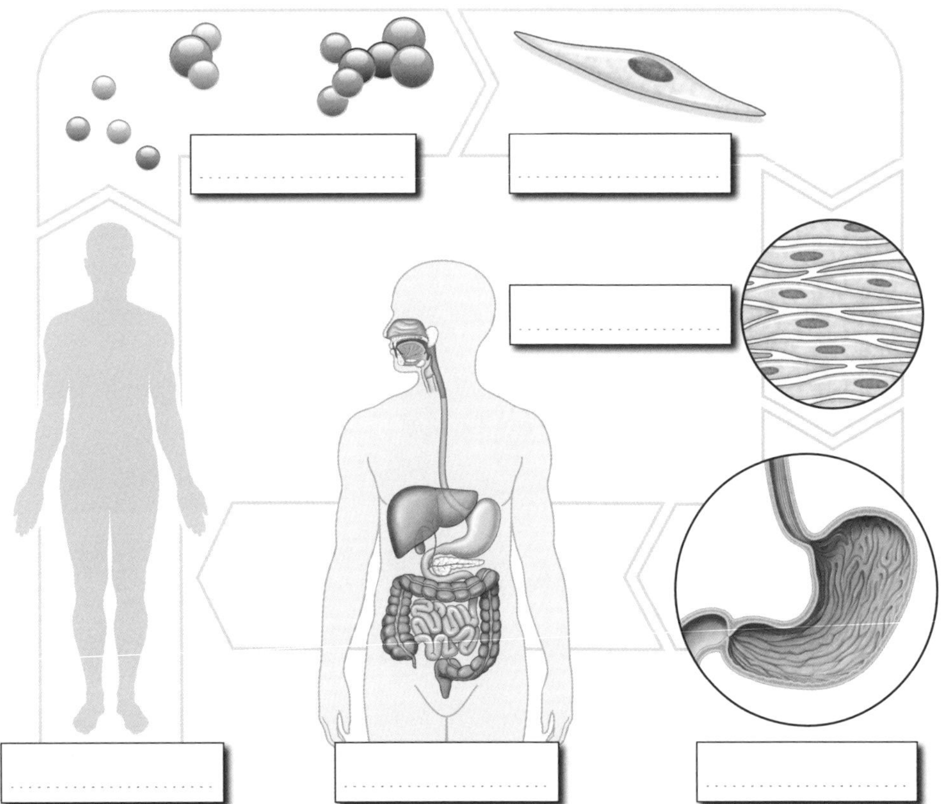

Figure 1.1 The levels of structural complexity

2. Using the list of key choices on previous page, complete Table 1.1.

Table 1.1 Levels of structural complexity and their characteristics

Level of structural complexity	Characteristics
	Comprises many systems that work interdependently to maintain health
	Carries out a specific function and is composed of different types of tissue
	Smallest independent units of living matter
	Consists of one or more organs and contributes to one or more survival needs of the body
	Atoms and molecules that form the building blocks of larger substances
	Group of cells with similar structures and functions

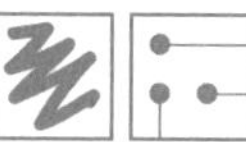

COLOURING AND LABELLING

3. Figure 1.2 shows two of the body's transport systems. Complete the captions below each one.

4. Colour and label the structures identified on Figure 1.2.

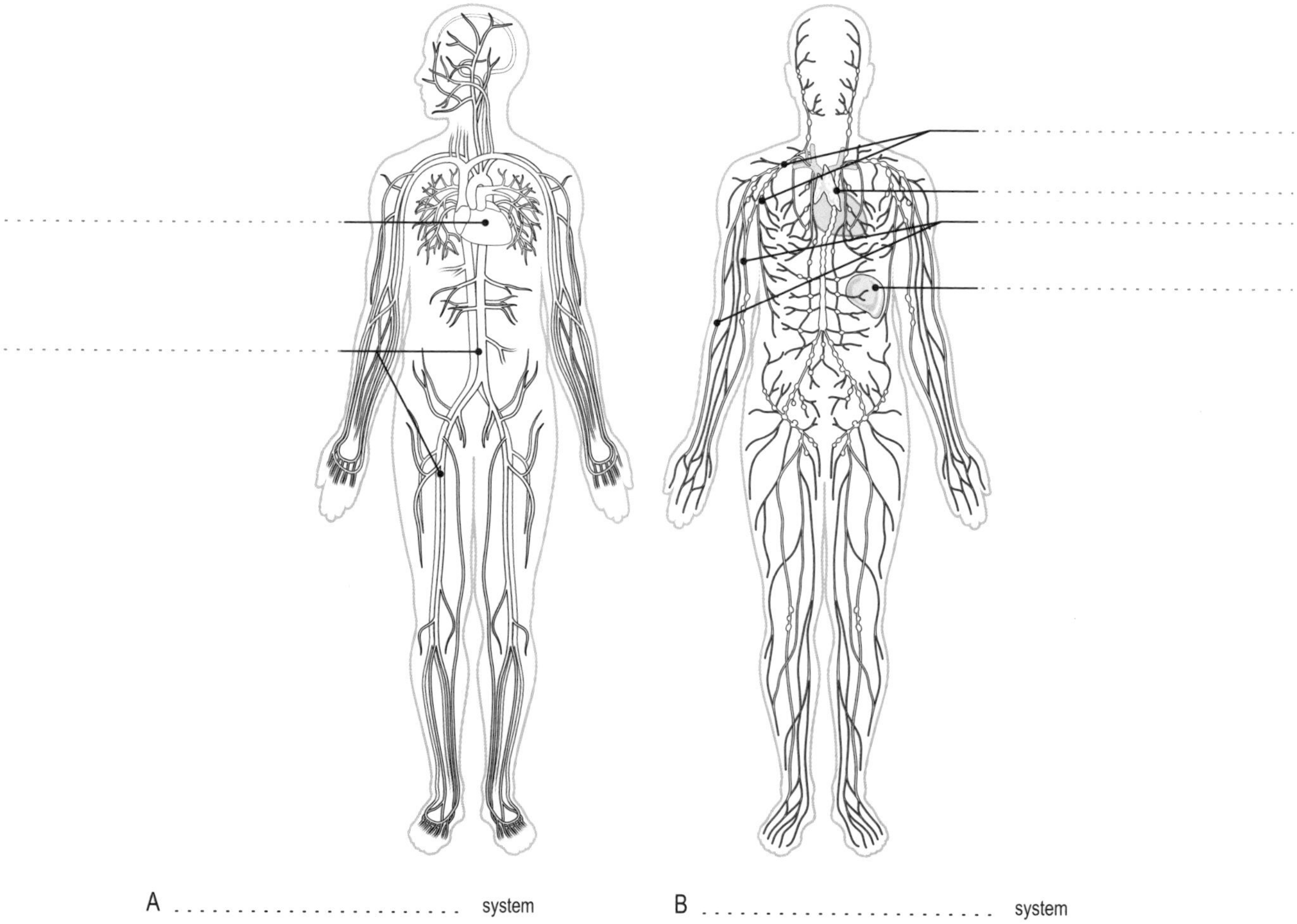

A .... system

B .... system

Figure 1.2 Body transport systems

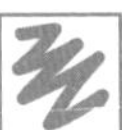 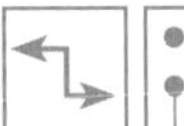

COLOURING, MATCHING AND LABELLING

5. Colour and match the following parts of the nervous system shown on Figure 1.3:

- ○ Central nervous system
- ○ Peripheral nervous system

6. Label the structures indicated on Figure 1.3.

7. The very fast withdrawal of a finger from a very hot surface is an example of a

_______________________________________.

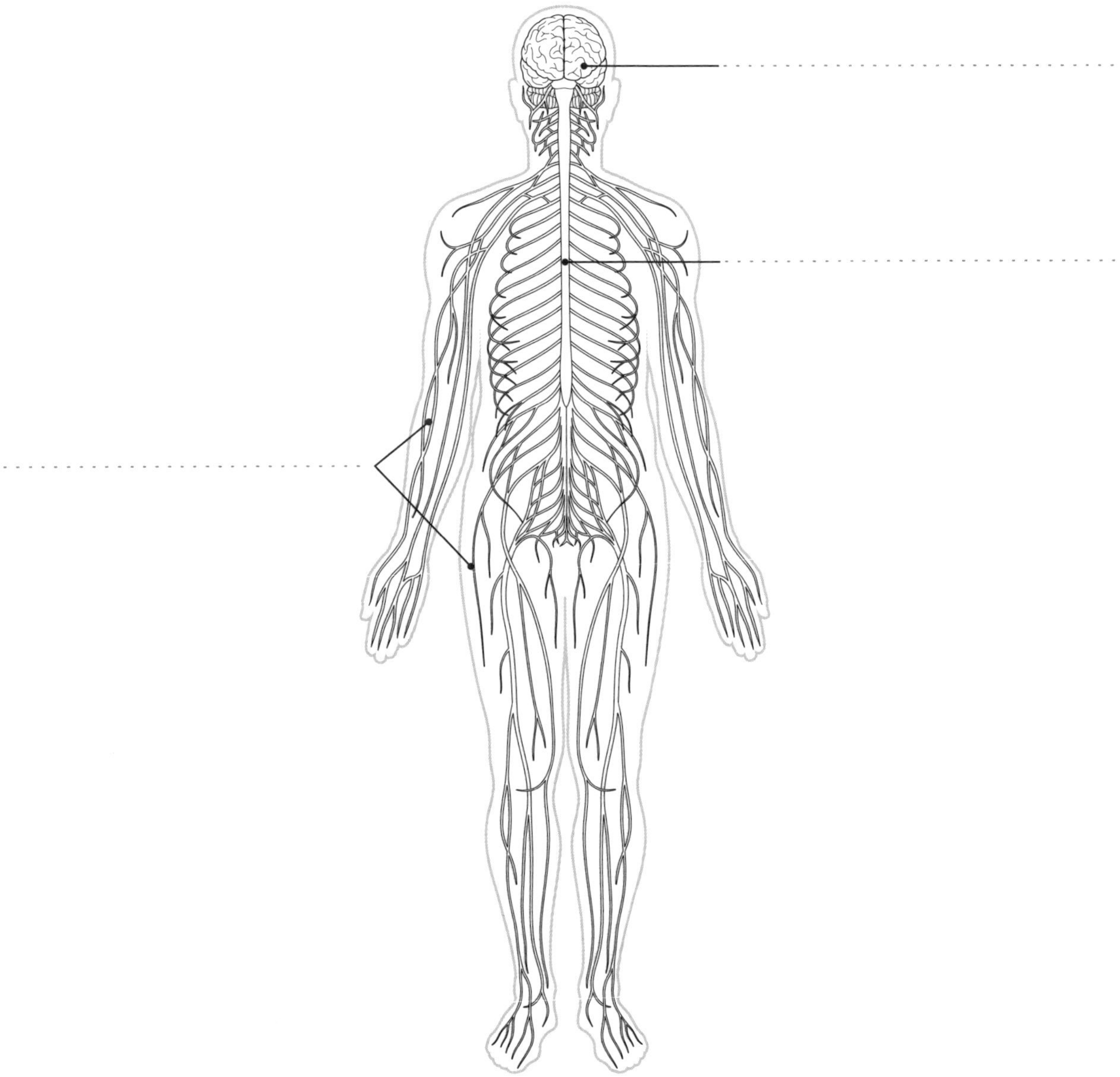

Figure 1.3 The nervous system

COLOURING, MATCHING AND LABELLING

8. Colour, match and label the structures listed below with those identified on Figure 1.4:

- ○ Bronchus
- ○ Left lung
- ○ Trachea
- ○ Larynx
- ○ Nasal cavity
- ○ Pharynx
- ○ Right lung
- ○ Alveoli

9. Name the two main gases exchanged in the lungs.

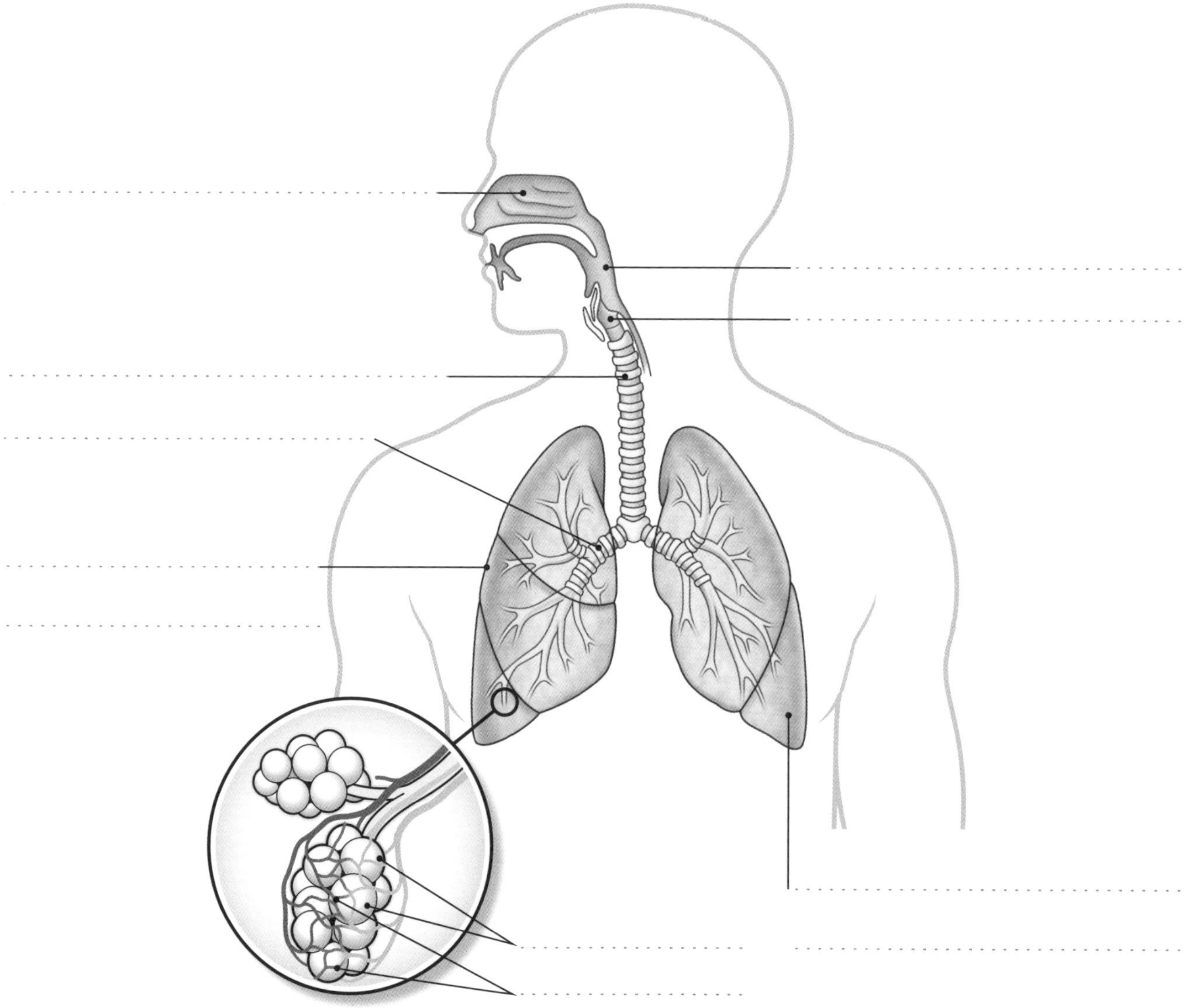

____

____

____

Figure 1.4 The respiratory system

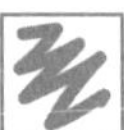 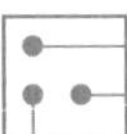

COLOURING AND LABELLING

10. Colour and label the organs of the digestive system shown on Figure 1.5.

11. Circle the accessory organs of the digestive system shown on Figure 1.5

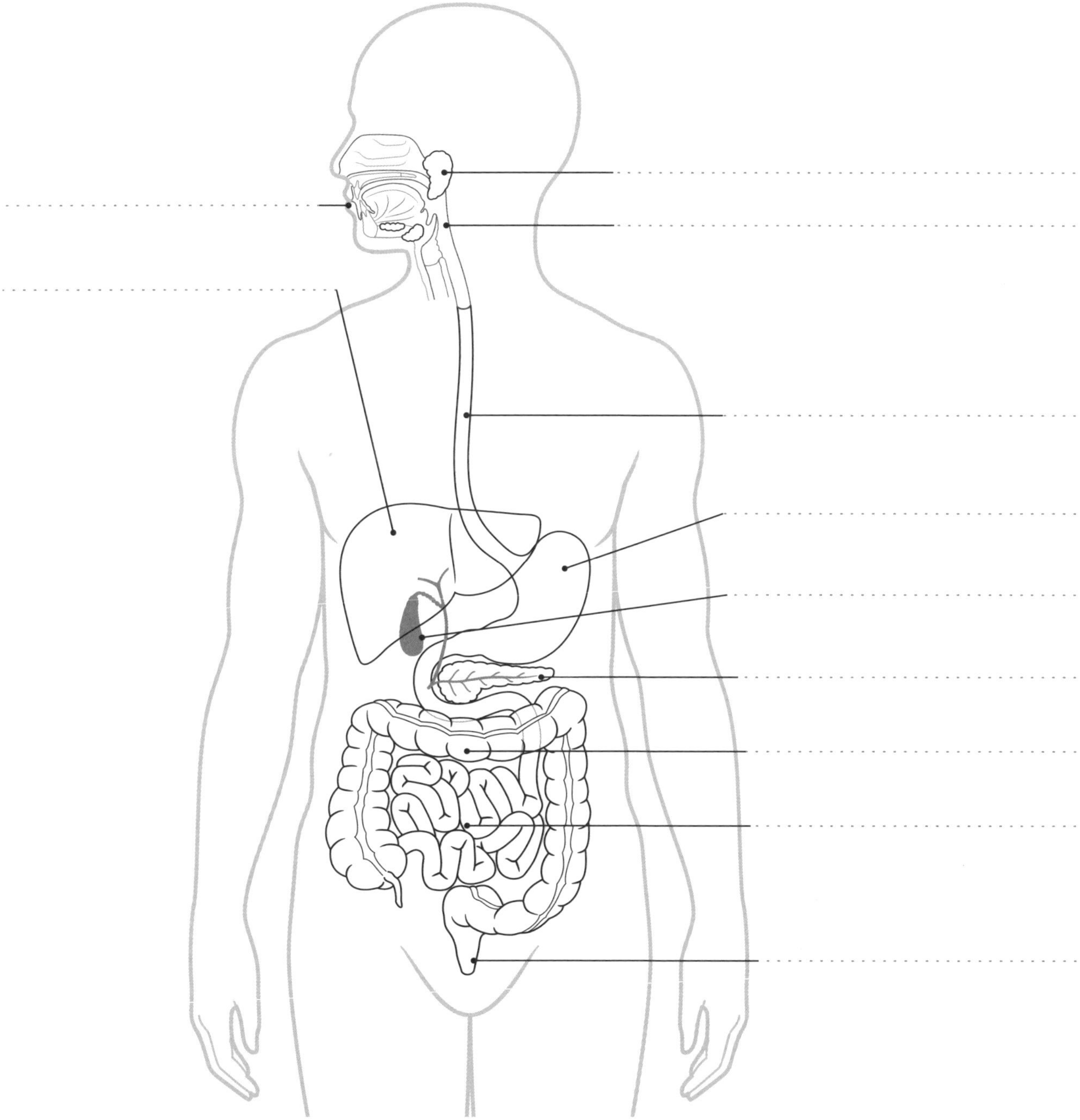

Figure 1.5 The digestive system

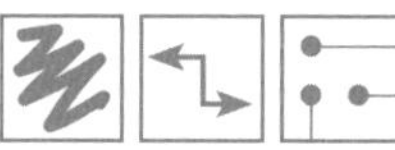

COLOURING, MATCHING AND LABELLING

12. Colour, match and label the organs of the urinary system shown on Figure 1.6:

- O Bladder
- O Kidney
- O Urethra
- O Ureter

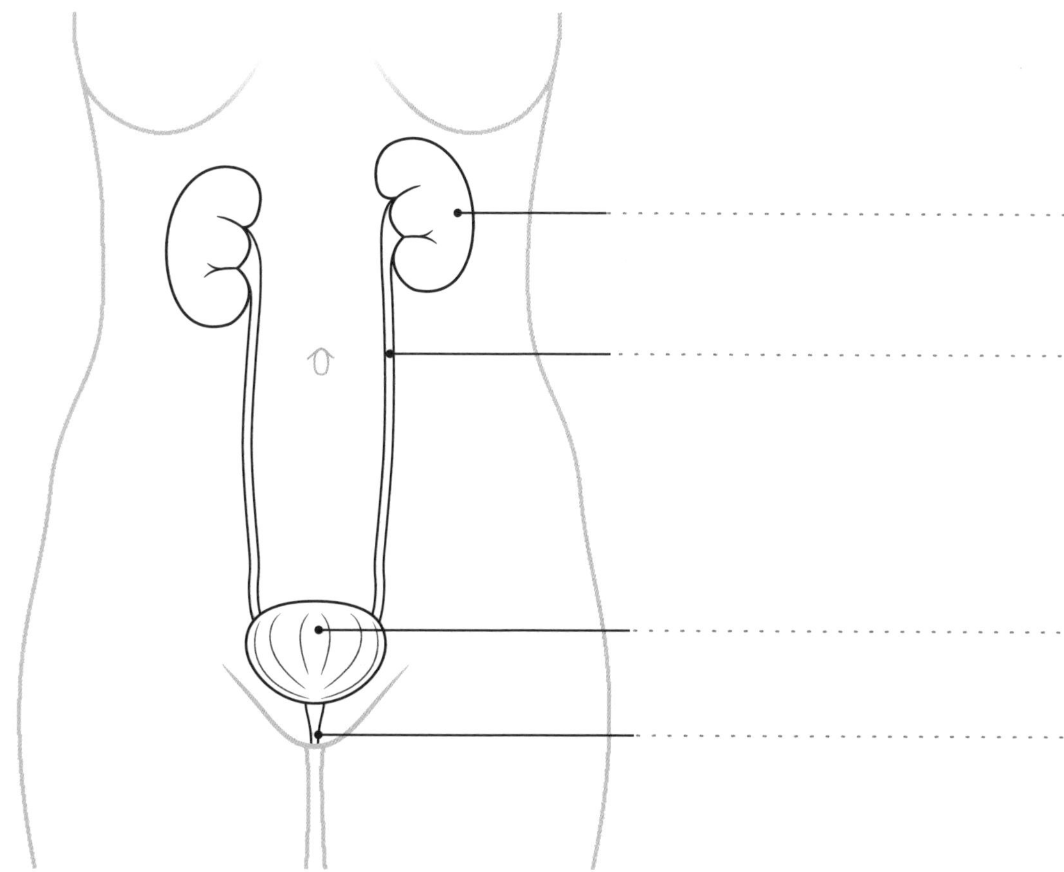

Figure 1.6 The urinary system

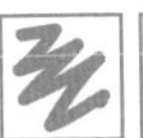 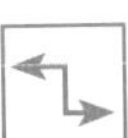 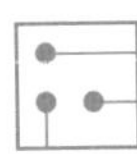

COLOURING, MATCHING AND LABELLING

13. Colour and match the following parts of the skeleton in Figure 1.7:

- ○ Axial skeleton
- ○ Appendicular skeleton

14. Label the bones identified on Figure 1.7.

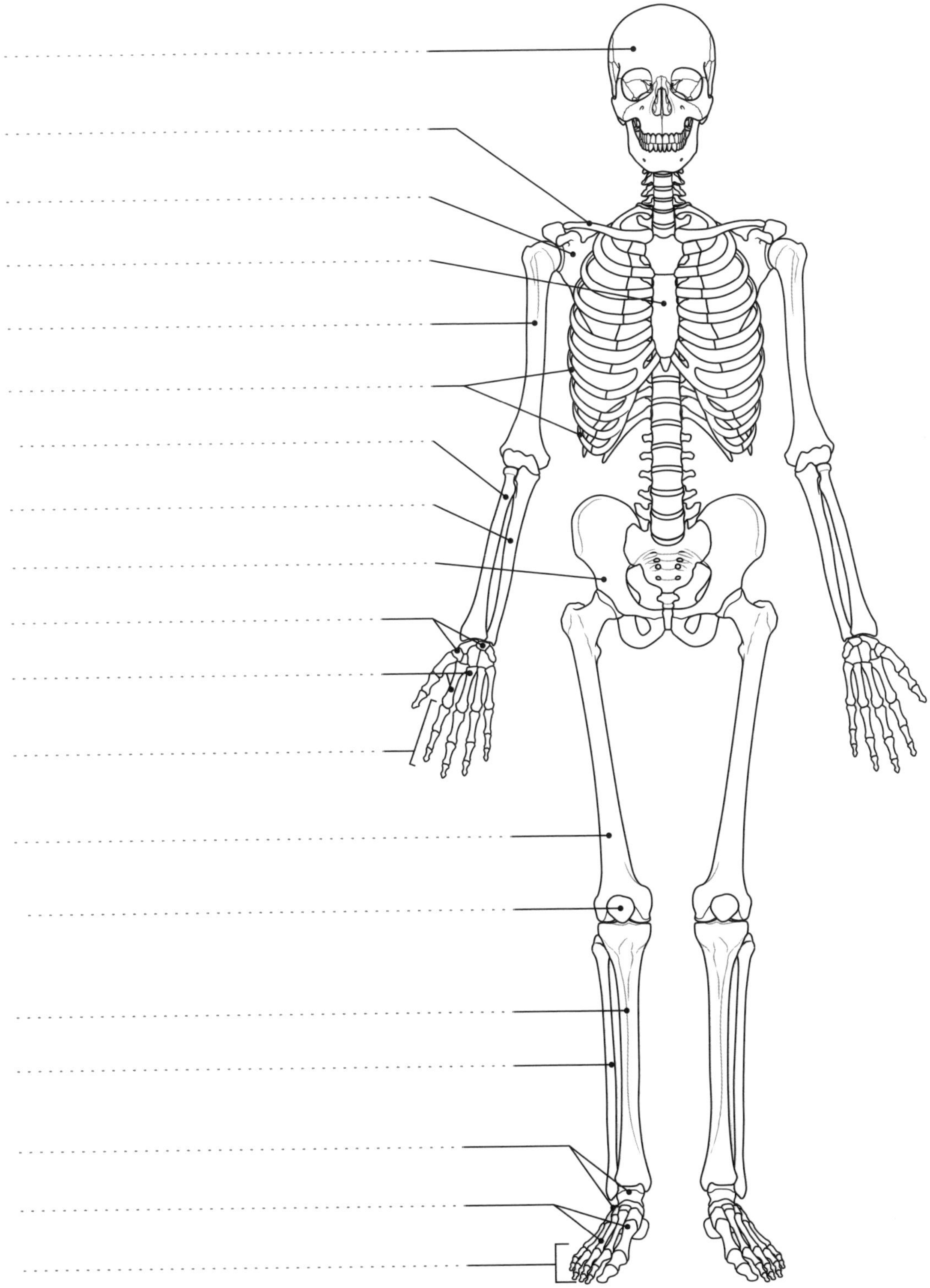

Figure 1.7 The skeleton

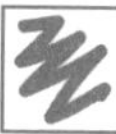

COLOURING AND MATCHING

15. Colour and match the structures listed below with those identified on Figure 1.8:

○ Vagina	○ Testis	○ Bladder
○ Ovary	○ Prostate gland	○ Urethra
○ Uterine tube	○ Penis	
○ Uterus	○ Deferent duct	

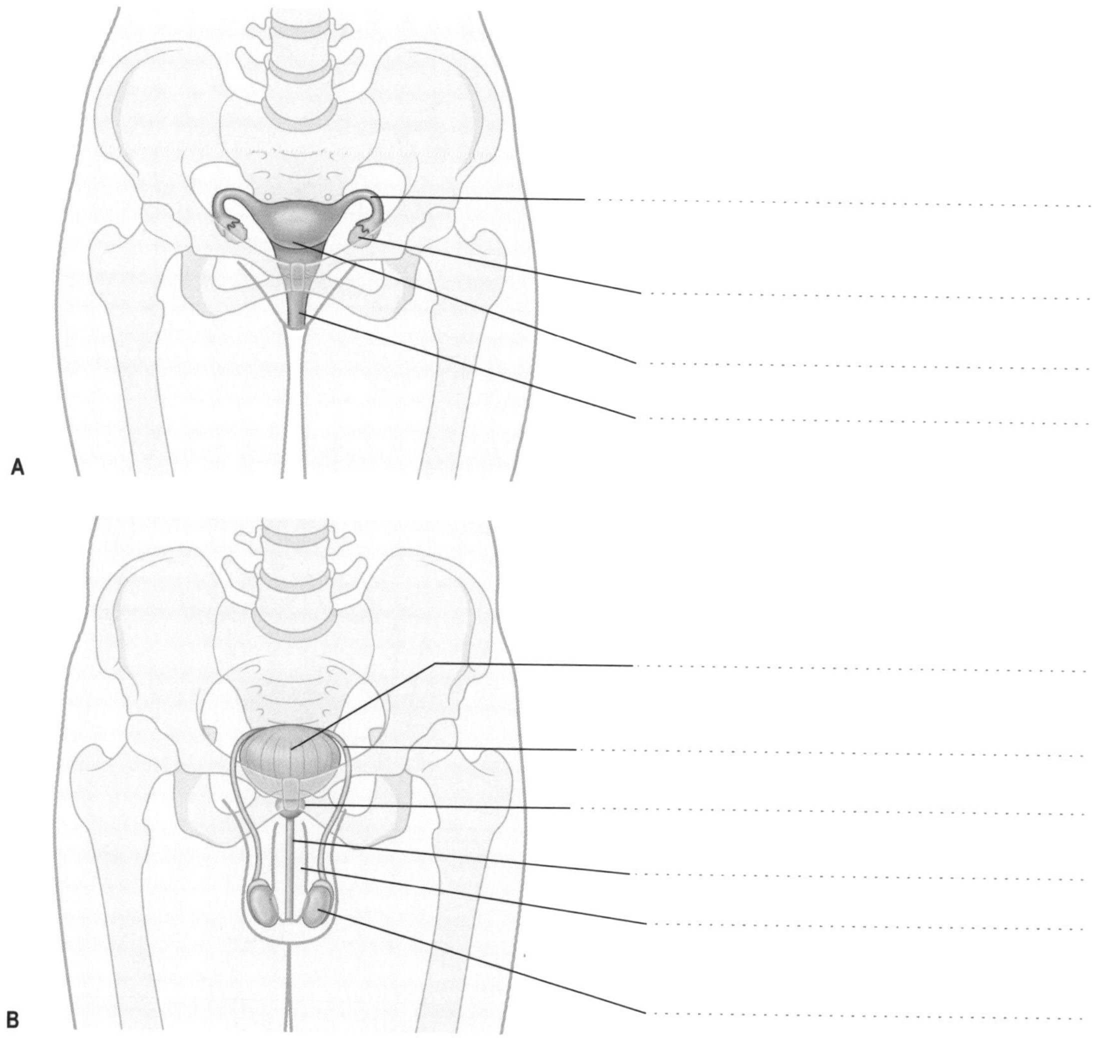

A

B

Figure 1.8 The reproductive systems. A. Female. B. Male.

COMPLETION

16. Complete the paragraph below describing the function of the female reproductive system.

The childbearing years begin at ______________________ and end at the ______________________. During this time, an ______________________ matures in the ovary about every ______________________ days. If ______________________ takes place, the zygote embeds itself in the ______________________ and grows to maturity during pregnancy, or ______________________, in about ______________________ weeks. If fertilisation does not occur, it is expelled from the body along with the ______________________, accompanied by bleeding, called ______________________.

17. Fill in the blanks in the paragraph below to provide an overview of the endocrine system.

The endocrine system consists of a number of ______________________ in various parts of the body. The glands synthesise and secrete chemical messengers called ______________________ into the ______________________. These chemicals stimulate ______________________. Changes in hormone levels are usually controlled by ______________________ mechanisms. The endocrine system, in conjunction with part of the ______________________ system, controls ______________________ body function. Changes involving the latter system are usually ______________________, whereas those of the endocrine system tend to be ______________________ and precise.

18. Complete Table 1.2 by listing the senses in the appropriate columns.

Table 1.2 The common and special senses

Common senses	Special senses

LABELLING

19. Identify the regional terms indicated on Figure 1.9.
20. Label the directional terms indicated on Figure. 1.9.

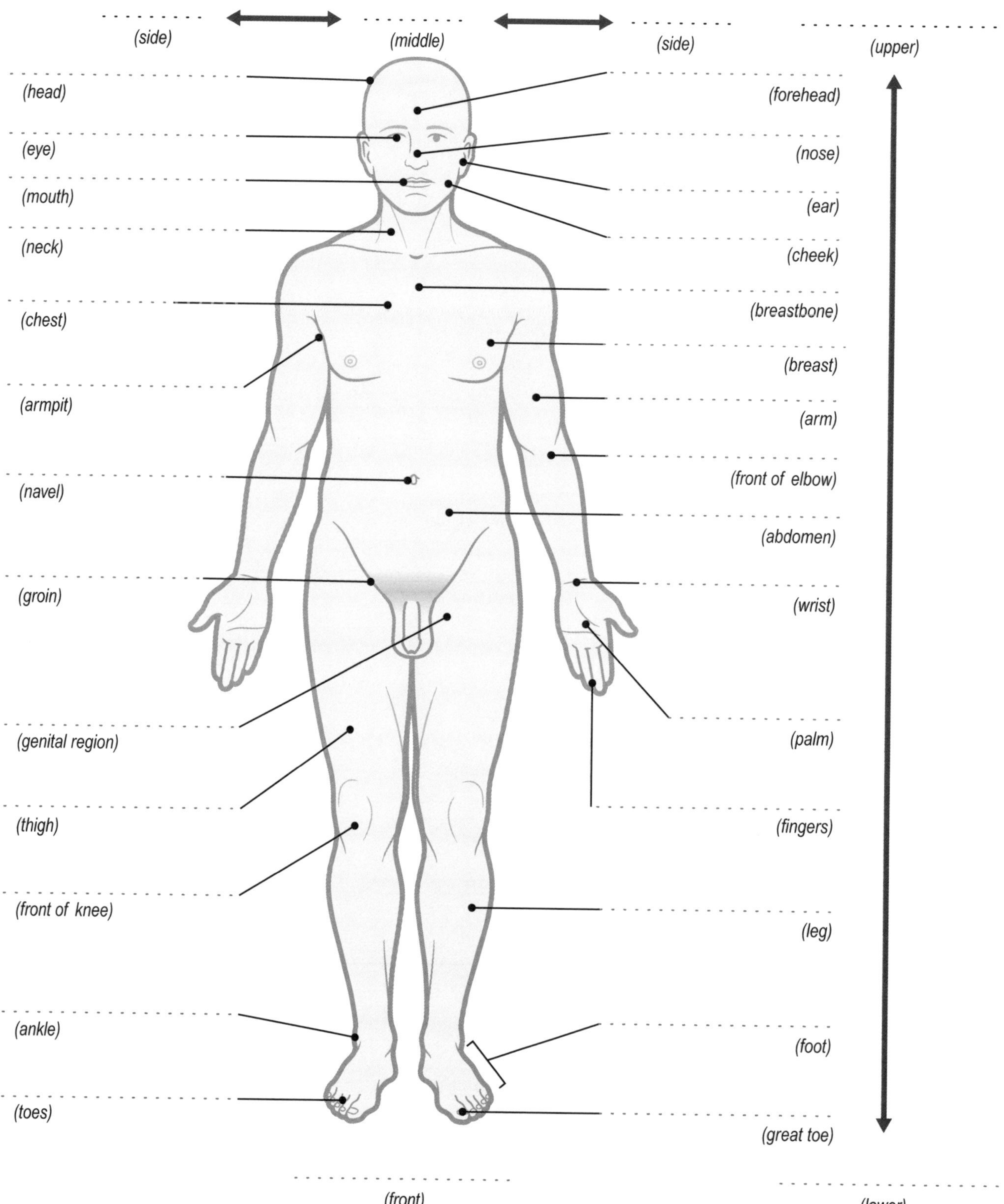

Figure 1.9 Regional and directional terms, two views

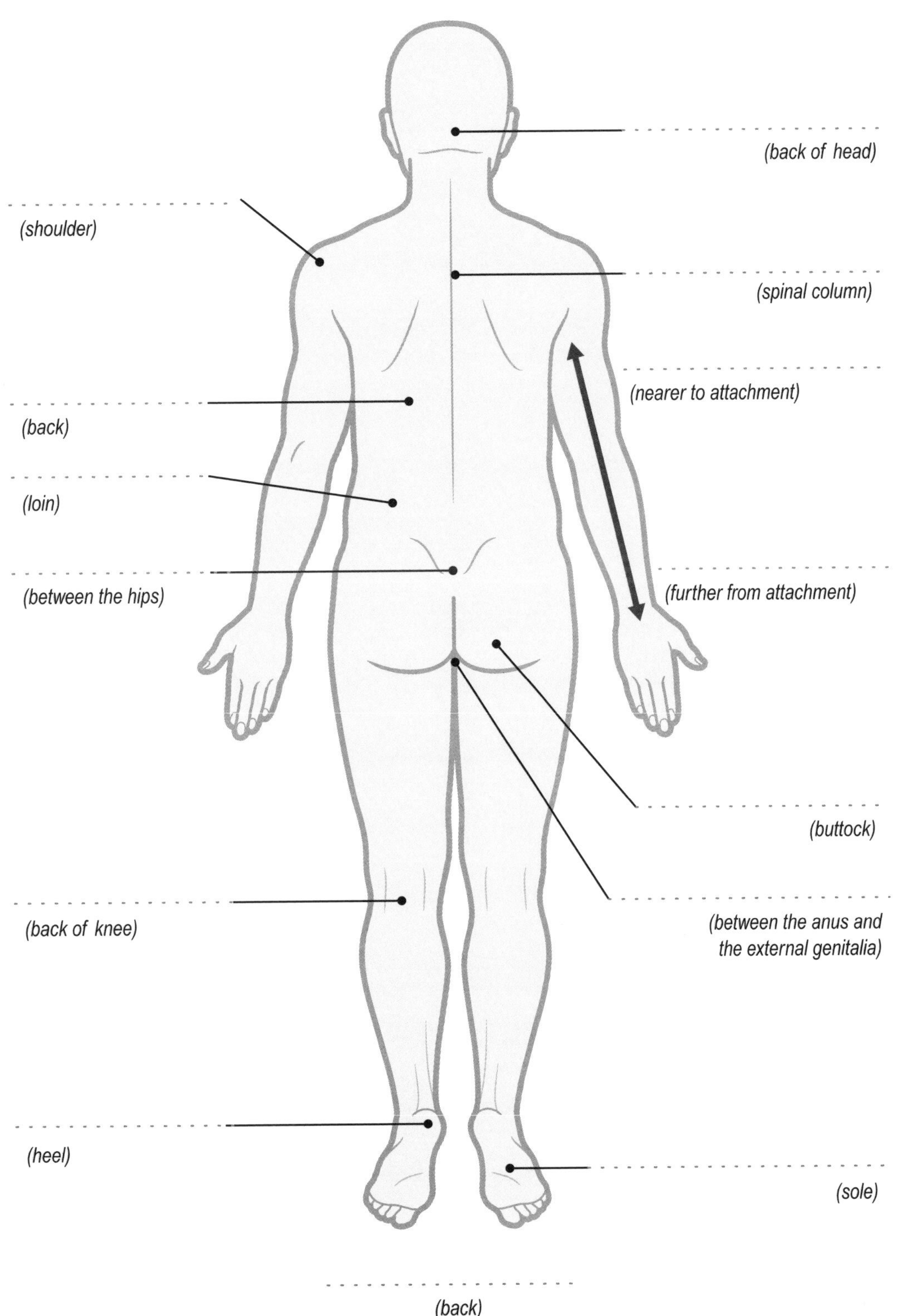
(back of head)
(shoulder)
(spinal column)
(nearer to attachment)
(back)
(loin)
(between the hips)
(further from attachment)
(buttock)
(back of knee)
(between the anus and the external genitalia)
(heel)
(sole)
(back)

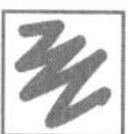 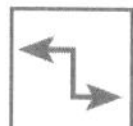 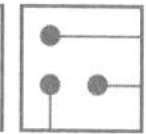

COLOURING, MATCHING AND LABELLING

21. Figure 1.10 shows the three body planes. Colour, match and label them.

- ○ A. ______________________ plane
- ○ B. ______________________ plane
- ○ C. ______________________ plane

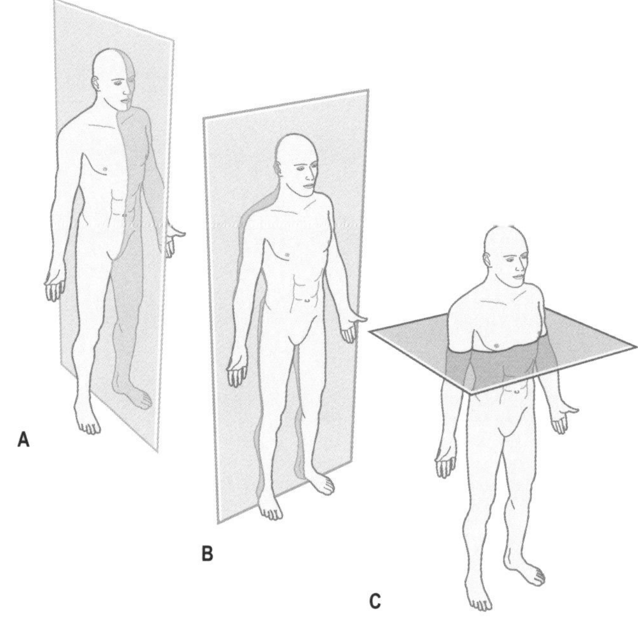

Figure 1.10 The three body planes

22. Colour and match the body cavities on Figure 1.11.

- ○ Thoracic cavity
- ○ Pelvic cavity
- ○ Abdominal cavity
- ○ Cranial cavity

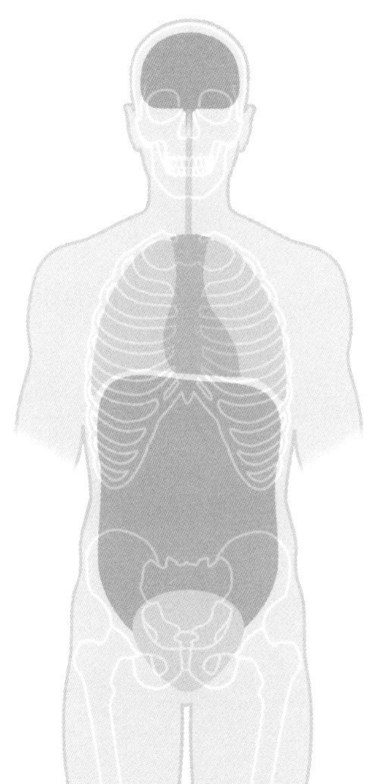

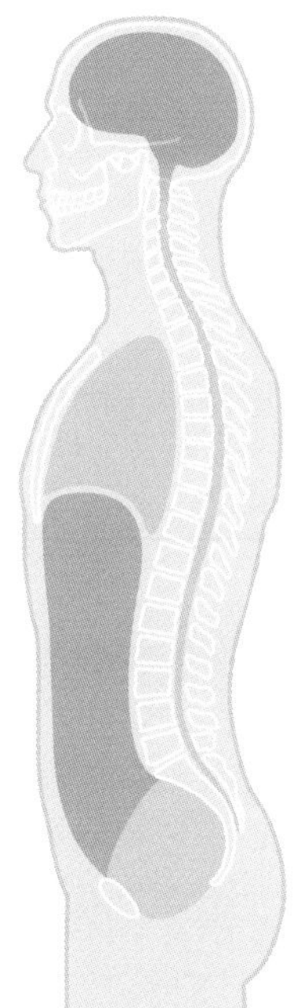

Figure 1.11 The body cavities

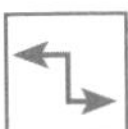

MATCHING

23. Complete Table 1.3 by matching the key choices with their corresponding body cavity.

Key choices	Heart	Spleen
Alveoli	Lungs	Sigmoid colon
Adrenal glands	Kidneys	Small intestine
Appendix	Liver	Stomach
Brain	Oesophagus	Transverse colon
Bronchi	Ovaries	Uterus
Duodenum	Pancreas	Urinary bladder
Gall bladder	Seminal vesicles	

Table 1.3 Contents of the body cavities

Cranial cavity	Thoracic cavity
Abdominal cavity	**Pelvic cavity**

POT LUCK

24. The fluid part of the blood is called ____________________.

25. Blood vessels that carry blood away from the heart are called ____________________.

26. The normal pulse rate in the healthy heart is around ____________________ beats per minute.

27. Name the two parts of the skull. ____________________

28. Which bones form the shoulder girdle? ____________________

29. Name the bones of the lower limb. ____________________

30. Outline the function of lymph nodes: ____________________

31. Briefly describe the difference between specific and nonspecific defence mechanisms.

32. Cross out the incorrect options to use the directional terms correctly.
    a. The humerus is **medial/lateral** to the heart.
    b. The vertebrae are **anterior/posterior** to the kidneys.
    c. The phalanges are **proximal/distal** to the ulna.
    d. The skull is **inferior/superior** to the vertebral column.
    e. The greater omentum is **anterior/posterior** to the small intestine.
    f. The appendix is **inferior/superior** to the stomach.
    g. The patella is **proximal/distal** to the tarsal bones.
    h. The scapulae are **medial/lateral** to the sternum.

33. Define the following terms:
    a. Anabolism ____________________
    b. Catabolism ____________________

MCQs

34. The blood volume in healthy adults is around: ______
    a. 3 litres
    b. 4 litres
    c. 5.5 litres
    d. 7 litres

35. The network of blood vessels that transport blood to and from the lungs is called the: _____
    a. Arterial circulation
    b. Capillary circulation
    c. Systemic circulation
    d. Pulmonary circulation

36. The white blood cells involved in immunity are: ___
    a. Lymphocytes
    b. Erythrocytes
    c. Thrombocytes
    d. Platelets

37. Organs of the lymphatic system include: (Choose all that apply) ____________
    a. Thymus
    b. Thyroid
    c. Adrenal glands
    d. Spleen

38. A nerve that transmits impulses from the spinal cord to the skin can be described as: _______
    a. Afferent
    b. Efferent
    c. Sensory
    d. Reflex

39. The gas that makes up about 21% of atmospheric air is: ____
    a. Carbon dioxide
    b. Hydrogen
    c. Oxygen
    d. Nitrogen

2 Physiological chemistry and processes

An understanding of the body's molecular structure underpins the study of all anatomy and physiology. This chapter covers basic chemistry, the structures and functions of important biological molecules, and some core physiological processes including homeostasis and fluid balance.

BIOLOGICAL CHEMISTRY

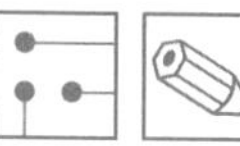

LABELLING AND COMPLETION

1. Figure 2.1 shows the basic structure of an atom. Label the three types of subatomic particles indicated as A, B and C.

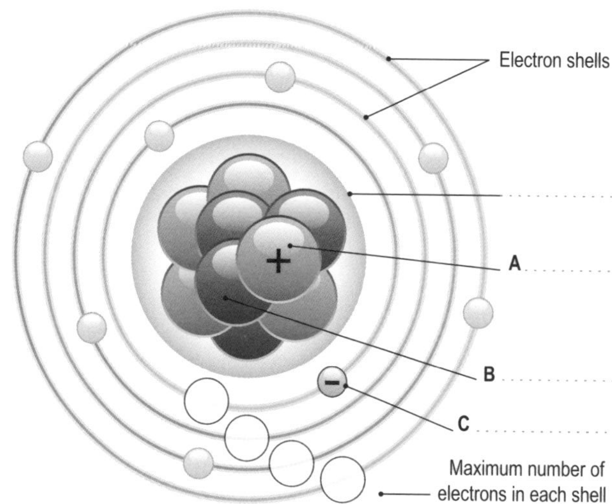

Figure 2.1 The atom

2. The central structure of the atom is called the ____________________________
3. Fill in the blank circles in Figure 2.1 to show the maximum number of electrons in each energy level.
4. Table 2.1 refers to characteristics of the main types of subatomic particle. Complete the table by filling in the blank spaces.

Table 2.1 Characteristics of subatomic particles

Particle	Mass	Electric charge	Location in atom
Proton			
Neutron			
Electron			

5. Ionic bonds and covalent bonds are two important types of chemical bond. Complete Table 2.2 by ticking the appropriate box for each of the descriptive phrases given.

Table 2.2 Chemical bonds

Characteristic	Ionic bonds	Covalent bonds
Gives rise to charged particles (ions)		
Most common bond		
Atoms transfer their electrons		
Links sodium and chloride in a molecule of sodium chloride		
Stable bond		
Atoms share their electrons		
There is no change in the number of protons or neutrons		
The weaker of the two bonds		
Links hydrogen and oxygen in a water molecule		

6. Table 2.3 lists some characteristics of the four main groups of biological substances. For each characteristic, decide to which of the classes of biological molecules it applies (it may apply to more than one), and tick the appropriate boxes in the table.

Table 2.3 Characteristics of some important biological molecules

Characteristic	Carbohydrates	Proteins	Nucleotides	Lipids
Building blocks are amino acids				
Contain carbon				
Molecules joined with glycosidic linkages				
Used to build genetic material				
Building blocks are monosaccharides				
Contain glycerol				
Contain hydrogen				
Molecules joined together with peptide bonds				
Strongly hydrophobic				
Built from sugar unit, phosphate group and base				
Enzymes are made from these				
Contain oxygen				

7. The following paragraph describes carbohydrate biology. Complete it by filling in the blanks.

Carbohydrates are mainly used to provide ________________ for body cells. The carbohydrate used by cells for this purpose is the monosaccharide ________________, which is carried to all body cells in the ________________. An excess of this monosaccharide can be stored as ________________, mainly in the liver. It can also be converted to ________________ and stored in adipose tissue. The carbohydrates ________________ and ________________ are integral components of DNA and RNA, respectively. Some carbohydrates are exposed on cell membranes as recognition and binding molecules called ________________, which allow the cell to interact with other cells and extracellular molecules.

8. The following paragraphs describe the biology of lipids. Complete them using the key choices supplied. Note that you may not use any key choice more than once, and you will not need them all.

The lipids are a varied group of substances and include certain ________________, such as steroids. Chemically, they are all ________________, meaning water repelling. In the form of ________________, they are the main component of the cell membrane, making a ________________ layer separating the cell contents from the extracellular environment. The steroid derivative ________________ stabilises cell membranes. Vitamins __________, __________, __________ and __________ are lipids.

Fats are a form of lipid and store energy in ________________ tissue. The alternative name for fats is ________________. Compared to energy release from a molecule of glucose, breaking down fat produces ________________ energy. Subcutaneous fat ________________ the body, and internal fat ________________ internal organs. Fats from animal sources are classified as ________________ and are usually ________________ at room temperature.

Key choices:

A	E	K	Protects
Adipose	Enzymes	Less	Saturated
B	Epithelial	Lipids	Single
C	Fluid	More	Solid
Cholesterol	Hormones	Nourishes	Triglycerides
D	Hydrophobic	Phospholipids	Unsaturated
Double	Insulates	Prostaglandins	

MATCHING

9. Match the correct pH in List A with the appropriate substance in list B.

List A	*List B*	
13	a. Distilled water	____
3.5	b. Gastric juice	____
3.0	c. Pancreatic juice	____
8.3	d. Oven cleaner	____
7.0	e. Aspirin	____
7.4	f. Blood	____
6.0	g. Breast milk	____
1.5	h. Cola	____

MCQs

10. Which of the following defines the atomic weight of an atom? __________
   a. Its total number of protons and electrons
   b. Its total number of neutrons, protons and electrons
   c. Its total number of neutrons and protons
   d. Its total number of protons

11. Which of the following defines the atomic number of an atom? __________
    a. Its total number of protons and electrons
    b. Its total number of neutrons, protons and electrons
    c. Its total number of neutrons and protons
    d. Its total number of protons

12. What is the definition of electron configuration? __________
    a. The type of atomic bond that an atom's electrons can form
    b. The number of electrons in each energy shell of the atom
    c. The number of electron energy shells in the atom
    d. The number of electrons available to form atomic bonds

13. Isotopes are atoms of the same element with different numbers of: ____________
    a. Protons and electrons
    b. Electrons
    c. Neutrons
    d. Protons and neutrons

14. Two isotopes of the same element will differ in atomic: __________
    a. Charge
    b. Weight
    c. Number
    d. Energy

15. An acid solution releases which ion when dissolved? __________
    a. Bicarbonate
    b. Hydroxyl
    c. Hydrogen
    d. Sodium

16. An alkaline solution is characterised by high levels of which ion? __________
    a. Bicarbonate
    b. Hydroxyl
    c. Hydrogen
    d. Sodium

17. Which of the following statements is true? __________
    a. An acid solution has a higher pH than an alkaline solution.
    b. A strongly acidic solution has a higher pH than a weaker one.
    c. There are no ions in a neutral solution.
    d. An alkaline solution has a higher pH than an acidic solution.

18. What is the function of an alkaline buffer in the body? __________
    a. It mops up hydroxyl ions and increases pH.
    b. It mops up hydrogen ions and decreases pH.
    c. It mops up hydroxyl ions and decreases pH.
    d. It mops up hydrogen ions and increases pH.

? POT LUCK

19. Which two organs are most important in maintaining the acid–base balance in the body by adjusting excretion of excess acid or base?

    - ______________________________
    - ______________________________

20. Define the term acidosis: ______________________________

21. Write down the equation that represents the conversion of carbon dioxide to bicarbonate in body fluids.____

22. Proteins are used in the body in many ways. Circle those items in the following list that are composed (at least mainly) of protein.

Insulin	Vitamin K	Antibodies
Haemoglobin	Adenosine triphosphate	Enzymes
The cell membrane	Deoxyribonucleic acid	Sucrose
Glycogen	Adipose tissue	Collagen

23. The following paragraph relates to enzymes but contains nine errors. Find the errors and correct them.

Enzymes are lipids that are used in the body to decrease the reactivity of active chemicals on which the body's metabolism depends. They are not themselves normally used up in the reactions in which they participate and are usually fairly nonspecific in the reactions they control. They can either cause two or more molecules to bind together (a catabolic reaction) or cause the breaking up of a molecule into smaller groups (a synthetic reaction). The molecule(s) entering the reaction are called products and they bind to a reactive site on the enzyme molecule called the catalytic site. Some reactions require the presence of a catalytic converter, which promotes binding of the enzyme to the other participating molecules. They are bound for only a fraction of a second but, when they are released, the reaction has occurred, and the new forms of the reactants are now called substrates.

PHYSIOLOGICAL PROCESSES

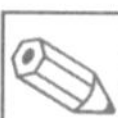

COMPLETION

24. Complete the paragraph correctly by crossing out the wrong words or statements.

The **internal/external** environment surrounds the body and provides the oxygen and nutrients its cells require. The **internal/external** environment is the medium in which the body cells exist. Cells are bathed in **intracellular/interstitial** fluid, also known as **lymph/tissue fluid**. The cell **membrane/tissue** provides a potential barrier to substances entering or leaving the cell. This property is known as **osmosis/selective permeability**.

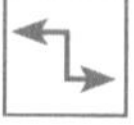

MATCHING

25. Match the key choices with the blanks in the paragraph below to describe how a negative feedback mechanism operates, using body temperature as an example.

Key choices:

Normal	Homeostasis	Reverses
Detectors	Control centre	Effector

The composition of the internal environment is maintained within narrow limits, and this fairly constant state is called ________________. In systems controlled by negative feedback mechanisms, the effector response ________________ the effect of the original stimulus. When body temperature falls below the preset level, specialised temperature-sensitive nerve endings act as ________________ and relay this information to cells in the hypothalamus of the brain that form the ________________. This results in the activation of ________________ responses, which raise body temperature. When body temperature returns to the ________________ range again, the temperature-sensitive nerve endings no longer stimulate the cells in the hypothalamus, and the heat-conserving mechanisms are switched off.

? POT LUCK

26. List two physiological responses that will counteract a fall in body temperature:

- ____
- ____

27. State four other physiological variables that are controlled by negative feedback systems:

- ________________
- ________________
- ________________
- ________________

28. Briefly outline how a positive feedback mechanism operates. ____

____

____

____

29. What percentage of body mass in an average adult is water? ________________________

30. Circle all of the following that are associated primarily with the intracellular environment.

Sodium	Urine	Synovial fluid
Cytoplasm	Glomerular filtrate	Plasma
Cerebrospinal fluid	Lymph	Saliva
Potassium	Blood	ATP

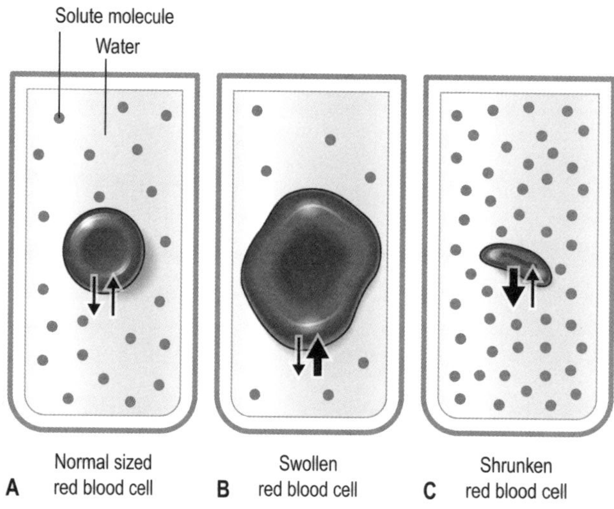

Figure 2.2 Red blood cells in three solutions of different concentrations demonstrating the effects of osmosis

31. The following paragraph describes Figure 2.2, which shows three red blood cells suspended in different water concentrations. Complete it by deleting the incorrect options in bold.

Figure 2.2 demonstrates osmosis, which refers specifically to the movement of **water/solute/diffusible** molecules down their **diffusion/concentration/pressure** gradient. The force driving this is called osmotic **pull/pressure/force.** In A, the red blood cell has not changed in size. This indicates that the solution is **hypotonic/isotonic/hypertonic** – that is, the concentration of water in the suspending solution is **the same as/less than/higher than** the cell, and **there is no net water movement/more water is moving into the cell than out of it/more water is moving out of the cell than into it**. In B, the red blood cell has swollen. This indicates that the solution is **hypotonic/isotonic/hypertonic** – that is, the concentration of water in the suspending solution is the **same as/less than/higher than** the cell, and **there is no net water movement/more water is moving into the cell than out of it/more water is moving out of the cell than into it**. In C, the red cell has shrunk. This indicates that the solution is **hypotonic/isotonic/hypertonic** – that is, the concentration of water in the suspending solution is the **same as/less than/higher than** the cell, and **there is no net water movement/ more water is moving into the cell than out of it/more water is moving out of the cell than into it**.
The movement of water in A, B and C will proceed until the **end point/equivalence/equilibrium** is reached, and water concentrations on either side of the red blood cell membrane are **equal/in flux/stable**.

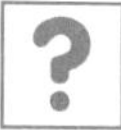

MCQs

32. Which of the following is true regarding a substance moving up its concentration gradient? _________
    a. It requires energy.
    b. Diffusion always involves such movement.
    c. Substances cannot move down a concentration gradient.
    d. It cannot occur across a barrier such as a cell membrane.

33. Which of the following physiological processes involves osmosis? _________
    a. Gas exchange in the alveoli
    b. Exchange of sodium and potassium
    c. Water movement in and out of cells
    d. Movement of molecules that requires a supply of ATP ions across cell membranes.

34. Oxygen molecules travel from the alveoli into the bloodstream by:_________
    a. Diffusion
    b. Active transport
    c. Dilution
    d. Osmosis.

35. Diffusion requires: ________
    a. A semipermeable membrane
    b. The presence of water
    c. Energy
    d. A concentration gradient.

36. Diffusion of molecules from one side of a semipermeable membrane to the other is speeded up when: _______
    a. The molecules of the diffusing substance are large.
    b. The temperature of the system is increased.
    c. The concentration of the diffusing substance is decreased.
    d. The pH of the system is as close to neutral as possible.

37. Figure 2.3 shows a collection of tissue cells, with blood capillaries and a lymphatic vessel. Colour and match:

- ○ All cell nuclei
- ○ All intracellular fluid
- ○ Blood plasma
- ○ Lymph
- ○ All interstitial fluid

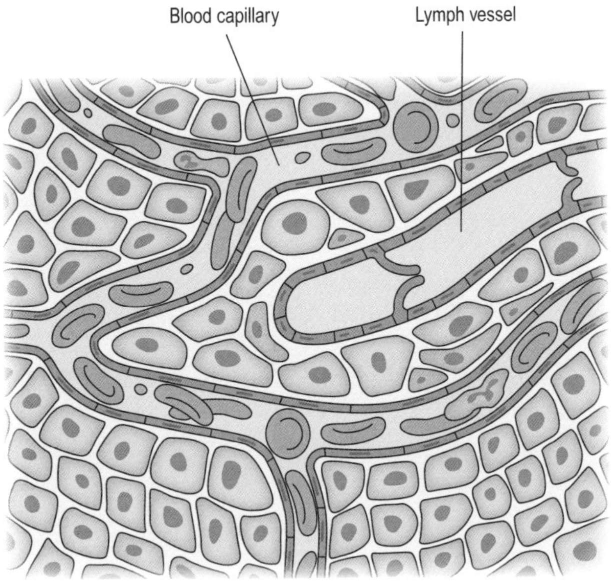

Figure 2.3 Distribution of intra- and extracellular fluid

38. The following fluids are all shown on Figure 2.3. Decide if each is intracellular or extracellular fluid.

- Fluid inside blood cells: ____________________
- Fluid inside lymph vessel: ____________________
- Fluid in blood plasma: ____________________
- Fluid inside tissue cells: ____________________
- Fluid between tissue cells: ____________________
- Fluid inside endothelial cells: ____________________

3 Cells and tissues

Cells are the smallest functional units of the body. Groups of similar cells form tissues, each of which has a distinct and specialised function. This chapter will help you learn about the structure of cells and the characteristics of different types of tissue.

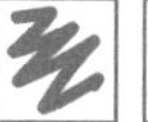

COLOURING AND LABELLING

1. Colour and label the intracellular structures identified on Figure 3.1.
2. Label the plasma membrane on Figure 3.1.

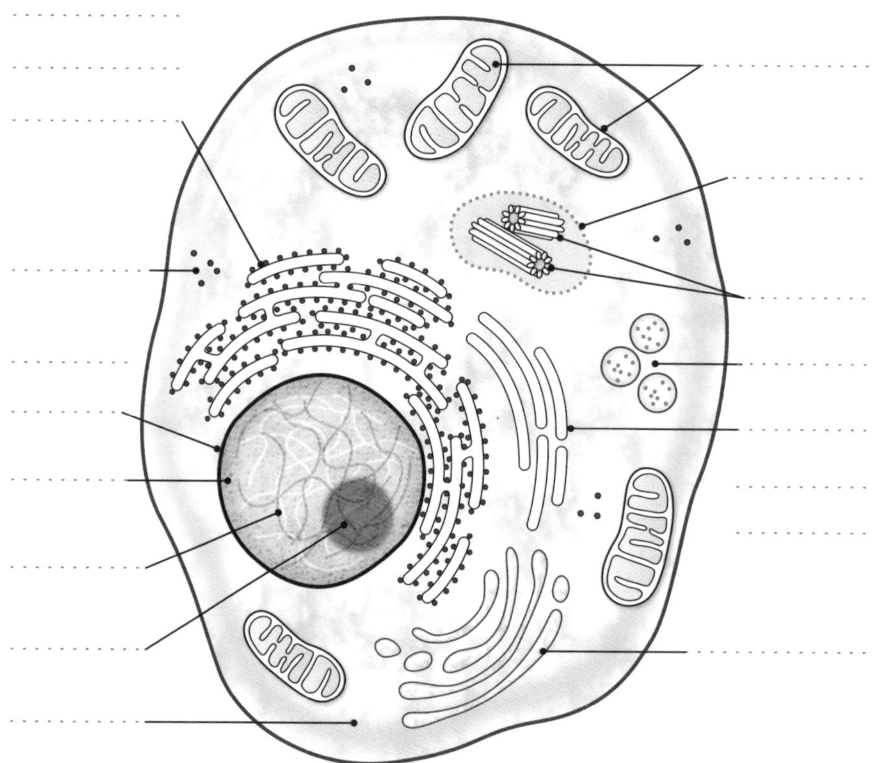

Figure 3.1 The simple cell

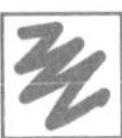 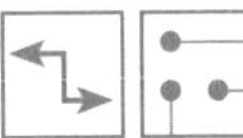

COLOURING, MATCHING AND LABELLING

3. Name the types of epithelial tissues shown in Figure 3.2.
4. On each type of epithelial tissue shown in Figure 3.2, colour and match where shown:

○ Epithelial cell ○ Basement membrane ○ Nucleus

5. Identify one organ where the tissue in Figure 3.2E is found. ____________________
6. Outline the function of the tissue shown in:

   a. Figure 3.2A ____________________

   b. Figure 3.2C ____________________

   c. Figure 3.2E ____________________

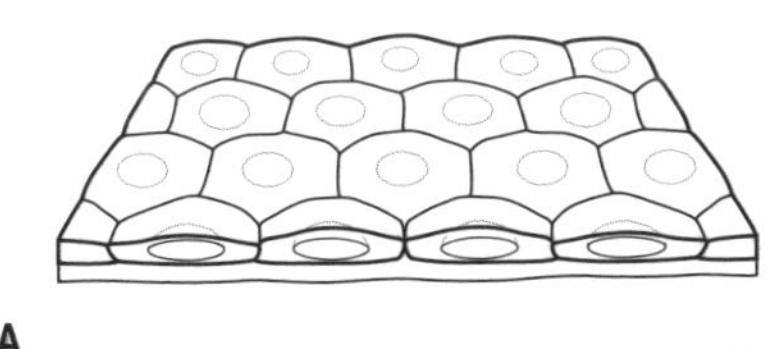

A ....

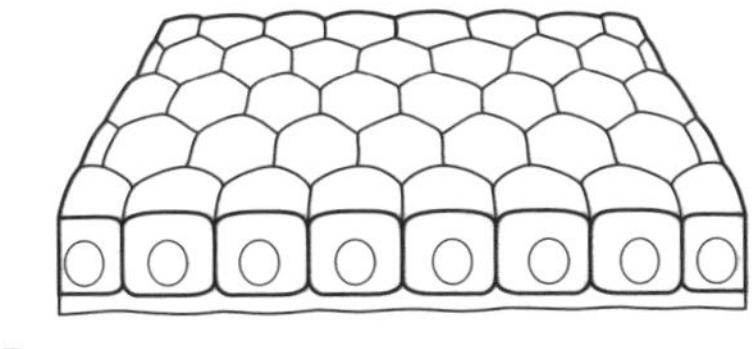

B ....

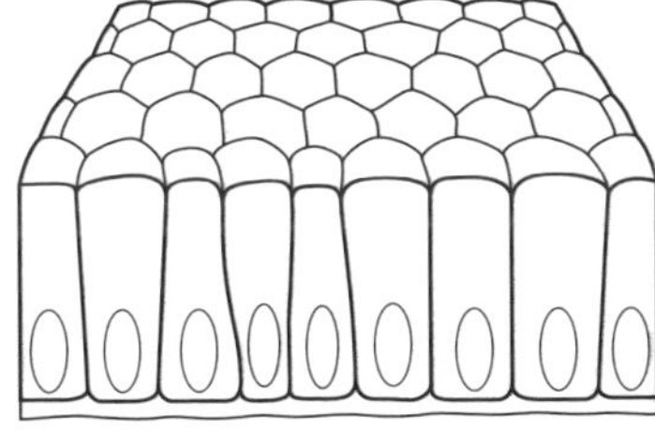

C ....

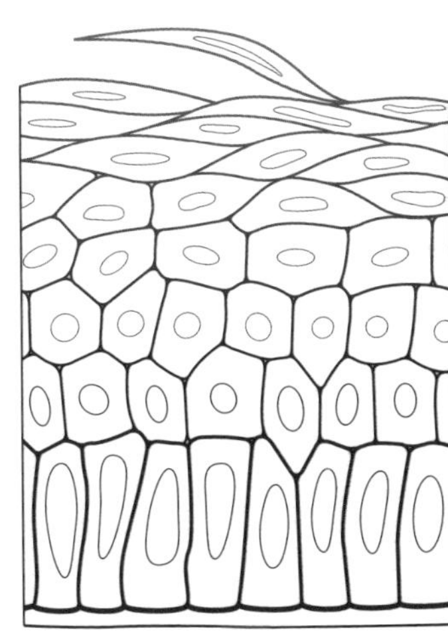

D ....

i ....

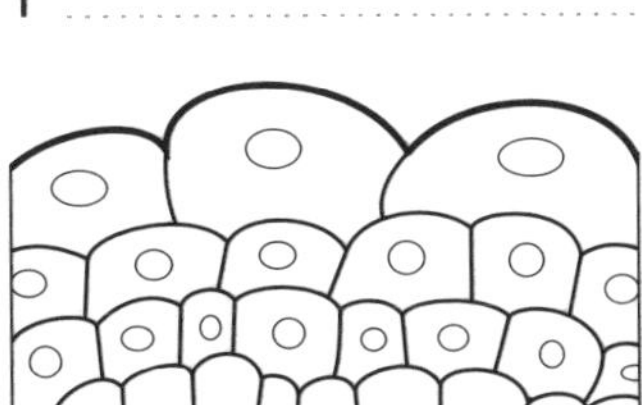

ii ....

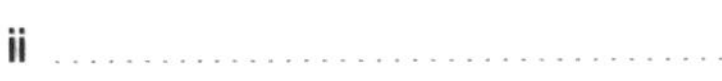

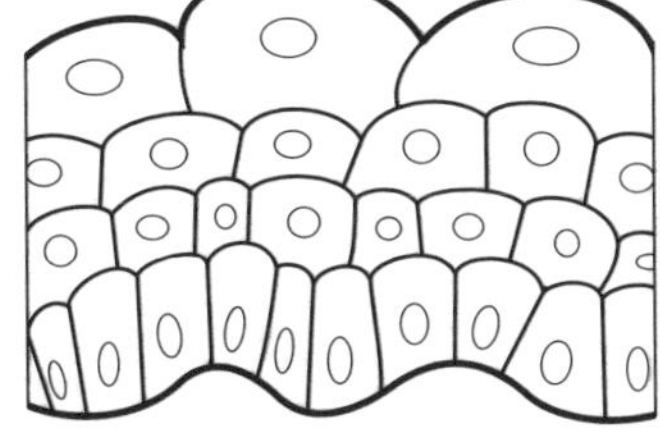

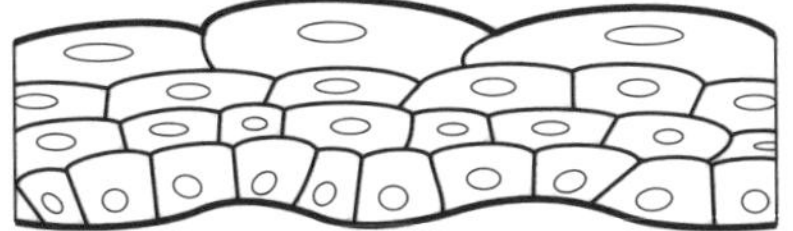

E ....

Figure 3.2 Types of epithelial tissue

 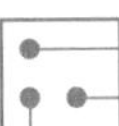

MATCHING AND LABELLING

7. Name each type of connective tissue shown in Figure 3.3.

8. Label the cells and fibres on each part of Figure 3.3.

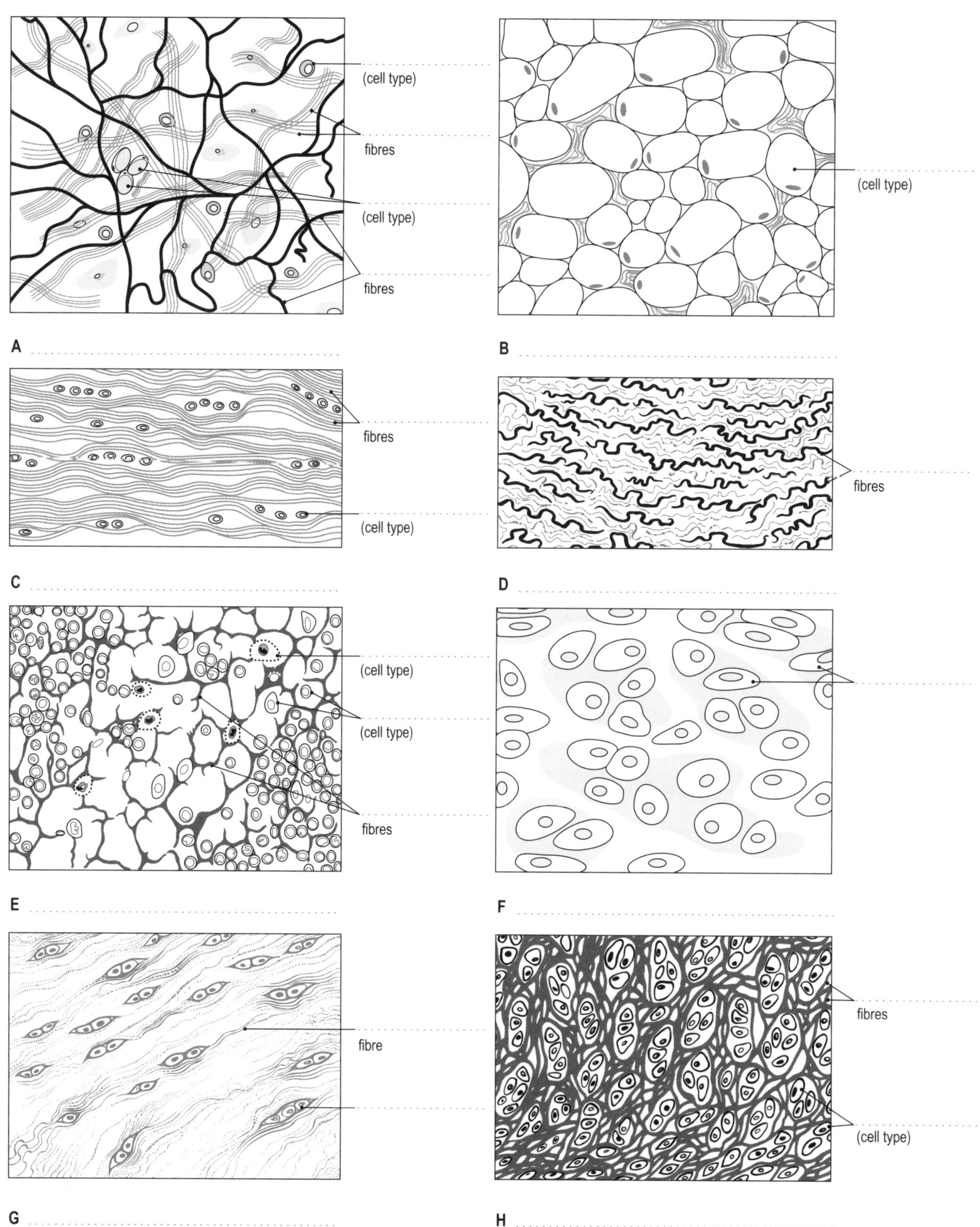

Figure 3.3 Types of connective tissue

9. Distinguish the exocrine glands on Figure 3.4 by colouring them to correspond with the key below.
10. Name the different types of exocrine glands on Figure 3.4.

○ Simple glands
○ Compound glands

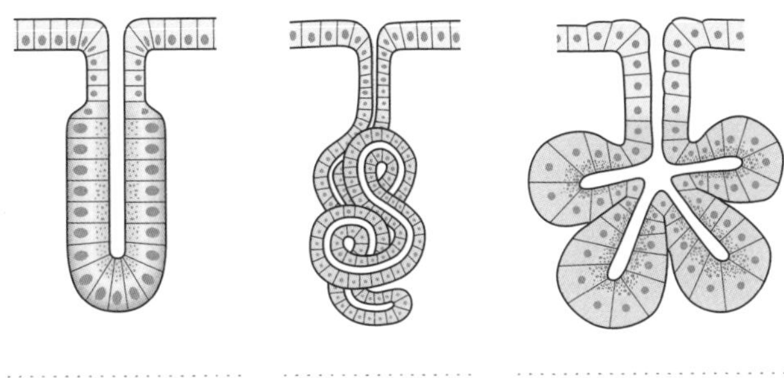

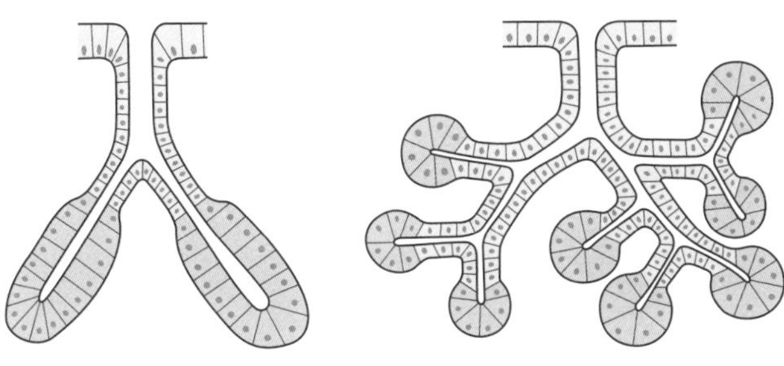

Figure 3.4 Exocrine glands

MATCHING

11. Match the organelles from the list of key choices with their functions in Table 3.1.

Key choices:
Lysosomes
Ribosomes
Golgi apparatus
Smooth endoplasmic reticulum
Rough endoplasmic reticulum
Nucleus
Microfilaments
Microtubules
Mitochondria

Table 3.1 Intracellular organelles and their functions

Organelle	Function
	The largest organelle; directs the activities of the cell
	Sites of aerobic respiration, often described as the powerhouse of the cell
	Tiny granules consisting of RNA and protein, which synthesise proteins for use within cells
	Manufactures proteins exported from cells
	Synthesise lipids and steroid hormones
	Flattened membranous sacs that form membrane-bound vesicles
	Vesicles that contain enzymes for the breakdown of substances, such as fragments of old organelles
	Tiny strands of protein that provide the structural support and shape of a cell
	Contractile proteins involved in the movement of cells and of organelles within cells

12. Match the key choices to the spaces in the paragraph below to describe bulk transport.

Key choices:	Pinocytosis	Plasma membrane
Exocytosis	Vacuole	Enzymes
Digest	Phagocytosis	Lysosomes

Transfer of large particles across the plasma membrane into the cell occurs by ________________, and smaller particles enter by ________________. The particles are engulfed by extensions of the ________________ that enclose them, forming a membrane-bound ________________. Then ________________ adhere to the cell membrane, releasing ________________ that ________________ the contents. Extrusion of waste materials by the reverse process is called ________________.

COMPLETION

13. Complete the paragraph about the cell cycle by crossing out the incorrect options.

Most body cells have **23/46** chromosomes and divide by **mitosis/meiosis**. The daughter cells of mitosis are genetically **identical/different**. The formation of gametes takes place by **mitosis/meiosis** and the daughter cells are genetically **identical/different**. The period between two cell divisions is known as the **chromosome/cell** cycle, which has two stages, the M phase and the interphase. **The M phase/interphase** is the longer stage. The interphase has **three/four** separate stages. Most cell growth takes place during the **first/second** gap phase; the chromosomes replicate during the **second gap phase/S phase**.

14. Complete the blanks in the paragraph below to describe the structure and functions of muscle tissue.

Muscle cells are also called ________________. Muscle tissue has the property of ________________, which brings about movement, both within the body and of the body itself. This requires a blood supply to provide ________________, ________________ and ________________ and to remove ________________. The chemical energy needed is derived from ________________.Skeletal muscle is also known as ________________ muscle because ________________ is under conscious control. When examined under the microscope, the cells are roughly ________________ in shape and may be as long as ________________ cm. The cells show a pattern of clearly visible stripes, also known as ________________.

Skeletal muscle is stimulated by ________________ nerve impulses that originate in the brain or spinal cord and end at the ________________.

Smooth muscle has the intrinsic ability to ________________ and ________________, a property known as automaticity (e.g. ________________), but it can also be stimulated by ________________ nerve impulses, some ________________ and ________________.

Cardiac muscle is found only in the wall of the ________________________, which has its own ________________________ system, meaning that this tissue contracts in a coordinated manner without external stimulation. ________________________ nerve impulses and some ________________________ influence the activity of this type of muscle.

15. Complete the paragraph below to describe characteristics of mucous membranes.

Mucous membrane is sometimes referred to as the ____________. It forms the moist lining of body tracts, such as the ________________, ________________ and ____________________ tracts. The membrane consists of ______________ cells, some of which produce a secretion called ______________. This sticky substance is present in the alimentary tract, where it ________________________ the contents, and in the respiratory system, where it traps ____________________.

? POT LUCK

16. There are six errors in the paragraph below describing the structure of cell membranes. Find the errors and correct them.

The plasma membrane consists of two layers of phospholipids, with some carbohydrate molecules embedded in them. The hormone cholesterol is also present. Membrane carbohydrates are involved in the transport of substances across the plasma membrane. The phospholipid molecules have a head that is electrically charged and hydrophilic (meaning water hating) and a tail that has no charge and is hydrophobic. The phospholipid bilayer is arranged like a sandwich, with the hydrophilic heads on the inside and the hydrophobic tails on the outside. These differences also influence the passage of substances across the cell membrane.

17. Define the following terms:

a. Hypertrophy ____

b. Hyperplasia ____

c. Atrophy ____

18. Explain the difference between cell death by apoptosis and necrosis. ______________________________

MCQs

19. Which forms of transport across cell membranes require energy? (Choose all that apply.) __________
    a. Active transport
    b. Facilitated diffusion
    c. Osmosis
    d. Bulk transport

20. The number of membrane carrier molecules determines the rate of: __________
    a. Active transport
    b. Facilitated diffusion
    c. Osmosis
    d. Bulk transport

21. Movement of water across a cell membrane down its concentration gradient is by: __________
    a. Active transport
    b. Facilitated diffusion
    c. Osmosis
    d. Bulk transport

22. Movement of a small molecule up its concentration gradient occurs during: __________
    a. Active transport
    b. Diffusion
    c. Osmosis
    d. Bulk transport

23. Which forms of transport only take place across membranes? (Choose all that apply.) __________
    a. Active transport
    b. Diffusion
    c. Osmosis
    d. Bulk transport

24. Gas molecules move across a cell membrane by: __________
    a. Active transport
    b. Diffusion
    c. Osmosis
    d. Bulk transport

25. The transport maximum determines the maximum rate of: __________
    a. Filtration
    b. Facilitated diffusion
    c. Osmosis
    d. Diffusion

26. Epithelial tissue that lines structures subject to wear and tear is: __________
    a. Ciliated
    b. Columnar
    c. Stratified
    d. Transitional

27. Epithelial tissue found on dry surfaces is relatively waterproof because it contains: _____
    a. Collagen
    b. Melanin
    c. A semisolid matrix
    d. Keratin

28. Which connective tissue cells secrete collagen? __________
    a. Fibroblasts
    b. Adipocytes
    c. Macrophages
    d. Mast cells

29. Periosteum, the membrane that covers bone, is formed from: __________
    a. Elastic tissue
    b. Fibrous tissue
    c. Fibrocartilage
    d. Hyaline cartilage

30. The intervertebral discs are formed from: __________
    a. Connective tissue
    b. Hyaline cartilage
    c. Fibrocartilage
    d. Elastic fibrocartilage

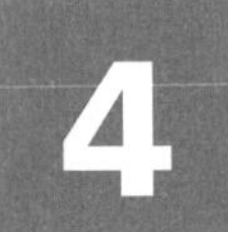

The blood

The blood is a fluid connective tissue, which travels within the closed circulatory system. It carries nutrients, wastes, respiratory gases and other substances important to body function. This chapter will test your understanding of the physiology of blood.

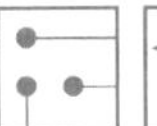 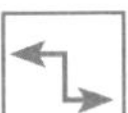 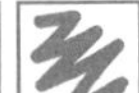

LABELLING, MATCHING AND COLOURING

1. Figure 4.1A shows whole blood that has been prevented from clotting and allowed to stand for some time. Label and colour the two layers A and B.
2. Figure 4.1B shows whole blood that has been allowed to clot. Label and colour the parts A and B.
3. What is present in the fluid portion in Figure 4.1A that is absent from Figure 4.1B? ______________________

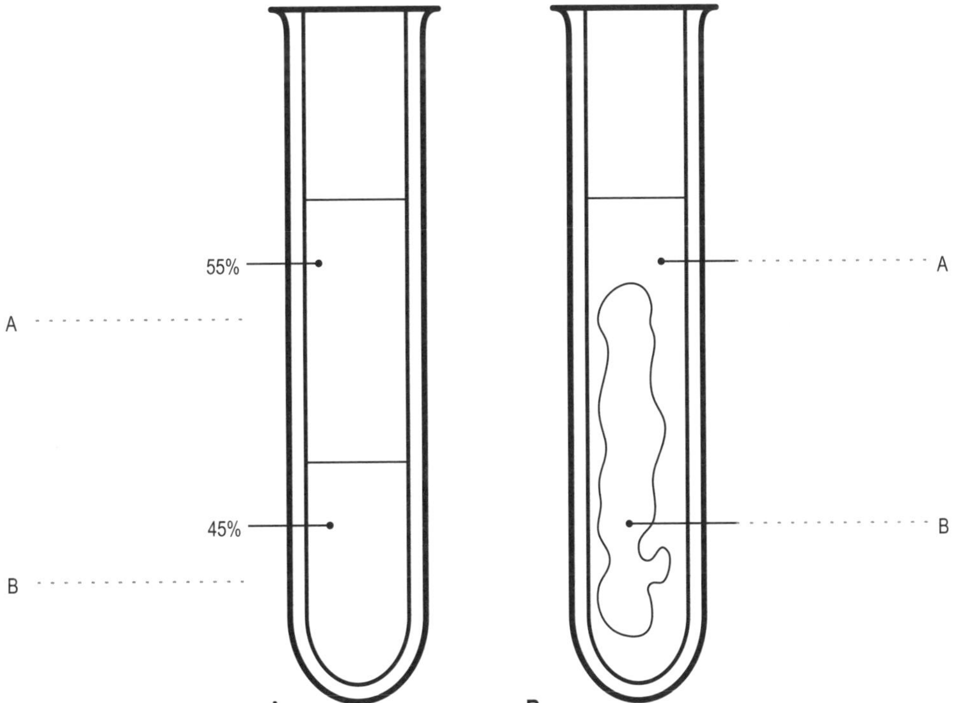

Figure 4.1 The proportions of blood cells and plasma in whole blood separated by gravity. (A) Blood prevented from clotting. (B) Blood allowed to clot.

4. Figure 4.2 shows the eight main types of blood cell. Name each type in the space provided. Cells C to H are white blood cells.

5. In Figure 4.2, colour and label the granules in the cytoplasm of those white cells that contain them and the nuclei of the cells that have them.

6. Explain why cell A does not have a nucleus.

____

____

7. The letters in list A correspond with the blood cells in Figure 4.2. The box on the next page lists 20 numbered key choices that can be used to describe each blood cell. Match each cell type with the relevant key choices. (Be careful, you can use each key choice more than once)

List A. List the numbers of the key choices here.
a. ______________________
b. ______________________
c. ______________________
d. ______________________
e. ______________________
f. ______________________
g. ______________________
h. ______________________

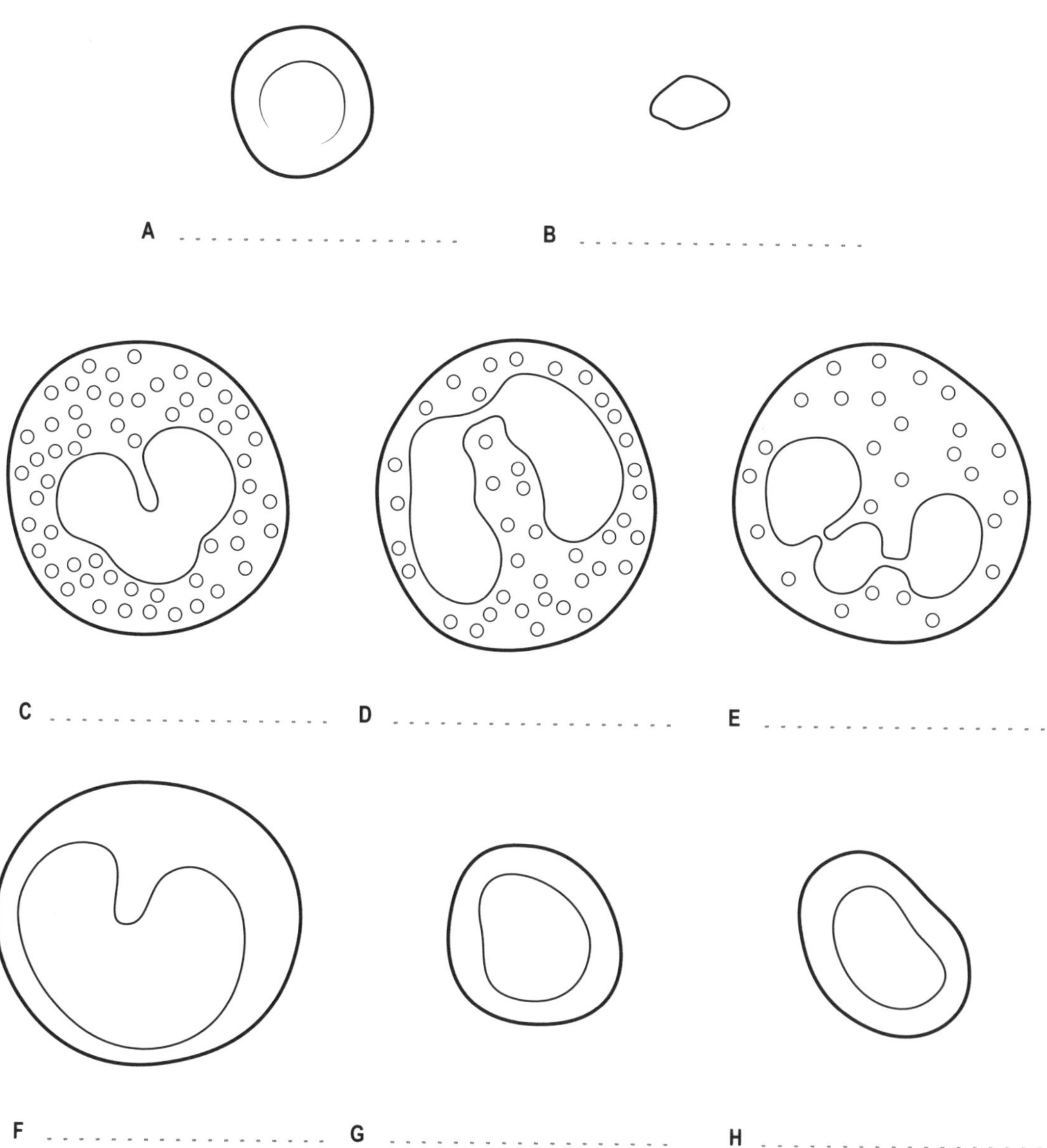

Figure 4.2 (A–H) Blood cells

Key choices box for question 7:
1. Circulating mast cell
2. Makes antibodies
3. Important in clotting
4. Granulocyte
5. Agranulocyte
6. Most common blood phagocyte
7. 1%–6% of total white blood cells
8. Cell fragment
9. Large single nucleus
10. Involved in immunity
11. Diameter of about 7 microns
12. Has no nucleus
13. Contains haemoglobin
14. 0.04–0.44 × 10^9 cells/litre
15. Smallest white blood cell(s)
16. 2%–10% of total white cells
17. Made in red bone marrow
18. Originate from pluripotent stem cells
19. Synthesis is called erythropoiesis
20. Biconcave in shape

8. Table 4.1 lists various descriptive phrases. Match them with the suggested components of blood plasma in list A. (Be careful, not everything in list A is actually found in plasma!)

List A

Haemoglobin	Hormones
Amino acids	Water
Electrolyte	Albumin
Glucose	Bile
Rhesus antigens	Antibodies
Intrinsic factor	Bicarbonate ion
Calcium	Iron

9. Figure 4.3 is a flow chart describing the control of red blood cell synthesis. Complete it by putting the statements below into the diagram in the correct order.

Statements:
Bone marrow increases erythropoiesis.
Increased blood oxygen-carrying capacity reverses tissue hypoxia.
Red blood cell numbers rise.
Kidneys secrete erythropoietin into the blood.

Table 4.1 Components of plasma

Descriptive phrase	Component
These chemicals travel from the gland of origin to distant tissues.	
These provide the building blocks for new tissue proteins.	
These molecules are also called immunoglobulins.	
90%–92% of plasma is this.	
This substance is needed for haemoglobin synthesis.	
An important non-nitrogenous waste is carried as this.	
A general term for ions, such as phosphate in body fluids.	
This is needed for healthy bones and teeth.	
This is the principal fuel source for body cells.	
This is mainly responsible for blood viscosity.	

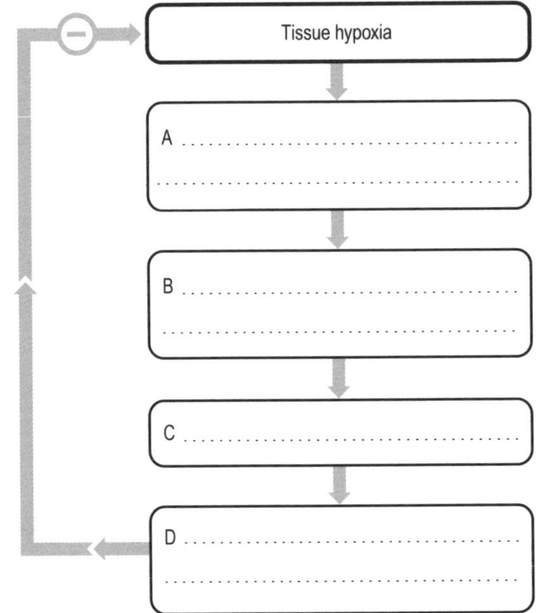

Figure 4.3 Control of erythropoiesis

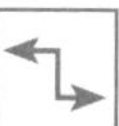 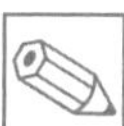

MATCHING AND COMPLETION

10. Complete Table 4.2, which describes the ABO system of blood grouping.

Table 4.2 The ABO system of blood grouping

Blood group	Type of antigen present on red cell surface	Type of antibody present in plasma	Can safely donate to:	Can safely receive from:
A				
B				
AB				
O				

11. Table 4.3 represents results from a test plate used to cross-match blood. Blood samples from Harold, Amanda, Hassan and Ayesha have been mixed with anti-A or anti-B antibodies and examined for agglutination. Study the results and answer the questions that follow.

Table 4.3 Test results from mixing blood samples from four individuals with anti-A and anti-B antibodies

Name of subject	Mixed with anti-A antibodies:	Mixed with anti-B antibodies:
Harold	Agglutinates	Agglutinates
Amanda	No reaction	Agglutinates
Hassan	No reaction	No reaction
Ayesha	Agglutinates	No reaction

a. Who is blood group A? ________________

b. Which antigens, if any, does Harold have on his red blood cells? ____________________

c. Who, if anyone, could donate to Harold? ______________________

d. Can Ayesha give to Hassan and, if not, why not? ____

____

____

e. What blood group is Amanda? ________________________________

f. Which of the four people could donate to all the others? ______________________________________

COMPLETION

12. Write the equation representing the binding between haemoglobin and oxygen. ________________________

13. The following paragraph describes the destruction of red blood cells. Complete it by filling in the blanks.

The life span of red blood cells is usually about _______ days. Their breakdown, also called _____________, is carried out by phagocytic ________________ cells found mainly in the _________, __________ and ______________. Their breakdown releases the mineral _________, which is kept by the body and stored in the _________. It is used to form new _____________. The protein released is converted to the intermediate ______________, and then to the yellow pigment _____________, before being bound to plasma protein and transported to the ___________, where it is excreted in the __________.

MCQs

14. Red blood cells are released into the circulation as which type of immature cell? __________
    a. Erythrocyte
    b. Reticulocyte
    c. Proerythroblast
    d. Erythroblast

15. What is the normal erythrocyte count per cubic millimetre (mm^3) of blood in a healthy adult male? __________
    a. $3.8–5 \times 10^4$
    b. $2–4.5 \times 10^5$
    c. $8.3–9.3 \times 10^7$
    d. $4.5–6.5 \times 10^6$

16. What proportion of all body cells is made up of red blood cells? __________
    a. 25%
    b. 30%
    c. 10%
    d. 5%

17. How many million haemoglobin molecules does a single red blood cell carry? __________
    a. 2.8
    b. 28
    c. 280
    d. 2800

18. Which vitamin, along with folic acid, is essential for red blood cell maturation? __________
    a. B_1
    b. B_2
    c. B_6
    d. B_{12}

19. Production of new red blood cells takes place in the: __________
    a. Liver
    b. Red bone marrow
    c. Kidneys
    d. Spleen

20. In the bloodstream, red blood cells transport: __________
    a. Oxygen and glucose
    b. Oxygen, carbon dioxide and glucose
    c. Oxygen, carbon dioxide and other wastes
    d. Oxygen and carbon dioxide

21. One consequence of a reduction in plasma protein levels may be: __________
    a. Increased blood viscosity
    b. Reduced blood oxygen carrying capacity
    c. Increased likelihood of clotting
    d. Development of oedema

22. Which white blood cell releases histamine in an allergic reaction? __________
    a. Eosinophil
    b. Basophil
    c. Neutrophil
    d. Monocyte

23. Which of the following conditions increases the binding of oxygen to haemoglobin? __________
    a. Increased tissue temperature
    b. Increased tissue carbon dioxide levels
    c. High oxygen levels
    d. An acidic tissue environment

24. Which of the following conditions increases the release of oxygen from oxyhaemoglobin? __________
    a. Tissue hypoxia
    b. Low carbon dioxide levels
    c. A rising tissue pH
    d. Cooler tissue temperature

25. Thrombin: __________
    a. Activates fibrinogen
    b. Breaks down blood clots
    c. Activates prothrombin
    d. Activates platelets

5 The cardiovascular system

The cardiovascular system consists of the heart, which is a pump, and a vast network of vessels, which are the transport system for the blood. Together, they supply all body tissues with nutrients and carry away wastes. This chapter will test your understanding of the structure and function of the heart and the different types of blood vessels, as well as key aspects of cardiovascular function.

THE HEART

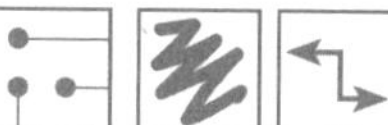

LABELLING, COLOURING AND MATCHING

1. Name the chambers of the heart shown on Figure 5.1.

A: ____________	C: ____________
B: ____________	D: ____________

2. Label all the structures indicated on Figure 5.1.

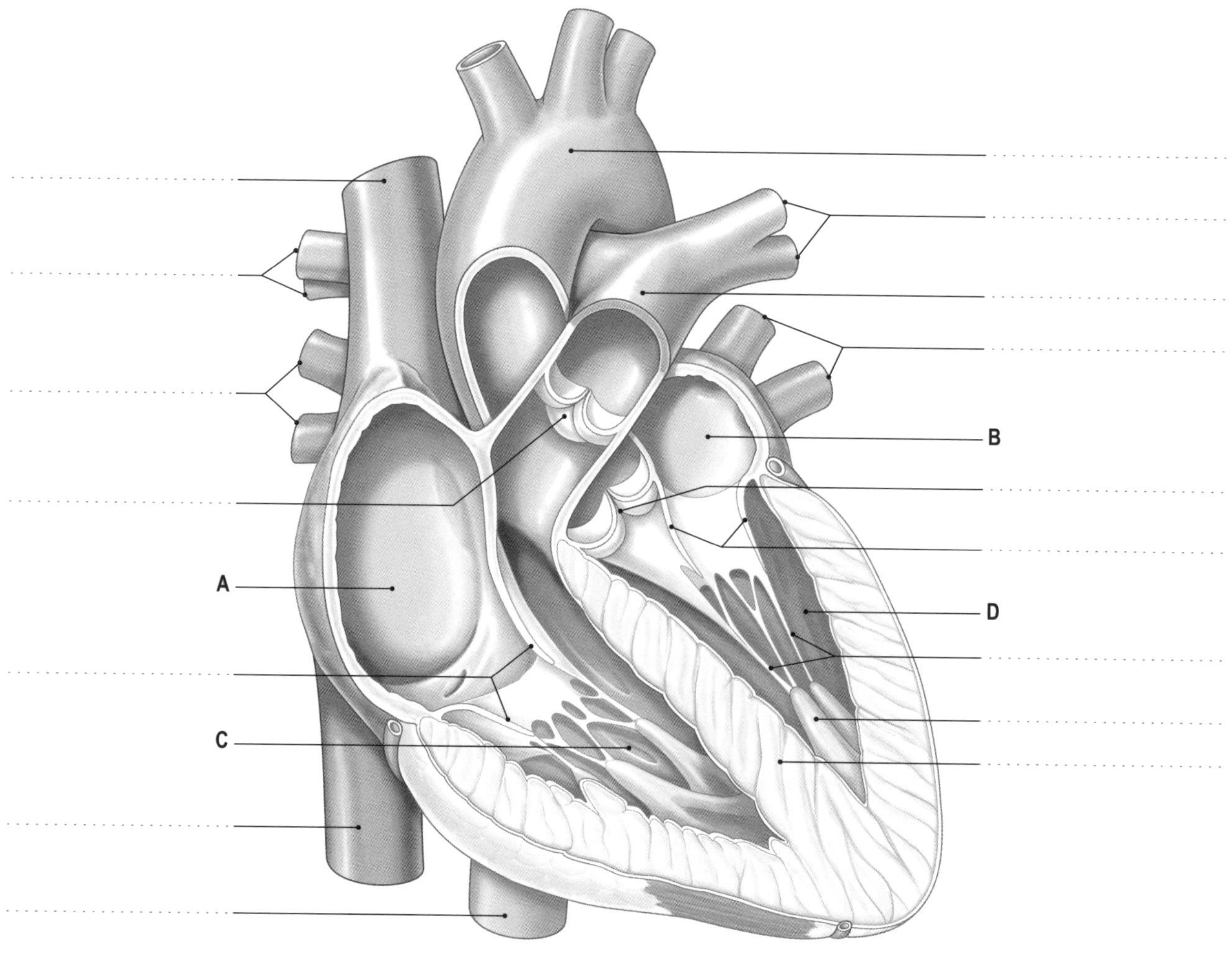

Figure 5.1 Interior of the heart

3. Figure 5.2 shows the main layers and tissues of the heart wall. Colour and label the structures shown.

4. In which heart chamber is the myocardium thickest, and why? ______________________

____

5. Match each of the statements in list A with the appropriate item in list B. (You will need to use the items in list B more than once.)

List A

a. Junctions between the cells here are called intercalated discs: ______________________

b. Secretes pericardial fluid: ______________________

c. Fibrous and inelastic tissue: | ______________________

d. Made up of endothelial cells: ______________________

e. Is a double membrane, folded back on itself: ______________________

f. Prevents the heart from overdistention: ______________________

g. Covers the valves of the heart: ______________________

h. The muscle here that is found only in the heart: ______________________

i. Contains the pericardial space: ______________________

j. Thickest in the left ventricle and at the base of the heart: ______________________

k. Continuous with the lining of the blood vessels leaving and entering the heart: ______________________

l. Lines the heart chambers: ______________________

List B	
Myocardium	Fibrous pericardium
Endocardium	Serous pericardium

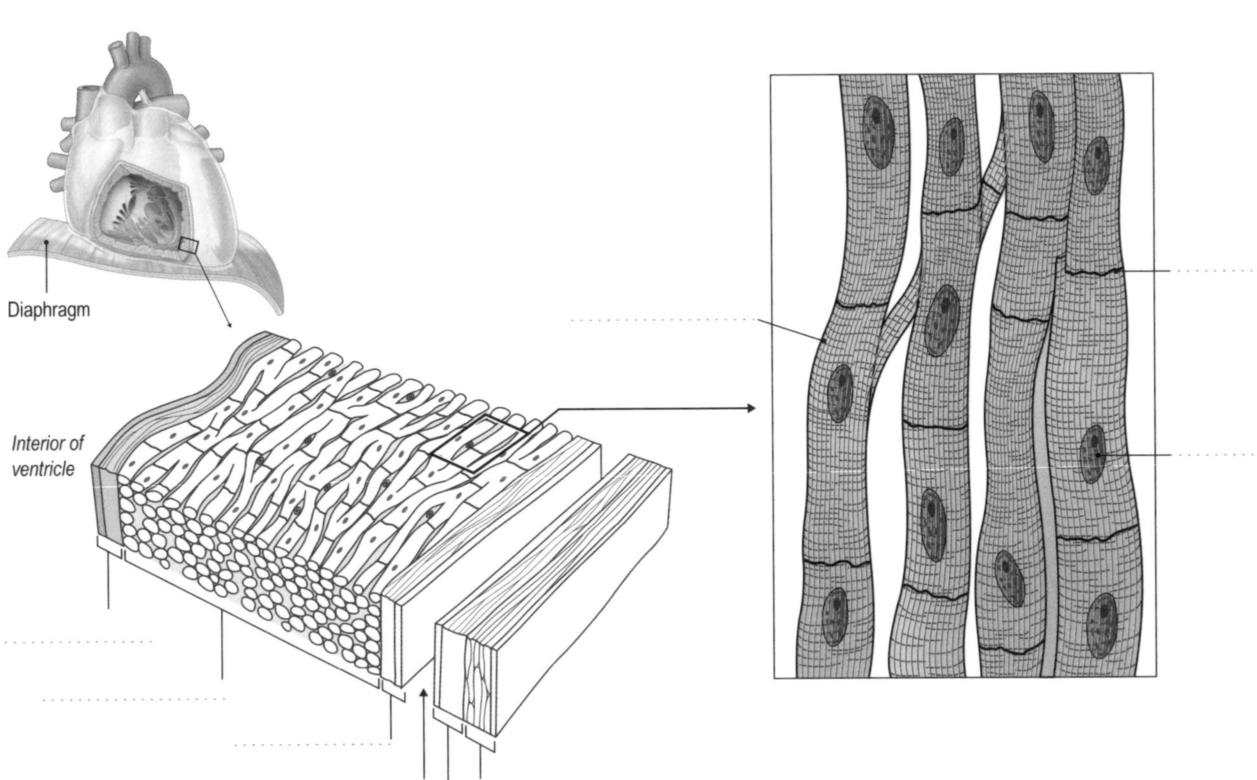

Figure 5.2 Layers of the heart wall

6. The double-membrane arrangement of the serous pericardium is found in which two other locations in the body?

- ______________________
- ______________________

7. Label the structures indicated on Figure 5.3, which shows the conducting system of the heart, and colour the conducting tissue.

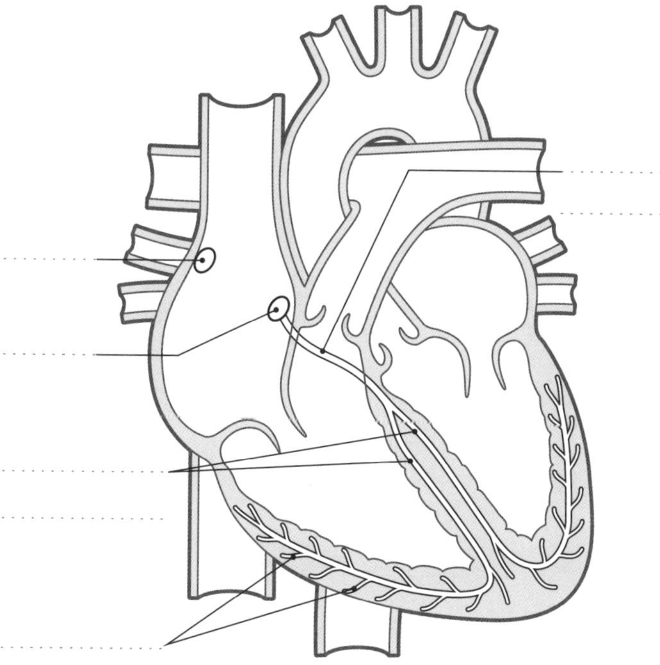

Figure 5.3 Conduction system of the heart

MCQs

8. The chordae tendineae prevent regurgitation from: ________
   a. The atria into the vena cavae
   b. The ventricles into the atria
   c. The pulmonary artery and aorta into the ventricles
   d. The atria into the ventricles

9. The atria: ________
   a. Have fewer layers in their walls than the ventricles
   b. Do not require muscle in their walls
   c. Have thinner walls than the ventricles
   d. Contract sequentially, with the left following the right

10. How is the heart muscle supplied with oxygen and nutrients? ________
    a. From the blood that circulates through the heart chambers
    b. By the coronary arteries, which branch from the aorta
    c. By the pulmonary arteries, which also supply the lungs
    d. From the cardiac arteries, which are more extensive on the left side of the heart than the right

11. How is blood drained from the tissues of the heart? ________
    a. By venous channels that open into the inferior vena cava
    b. Into the vena cava directly
    c. Mainly into the coronary sinus, which empties into the right atrium
    d. Directly into the pulmonary artery, for oxygenation

12. What proportion of the cardiac output does the heart itself receive? ________
    a. 30%
    b. 20%
    c. 10%
    d. 5%

13. Which chamber of the heart has the largest blood supply? ________
    a. Right atrium
    b. Right ventricle
    c. Left atrium
    d. Left ventricle

14. The heart rate is regulated by the cardiovascular centre, found where in the brain ________?
    a. In the cerebral cortex
    b. In the hypothalamus
    c. In the medulla oblongata
    d. In the cerebellum

BLOOD VESSELS AND THE CIRCULATION OF THE BLOOD

COMPLETION

15. Complete the following paragraph, which describes the two circulation systems of the blood, by inserting the correct word in the spaces provided.

The heart pumps blood into two separate circulatory systems, the ______________ circulation and the ___________ circulation. The __________ side of the heart pumps blood to the lungs, whereas the _________ side of the heart supplies the rest of the body. The ____________ are the sites of exchange of nutrients, gases and wastes. Tissue wastes, including carbon dioxide, pass into the _____________ and the tissues are supplied with ____________ and _____________. By definition, a blood vessel returning blood to the heart is called a ___________ and a blood vessel carrying blood from the heart is an ___________.

16. The following paragraph describes the flow of blood through the pulmonary circulation. Complete it by crossing out the incorrect option in bold.

Blood leaving the right ventricle first enters the **pulmonary artery/pulmonary trunk/pulmonary vein**, which passes upwards close to the aorta and divides into the right **pulmonary artery/pulmonary trunk/pulmonary vein** and the left **pulmonary artery/pulmonary trunk/pulmonary vein** at the level of the fifth thoracic vertebra. Each of these branches goes to the corresponding **ventricle/lung/atrium** and enters these organs in the area called the **hilum/insertion/notch/root**. Within the tissues, the vessels divide and subdivide, giving a network of many millions of tiny **capillaries/venules/arterioles**, across the walls of which gases exchange. Blood draining these structures then passes through veins of increasing diameter, which finally unite in the **pulmonary artery/pulmonary vein / pulmonary trunk**, which carries the blood back to the **left atrium/left ventricle/right atrium** of the heart.

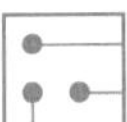 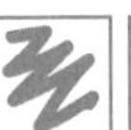 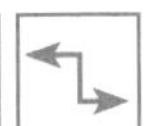

LABELLING, COLOURING AND MATCHING

17. Label and colour the layers of the blood vessel wall shown in Figure 5.4.

18. Match each of the three layers B, C and D identified in Figure 5.4 with the two most appropriate descriptive phrases given in the list of key choices below.

Key choices
- i. Composed of squamous epithelium
- ii. Rich in elastic tissue
- iii. Contains smooth muscle
- iv. This is also called the endothelium
- v. Contains mainly fibrous tissue
- vi. This layer is mainly for protection

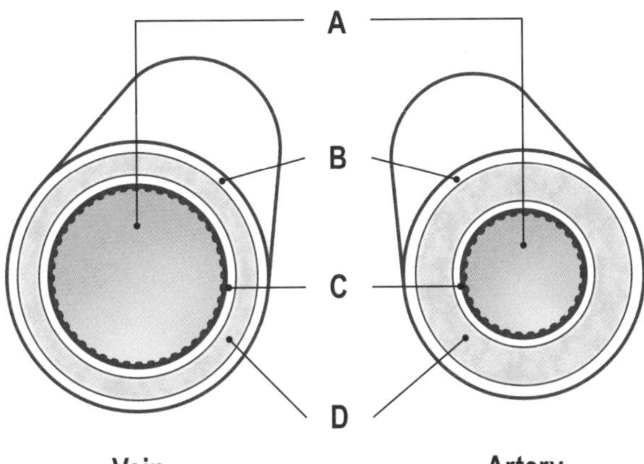

Figure 5.4 Structures of an artery and a vein

Layer A: ______________________________

Layer B: ______________________________

Layer C: ______________________________

Layer D: ______________________________

19. Figure 5.5 shows the interior of the heart. Label the structures shown.

20. On Figure 5.5, draw red arrows to indicate the direction of flow of oxygenated blood through the appropriate chambers and vessels. Using blue arrows, do the same for deoxygenated blood.

21. In the flowchart, put the terms supplied in the box in the correct order so that they correctly describe the flow of blood through the pulmonary and systemic circulations, beginning and finishing with the aorta. You will only need each term once.

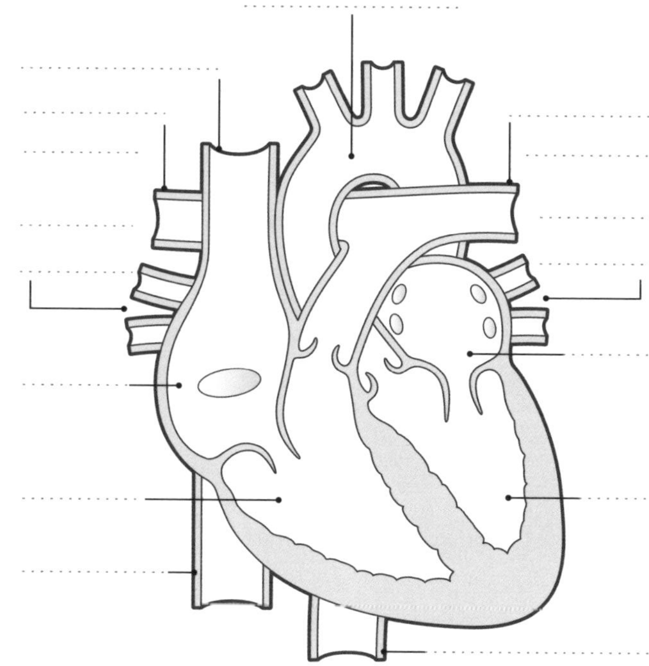

Figure 5.5 Direction of blood flow through the heart

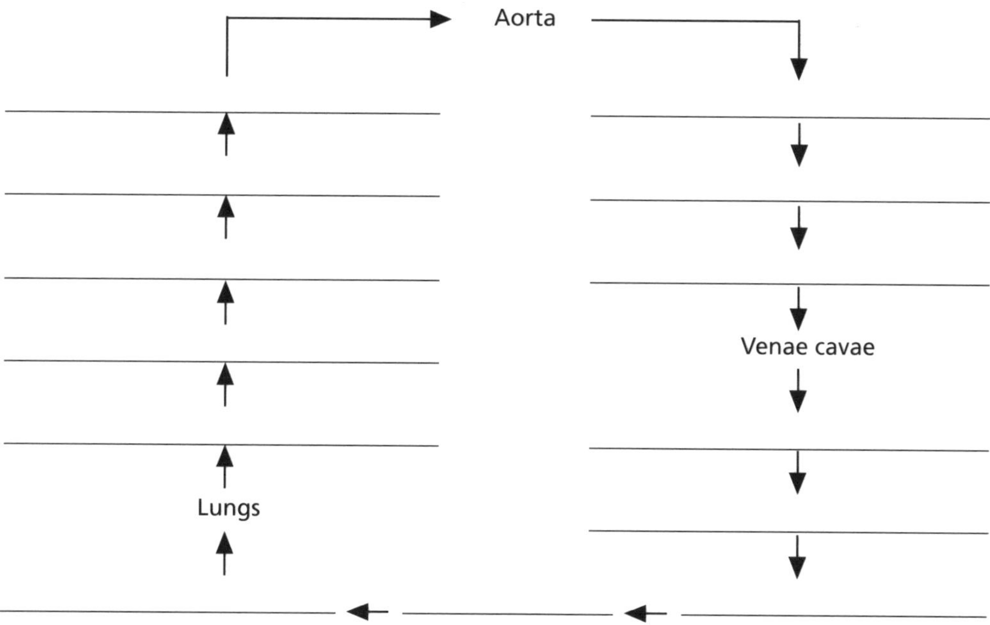

Left atrium	Left atrioventricular (mitral) valve
Right atrioventricular (tricuspid) valve	Right ventricle
Right atrium	Pulmonary arteries
Systemic arterial network	Capillaries of body tissues
Systemic venous network	Aortic valve
Left ventricle	Pulmonary veins
Pulmonary valve	

22. Figures 5.6 and 5.7 show the main arteries and veins of the limbs. Label the vessels shown and colour the arteries in red and the veins in blue.

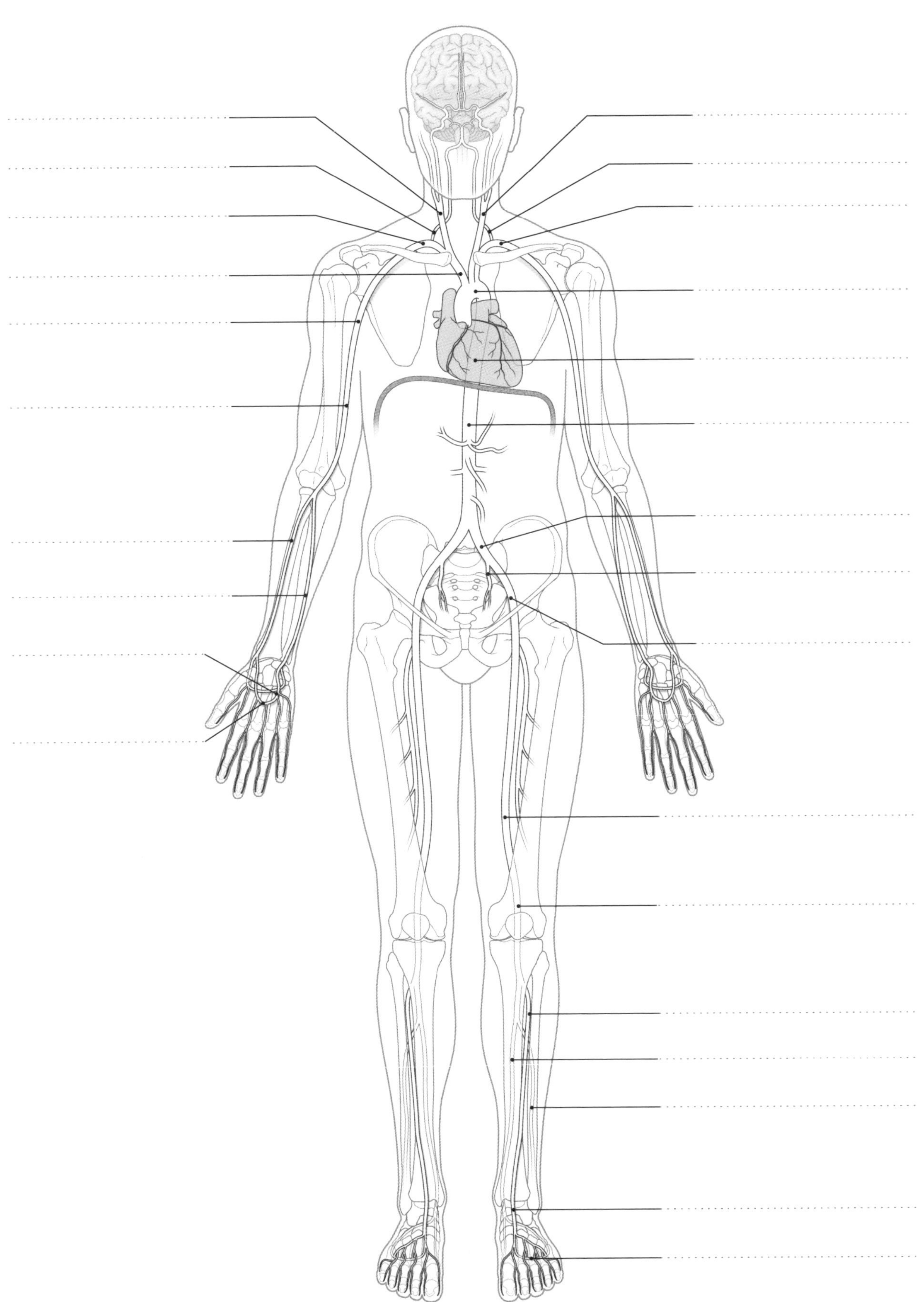

Figure 5.6 Aorta and main arteries

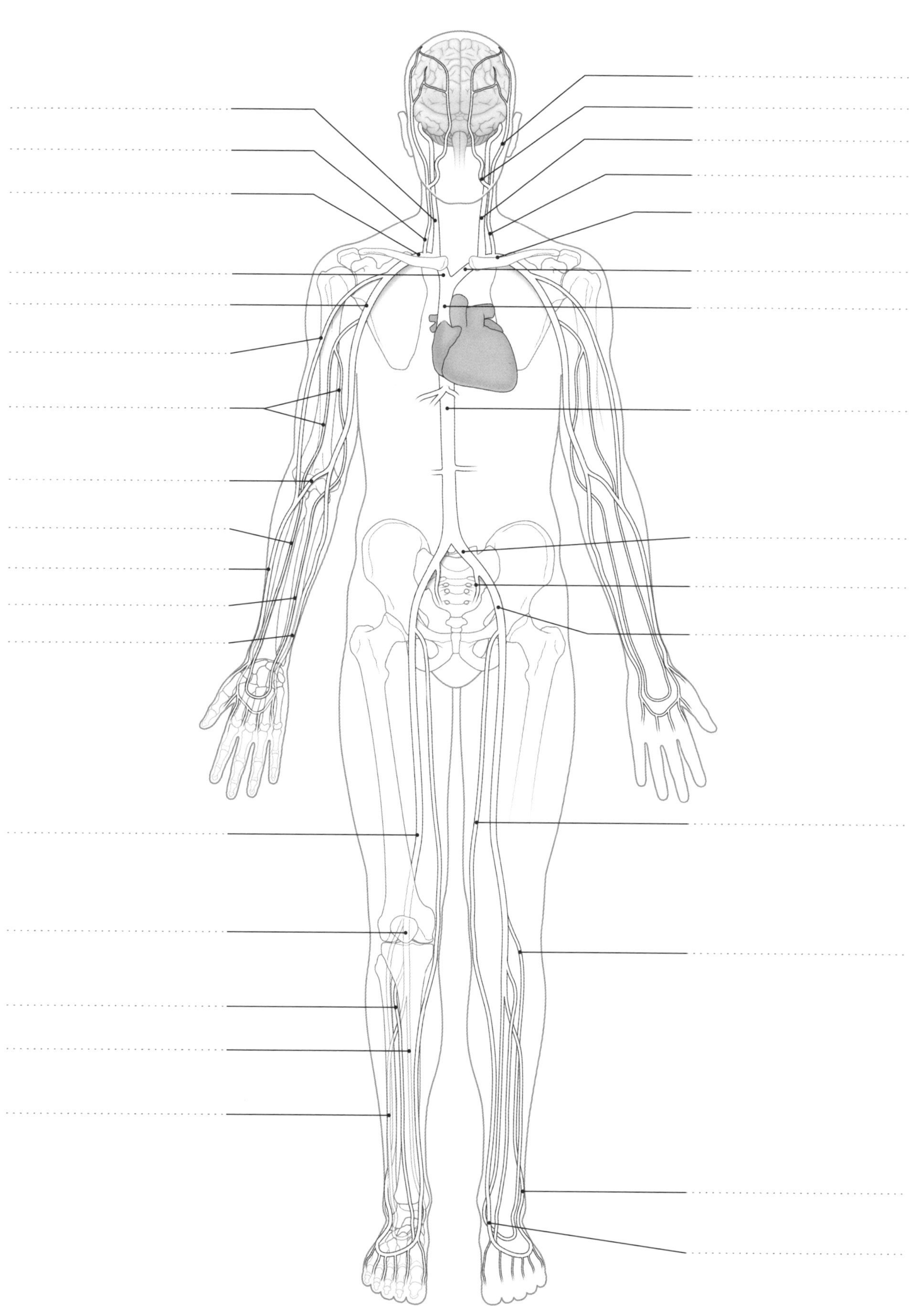

Figure 5.7 The venae cavae and main veins

23. Figure 5.8 shows the pressures across the capillary wall that control net water movement in and out of the capillary. Colour and match the arrows to represent hydrostatic and osmotic pressures at each end of the capillary.

24. In the spaces provided on Figure 5.8 insert the correct values for the pressures represented by each arrow.

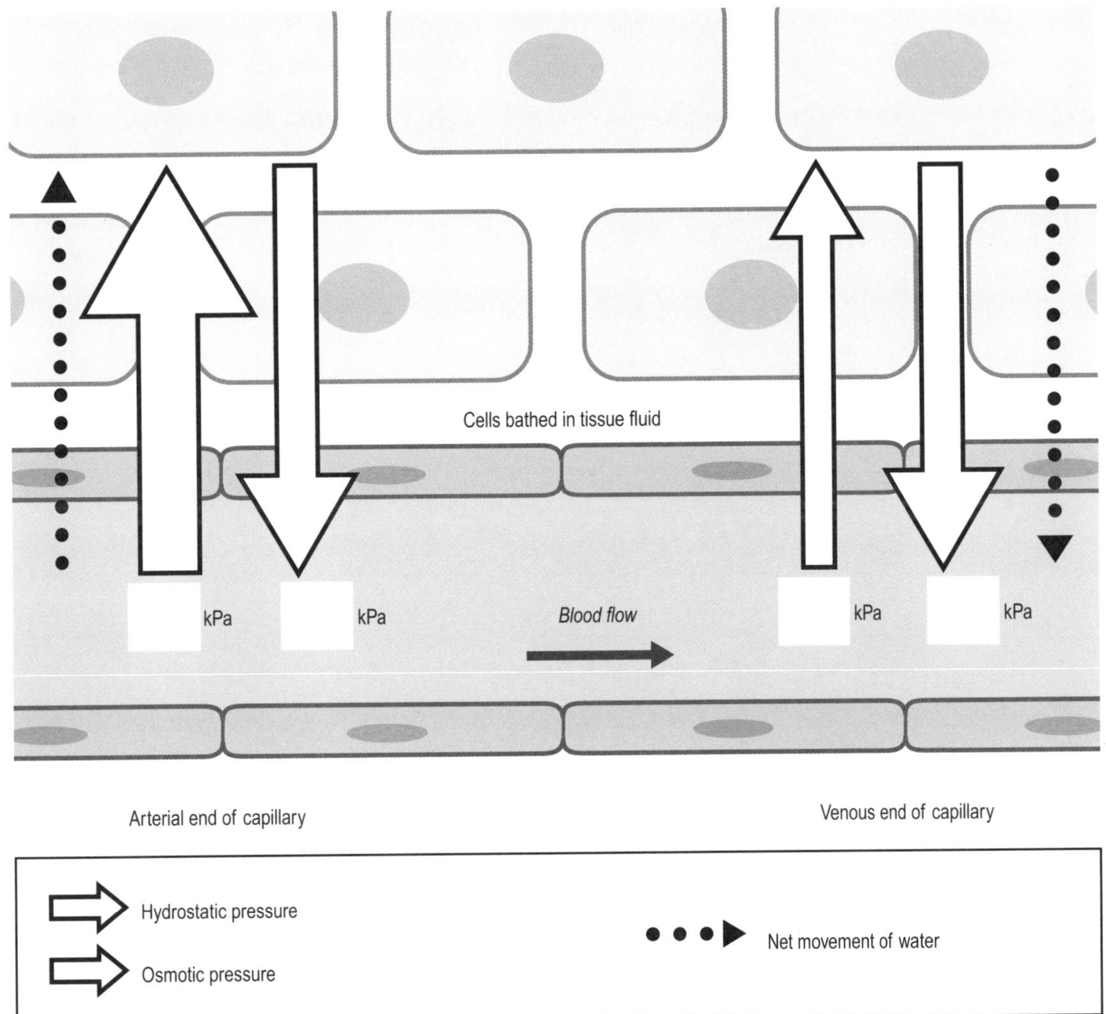

Figure 5.8 Effect of capillary pressures on water movement across capillary walls

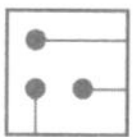

LABELLING

25. Figure 5.9 illustrates the fetal circulation. Label the structures indicated using the key choices provided.

Key choices:	Placenta	Ductus venosus
Abdominal aorta	Superior vena cava	Umbilical cord
Left ventricle	Pulmonary artery	Pulmonary veins
Inferior vena cava	Umbilical vein	Umbilical arteries
Right ventricle	Ductus arteriosus	Left atrium
Foramen ovale	Aortic arch	Internal iliac artery
Hepatic portal vein	Common iliac artery	
Umbilicus	Right atrium	

26. On Figure 5.9, insert arrows on the umbilical arteries and vein and the pulmonary arteries and veins, the right and left sides of the heart, in the aorta and through the foramen ovale and ductus arteriosus to show the direction of blood flow through the fetal circulation.

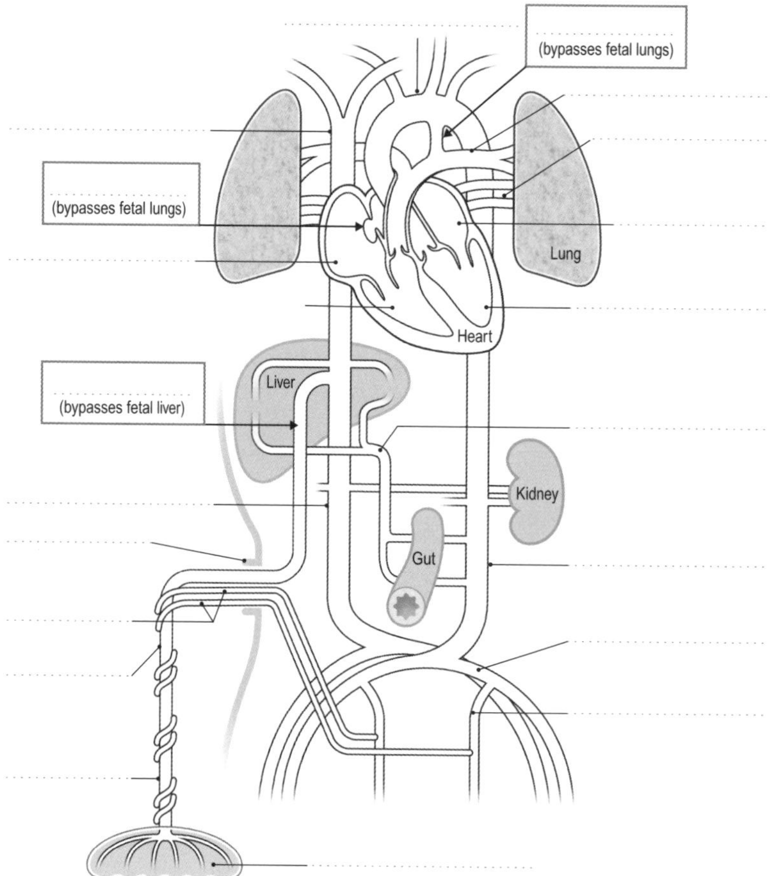

Figure 5.9 The fetal circulation

27. Trace the flow of blood from the heart through the leg by putting the vessels listed in the key choices below in the correct order, starting with the aorta and finishing with the inferior vena cava.

Key choices:	Digital arteries	Popliteal artery
Femoral vein	External iliac vein	Common iliac vein
Anterior tibial vein	Common iliac artery	Anterior tibial artery
Dorsalis pedis artery	Popliteal vein	
Femoral artery	Dorsal venous arch	

Descending aorta		Inferior vena cava
↓		↑
____________		____________
↓		↑
External iliac artery		____________
↓		↑
____________		____________
↓		↑
____________		____________
↓		↑
____________		____________
↓		↑
____________		____________
↓		↑
____________	→	Digital veins

28. Figure 5.10 shows the circulus arteriosus (circle of Willis), which lies on the base of the brain and is important in supplying most brain areas. Label and colour the arteries indicated.

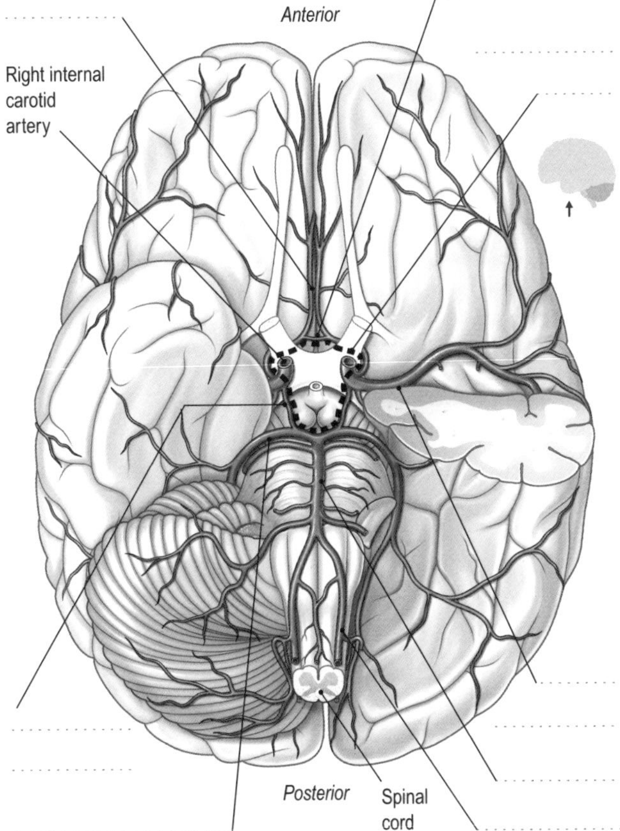

Figure 5.10 The circulus arteriosus (circle of Willis), viewed from below

MCQs

29. Veins have thinner walls than arteries because they: ________
    a. Carry less blood than arteries
    b. Carry blood at lower pressures than arteries
    c. Unlike arteries, have no muscle in their walls
    d. Are the vessels where gas and nutrient exchange takes place
30. Collateral circulation is: ________
    a. More than one artery supplying an area
    b. Venous drainage from the tissues
    c. The relationship of the systemic and pulmonary circuits
    d. Lymphatic vessels running alongside arteries
31. What is the function of valves in blood vessels? ________
    a. To keep the blood flowing in one direction
    b. To control the rate of blood flowing back to the heart
    c. To support the blood vessel walls
    d. To shut off blood flow in a damaged vessel
32. Valves are formed from which kind(s) of tissue? (Choose all that apply.) ________
    a. Muscle
    b. Adipose
    c. Endothelial
    d. Connective
33. Which are the capacitance vessels? ________
    a. The arteries, capable of withstanding high pressures
    b. The capillaries, because they are so tiny and numerous that their capacity is large
    c. The veins, whose soft walls allow easy expansion
    d. The arterioles, whose constriction and dilation control blood volume in the tissue beds
34. Sinusoids are found in areas of the body where: ________
    a. Large blood flow is required
    b. Rapid exchange between the blood and extracellular fluid is needed
    c. There is no lymphatic supply
    d. There are no blood vessels, such as the cornea of the eye
35. Flow along a blood vessel is determined in health primarily by: ________
    a. Blood vessel length
    b. Blood vessel diameter
    c. Blood viscosity
    d. Blood volume
36. Which of the following exchanges freely across capillary walls (tick all that apply)? ________
    a. Glucose
    b. Water
    c. Fibrinogen
    d. Sodium ions
37. The inferior vena cava is formed by the union of which veins? ________
    a. Left and right common iliac veins
    b. Internal and external iliac veins
    c. Femoral vein and saphenous vein
    d. Common iliac vein and femoral vein
38. What unusual arrangement of blood vessels is associated with the hepatic portal circulation? ________
    a. Capillaries in the liver drain directly into the portal vein
    b. Arterial blood passes through two sets of capillaries before returning to the venous circulation
    c. The portal vein is formed by the union of several other veins
    d. The portal vein links the arterial and venous circulations without an intervening capillary bed

CARDIOVASCULAR FUNCTION

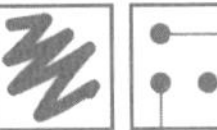

MATCHING, COLOURING AND LABELLING

39. Figure 5.11 shows the events of one complete cardiac cycle of a total duration of 0.8 second. Indicate the three events of the cardiac cycle by matching, colouring and labelling the boxes at A, B and C, and the arrows at i, ii and iii, using the key provided.

- O Complete cardiac diastole
- O Ventricular systole
- O Atrial systole

A

B

C

i

ii

iii

0.8 s

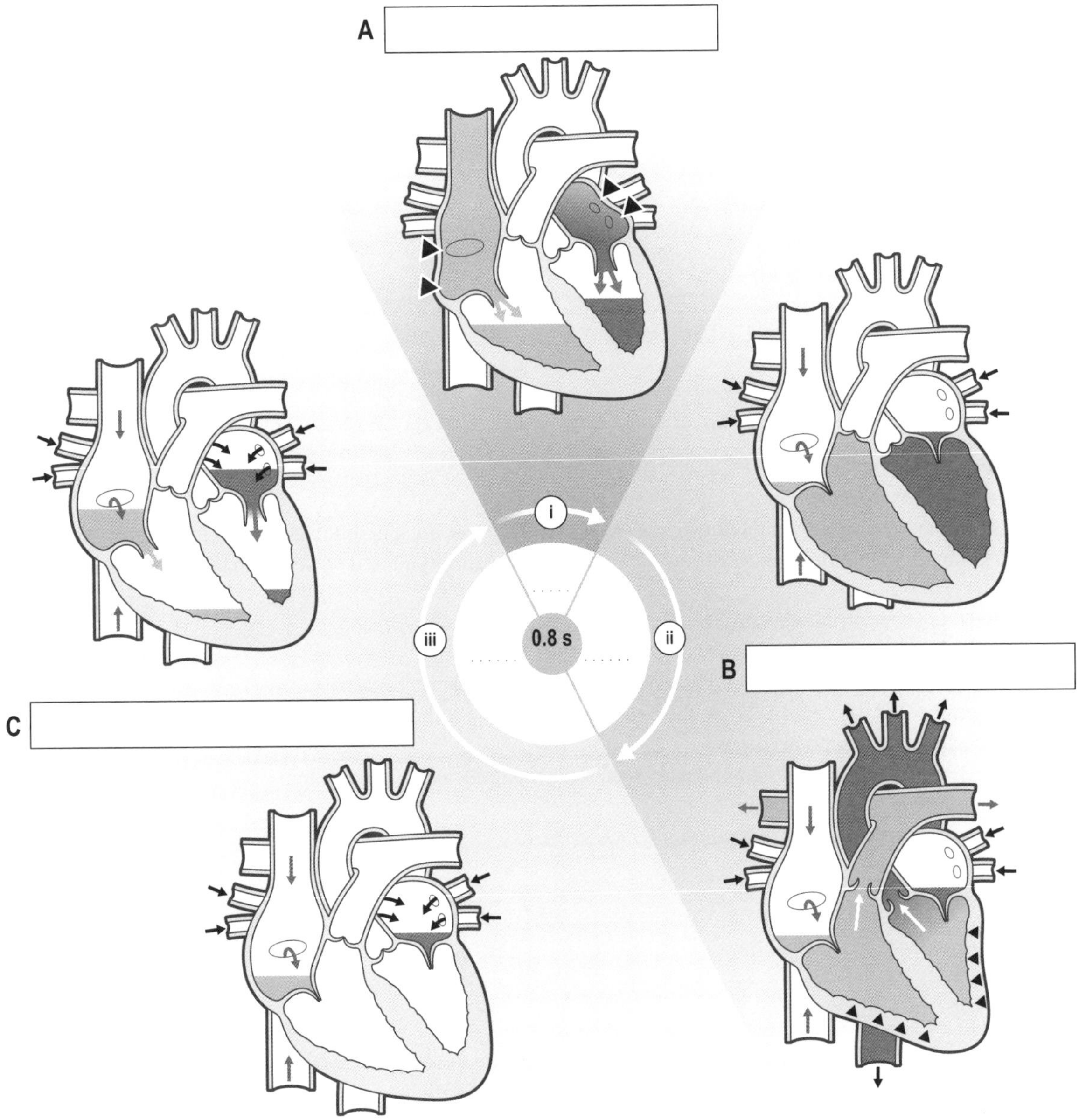

Figure 5.11 One complete cardiac cycle

40. On Figure 5.11 show the duration of each event by inserting the appropriate values at i, ii and iii.

41. From list A, match the events taking place during A, B and C by writing the appropriate key choices against each one.

A: ______________________________

B: ______________________________

C: ______________________________

List A
Atrioventricular valves open
Ventricles relaxed
Aortic/pulmonary valves open
Atria and ventricles relaxed
Atria contract
Ventricles contract
Aortic/pulmonary valves closed
Atrioventricular valves open
Atria relaxed
Aortic/pulmonary valves closed
Atrioventricular valves closed

42. Figure 5.12 shows a typical electrocardiogram (ECG) of one cardiac cycle. Label the individual waves.

43. On Figure 5.12, mark with an X where the impulse is passing through the atrioventricular node.

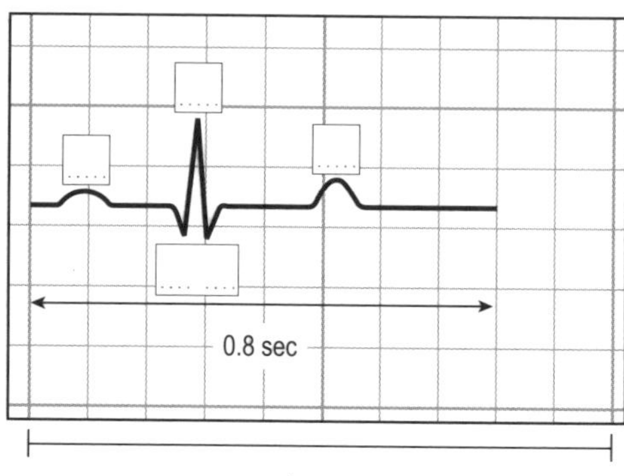

Figure 5.12 The electrocardiogram (ECG)

POT LUCK

44. The following statements relate to the ECG, but five of them are not correct. Identify the incorrect statements and write the correct versions in the spaces below.
    a. The QRS complex is bigger than the P wave because there is more muscle in the atria than in the ventricles.
    b. The QRS complex represents passage of the electrical impulse through the interventricular bundle and the Purkinje fibres.
    c. The T wave represents atrial relaxation.
    d. The P wave is initiated when the sinoatrial node fires.
    e. The ECG gives information about heart rate as well as heart rhythm.
    f. The waves on the ECG are generated by the opening and closing of heart valves.
    g. The P wave shows atrial repolarisation.
    h. The delay between the P and QRS components represents the time taken for the impulse to spread from the right to the left atrium.

____

____

____

____

____

45. Which of the following would increase stroke volume, assuming that no other factor changes to compensate? Tick all that apply.

a. Sympathetic stimulation: ______
b. Increased preload: ______
c. Increased vagal tone: ______
d. Increased heart rate: ______
e. Decreased secretion of adrenaline: ______
f. Decreased afterload: ______
g. Increased blood volume: ______
h. Decreased venous return: ______

46. Which of the following is associated with increased venous return to the heart, assuming no other factor changes to compensate? Tick all that apply.

a. Standing up from a supine position: ______
b. Decreased blood volume: ______
c. The skeletal muscle pump: ______
d. Increased blood pressure: ______
e. Decreased heart rate: ______
f. The respiratory pump: ______
g. Venous congestion: ______
h. Increased preload: ______

47. Decide whether the following terms apply to vasoconstriction or vasodilation.

a. Vessel wall thins: ______
b. Volume of blood that is carried is increased: ______
c. Increases pressure inside the vessel: ______
d. Decreased resistance to blood flow: ______
e. Smooth muscle in vessel wall is contracted: ______
f. Usually follows a decrease in sympathetic stimulation: ______
g. Lumen of vessel is wider: ______
h. Vessel wall thickens: ______
i. Smooth muscle in vessel wall is relaxed: ______
j. Lumen of vessel is reduced: ______
k. Increased resistance to blood flow: ______
l. Volume of blood that is carried is decreased: ______
m. Reduces pressure inside the vessel: ______
n. Usually caused by sympathetic stimulation: ______

COMPLETION

48. The following paragraph discusses autoregulation. Complete it by deleting the incorrect options in bold.

Autoregulation means **systemic/local** control of blood flow. For example, **increased/decreased** metabolic activity increases blood flow to a tissue. Cooler tissues receive **more/less** blood than warmer ones and blood vessels in warmer tissues **dilate/constrict** to **increase/decrease** blood supply. Oxygen and carbon dioxide levels are important in autoregulation; hypoxia **increases/decreases** blood flow to a capillary bed. The changes in blood vessel diameter controlling blood flow are mediated by the release of chemicals such as histamine, which is **vasoconstricting/vasodilating** in action, and nitric oxide, a potent and **short-/long-**lived mediator that **increases/decreases** blood flow to organs. On the other hand, adrenaline, also called **noradrenaline/epinephrine**, from the adrenal **medulla/cortex** and angiotensin II are powerful **vasoconstrictors/vasodilators.**

49. Complete the following paragraphs, which describe the body's control of blood pressure, by crossing out the incorrect options in bold and thus leaving the correct words or phrases.

The baroreceptor reflex is important in the **moment to moment/long-term** control of blood pressure. It is controlled by the cardiovascular centre found in the **medulla oblongata/carotid bodies**, which receives and integrates information from baroreceptors, chemoreceptors and higher centres in the brain. Baroreceptors are receptors sensitive to blood pressure and are found in the **carotid arteries/heart wall/aorta**. A **rise/fall** in blood pressure activates these receptors, which respond by increasing the activity of **parasympathetic/sympathetic** nerve fibres supplying the heart; this **slows the heart down/ speeds the heart up** and returns the system towards normal. In addition to this, **sympathetic/parasympathetic** nerve fibres supplying the blood vessels are **activated/inhibited**, which leads to **vasoconstriction/vasodilation**, again returning the system towards normal (note that most blood vessels have little or no **sympathetic/parasympathetic** innervation).

On the other hand, if the blood pressure **falls/rises**, baroreceptor activity is decreased, and this also triggers compensatory mechanisms. This time, **sympathetic/parasympathetic** activity is increased which leads to a(n) **reduction/increase** in heart rate; in addition, cardiac contractile force is **increased/reduced**. The blood vessels respond with **vasoconstriction/vasodilation**; this is mainly due to **increased/decreased** activity in **sympathetic/ parasympathetic** fibres. These measures lead to a restoration of blood pressure towards normal.

In addition to the activity of the baroreceptors described above, chemoreceptors in the **carotid bodies/aorta/higher centres of the brain** measure the pH of the blood. An increase in **oxygen/carbon dioxide** content of the blood decreases pH and **stimulates/inhibits** these receptors, leading to an **increase/decrease** in stroke volume and heart rate and a general **vasoconstriction/vasodilation**; this **increases/decreases** blood pressure. Other control mechanisms include the renin–angiotensin system, which is involved in **long-term/short-term** regulation; activation **increases/decreases** blood volume, thereby **increasing/decreasing** blood pressure.

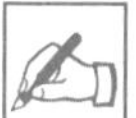

APPLYING WHAT YOU KNOW

50. If the heart rate is 75 beats per minute and the stroke volume is 75 mL, what is the cardiac output?

____

51. If the cardiac output is 5 litres/min and the pulse rate is 60 beats per minute, what is the stroke volume?

____

52. If the cardiac output is 5.5 litres/min and the stroke volume is 55 mL, what is the heart rate?

____

MCQs

53. Which of the following lists three effects which all increase heart rate? ________
    a. Sympathetic activation; reduced exercise; fear
    b. Rise in blood pressure; adrenaline (epinephrine) release; increased exercise
    c. Parasympathetic stimulation; fall in blood pressure; thyroxine release
    d. Adrenaline (epinephrine) release; active exercise; fall in blood pressure

54. Which of the following statements is true? ________
    a. Both the sympathetic and parasympathetic supply to the heart is via the vagus nerve
    b. The sympathetic supply to the heart increases the rate and force of the heartbeat
    c. The sinoatrial node is supplied only by sympathetic nerve fibres
    d. The heart rate slows during parasympathetic activity because of the release of noradrenaline

55. Blood pressure is usually expressed as: ________
    a. Diastolic pressure over systolic pressure
    b. Pulse pressure over diastolic pressure
    c. Systolic pressure over diastolic pressure
    d. Diastolic pressure over pulse pressure

56. Which of the following events can be measured as systolic blood pressure? ________
    a. Atrial contraction
    b. Ventricular contraction
    c. Pulse pressure
    d. Cardiac diastole

57. What are the two main factors in health determining blood pressure? ________
    a. Cardiac output and peripheral resistance
    b. Peripheral resistance and blood volume
    c. Blood volume and pulse pressure
    d. Pulse pressure and cardiac output

58. Which of the following is associated with the moment to moment control of blood pressure? ________
    a. The renin–angiotensin system
    b. Control of blood volume
    c. The baroreceptor reflex
    d. The Hering–Breuer reflex

59. When the atria contract, the atrioventricular valves open because: ________
    a. The pressure in the aorta is higher than the pressure in the ventricles
    b. The pressure in the ventricles is higher than the pressure in the pulmonary artery
    c. The pressure in the atria is higher than the pressure in the ventricles
    d. The pressure in the aorta is higher than the pressure in the atria

60. The cardiac valves ensure that flow of blood through the heart is one way. Where else in the cardiovascular system are there valves that are doing the same? ________
    a. Large veins such as the vena cava
    b. Capillaries
    c. Medium-sized veins
    d. Arteries

61. The second heart sound is due to: ________
    a. Rushing of blood into the aorta
    b. Contraction of the myocardium
    c. Discharge of the sinoatrial node
    d. Closing of the pulmonary and aortic valves

62. At which point in the cardiac cycle are the walls of the aorta stretched the most? ________
    a. During atrial systole
    b. When the atrioventricular valves open
    c. During the first heart sound
    d. During cardiac diastole

63. What is the function of the fetal ductus venosus? ________
    a. It bypasses the fetal liver
    b. It bypasses the fetal lungs
    c. It shunts blood from the right to the left side of the fetal heart
    d. It bypasses the fetal digestive tract

64. Which of the following is NOT TRUE of the placenta? ________
    a. Maternal blood flows into chambers called intervillous spaces.
    b. Maternal and fetal blood mixes to allow oxygenation of fetal red blood cells.
    c. Blood from the placenta is returned to the fetal heart in the umbilical vein.
    d. Endocrine cells in the placenta secrete oestrogen and progesterone to maintain pregnancy.

65. Which of the following is true of blood flow through the fetal lungs? ________
    a. There is no blood flow through the fetal lung, since the baby acquires all his oxygen from the mother
    b. The foramen ovale increases blood flow through the fetal pulmonary circulation to ensure growth of the fetal lungs
    c. The ductus arteriosus diverts blood from the fetal pulmonary artery into the fetal aorta because the fetal lungs are not functional
    d. At birth, when the baby takes his first breath, rising oxygen levels open the ductus arteriosus to allow blood to flow through the baby's pulmonary circulation

66. Which of the following is true of the ageing heart (choose all that apply)? ________
    a. The ventricles are slightly larger than in youth because the myocardial cells hypertrophy
    b. The compliance of the myocardium is usually higher than in youth because the connective tissue of the heart tends to degenerate
    c. The heart becomes more sensitive to sympathetic stimulation, increasing the resting heart rate
    d. The number of myocardial cells falls with age, as ageing cells die and are not replaced

67. When the body is upright, which of the following increase venous return to the heart (choose all that apply)? ________
    a. Gravity
    b. The respiratory pump
    c. The skeletal muscle pump
    d. Increased parasympathetic activity

6 The lymphatic system

The lymphatic system consists of a network of lymphatic vessels, the fluid that flows through them and various specialised organs and tissues. Its main functions are in tissue drainage and in the production and maintenance of immune cells.

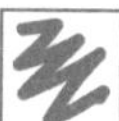 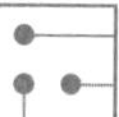 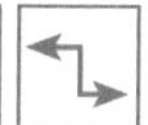

COLOURING, LABELLING AND MATCHING

1. Figure 6.1 shows the main structures of the lymphatic system. Label the structures indicated using the key choices listed.

Key choices:		
Inguinal nodes	Lymph follicles of the small intestine (Peyer's patches)	Right lymphatic duct
Lymphatic vessels of the lower limb	Submandibular nodes	Lymphatic vessels of the upper limb
Palatine tonsil	Cisterna chyli	Iliac nodes
Thoracic duct (twice)	Intestinal nodes	Popliteal nodes
	Axillary nodes	Cervical nodes

2. On Figure 6.1, colour and label the spleen, red bone marrow of the right femur and the thymus gland, using the key below.

- O Spleen
- O Thymus gland
- O Red bone marrow

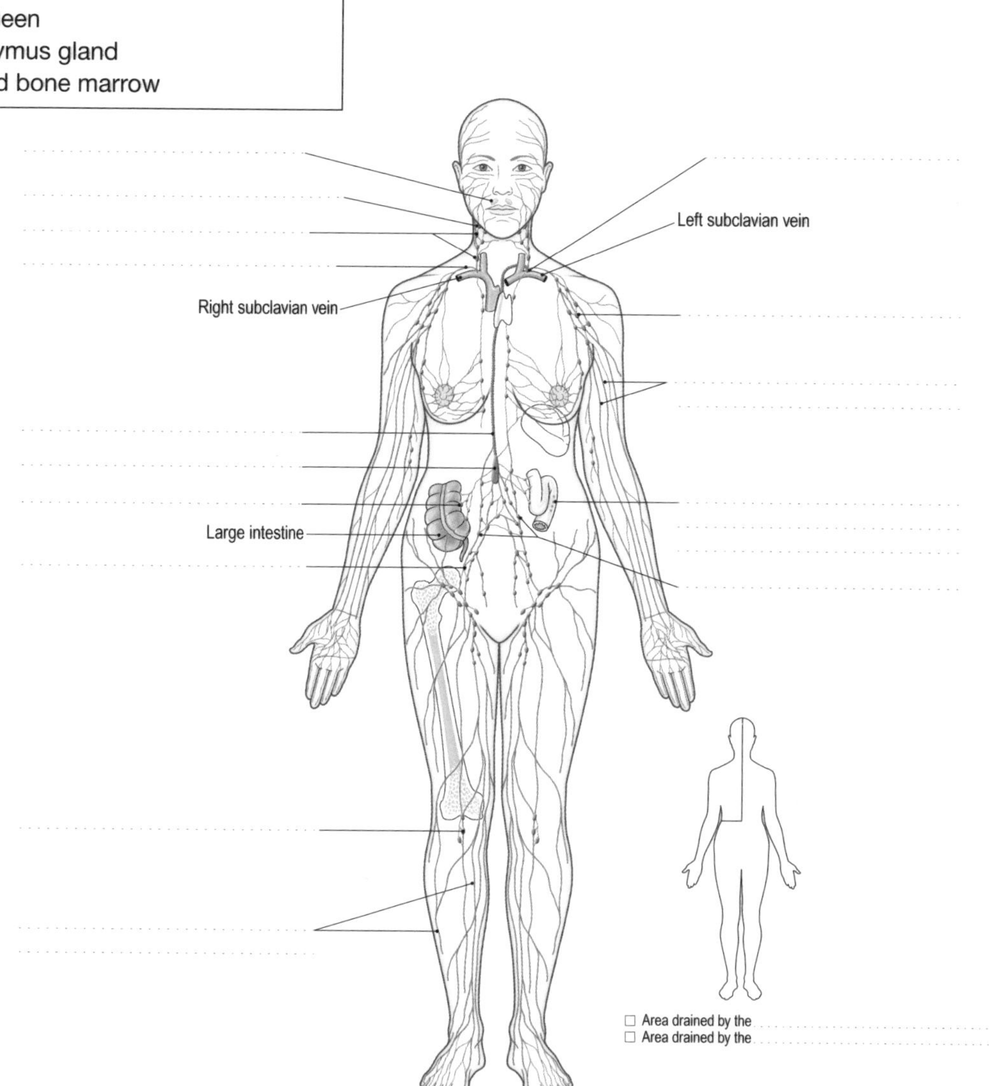

Figure 6.1 The lymphatic system

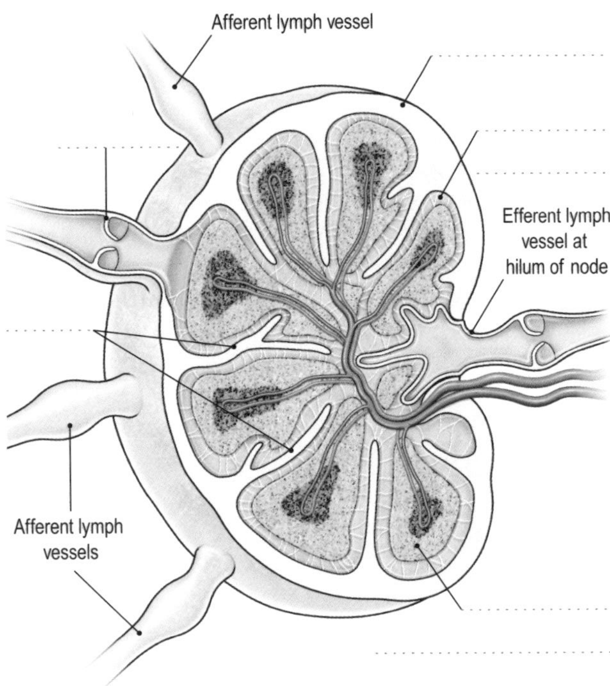

Figure 6.2 Section of a lymph node

3. Figure 6.2 shows the internal structure of a lymph node. Label the structures indicated and colour the capsule and associated trabeculae.
4. On Figure 6.2, insert arrows to show which way lymph will flow through this lymph node.
5. On average, lymph flows through how many lymph nodes before returning to the bloodstream? ____________________

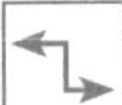

MATCHING

6. For each of the following key choices, decide whether it applies to the lymph nodes, the spleen or the thymus, and complete Table 6.1.

Key choices:

Where T-lymphocytes mature
Bean-shaped
Largest lymphatic organ
Site of multiplication of activated lymphocytes
Stores blood
Made up of two narrow lobes
Red blood cells destroyed here
Distributed throughout lymphatic system
Maximum weight usually 30–40 g
Lies immediately below the diaphragm
At its maximum size at puberty
Filters lymph
Oval in shape
Lies immediately behind the sternum
Size from pinhead to almond-sized
Secretes the hormone thymosin
Synthesises red blood cells in the fetus
Phagocytoses cellular debris

Table 6.1 Characteristics of lymph nodes, spleen and thymus

Spleen	Thymus	Lymph node

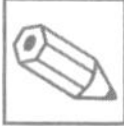

COMPLETION

7. The following paragraph describes lymphatic vessels. Complete it by scoring out the incorrect options in bold, leaving the correct option(s).

   The smallest lymphatic vessels are called **ducts/venules/capillaries**. One significant difference between them and the smallest blood vessels is that they are **only one cell thick/have permeable walls/originate in the tissues**; their function is to drain the lymph, containing **red blood cells/white blood cells/platelets**, away from the interstitial spaces. Most tissues have a network of these tiny vessels, but one notable exception is **bone tissue/muscle tissue/fatty tissue**. The individual tiny vessels join up to form larger ones, which now contain **two/three/four** layers of tissue in their walls, similar to veins in the cardiovascular system. The inner lining, the **endothelial/fibrous/muscular** layer, covers the valves, which **filter the lymph/store the lymph/regulate flow of lymph**. As vessels progressively unite and become wider and wider, eventually they empty into the biggest lymph vessels of all, the thoracic duct and the **right lymphatic duct/subclavian duct and the right lymphatic duct/thoracic duct and subclavian duct.** The first one of these drains the **left side of the body/ right side of the body above the diaphragm/lower limbs and pelvic area.** The second drains the **upper body above the pelvis/right side of the body/lower part of the body and the upper left side above the diaphragm.**

MCQs

8. Which important constituent of blood is absent from lymph? _______
   a. Glucose
   b. Erythrocytes
   c. Lymphocytes
   d. Antibodies

9. What is the difference between lymph and interstitial fluid? _______
   a. Lymph contains white blood cells and interstitial fluid does not
   b. Nothing; the two terms are interchangeable
   c. Interstitial fluid bathes the cells and lymph is found in the lymphatic vessels
   d. Lymph becomes interstitial fluid when it returns to the bloodstream

10. Which nutrient is absorbed into the lymphatic vessels of the small intestine? _______
    a. Glucose
    b. Amino acids
    c. Vitamins
    d. Fats

11. Which of the following does not contribute to lymph flow? _______
    a. Contraction of adjacent skeletal muscles
    b. Pulsation of nearby arteries
    c. Active propulsion by valves in the lymph vessel
    d. Peristalsis-like action of the lymph vessel wall

12. The thoracic duct empties lymph into the: _______
    a. Subclavian duct
    b. Subclavian vein
    c. Right lymphatic duct
    d. Superior vena cava

13. Which of the following lacks a network of lymphatic vessels? _______
    a. Brain and cornea
    b. Spinal cord and heart
    c. Liver and bones
    d. Epidermis and lungs

14. Which two types of tissue are found in a lymph node? _______
    a. Blood and lymphatic vessels
    b. Cartilage and smooth muscle
    c. Reticular and lymphatic tissue
    d. Lymphatic vessels in connective tissue

15. Which important protective cells are found within lymph nodes? _______
    a. Lymphocytes and macrophages
    b. Neutrophils and antibodies
    c. Red blood cells and monocytes
    d. Eosinophils and granulocytes

16. Which of the following statements is true concerning lymph nodes? _______
    a. The outer capsule of the node is formed of smooth muscle, to help propel lymph one-way through the system
    b. Each node has several efferent vessels but only one afferent vessel
    c. The cisterna chyli is the biggest lymph node in the body
    d. Each node has a concave surface called the hilum where various vessels enter and leave the node

17. Which group of nodes drains the arm? _______
    a. The mammary nodes
    b. The axillary nodes
    c. The inguinal nodes
    d. The cervical nodes

18. Mucosa-associated lymphoid tissue (MALT): _______
    a. Is enclosed within a protective capsule
    b. Filters lymph
    c. Contains T- and B-lymphocytes
    d. Is found only in the gastrointestinal tract

19. Tonsils are made up of lymphatic tissue and: _______
    a. Do not filter lymph
    b. Produce saliva
    c. Are well supplied with afferent lymphatic vessels
    d. Are found in a ring around the larynx

20. Aggregated lymph follicles (Peyer's patches) are found in the: _______
    a. Throat
    b. Lungs
    c. Gastrointestinal tract
    d. Lymph nodes

21. Thymosin: _______
    a. Is produced by the thyroid gland
    b. Is responsible for maturation of the thymus
    c. Is an essential cofactor in antibody production
    d. Levels increase with age

7 The nervous system

The nervous system detects and quickly responds to changes inside and outside the body. Together with the endocrine system, it controls important aspects of body function. Coordinated responses to changes in the body's internal environment maintain homeostasis and regulate its involuntary functions while responses to changes within the external environment maintain posture and other voluntary activities.

The nervous system consists of the brain, spinal cord and peripheral nerves organised to enable rapid communication between different parts of the body. This chapter is designed to help you learn more about the structure and functions of the nervous system and its components.

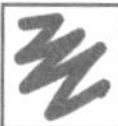 

COLOURING AND MATCHING

1. Figure 7.1 provides an overview of the nervous system. Colour and match:

   - ○ The central nervous system
   - ○ The peripheral nervous system.

2. Name the two main components of the central nervous system:

   - ________________________
   - ________________________

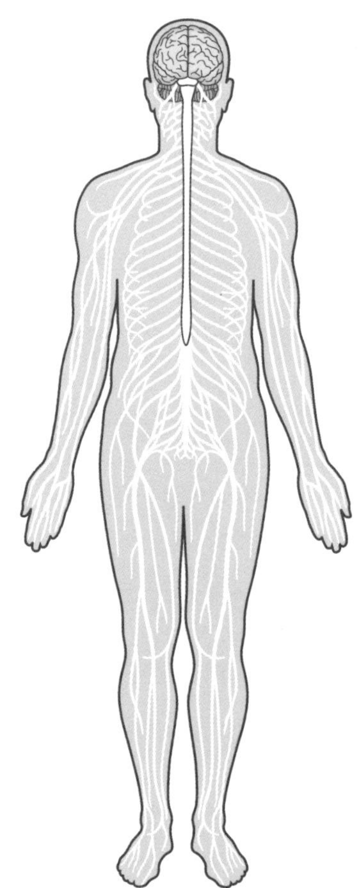

Figure 7.1 Overview of the nervous system

3. Match the key choices with their corresponding spaces in the paragraph below that describes the key components of the nervous system.

Key choices:
Afferent
Autonomic
Balance
Effector
Efferent
Glands
Motor
Movement
Parasympathetic
Sensory
Skeletal
Sympathetic

The peripheral nervous system has two functionally distinct divisions. One relays information along ________________ nerves towards the central nervous system; this is the ________________ division. The ________________ division transmits impulses from the brain and spinal cord to effector organs along ____________ nerves. Some of these nerves transmit impulses to ____________ or voluntary muscles enabling control of ________________ and maintenance of ____________. Smooth and cardiac muscle as well as ______________ are ________________ organs of the ____________ nervous system, which has two complementary divisions. The ______________ division prepares the body for 'fight or flight' while the ____________ division enables the body to 'rest and repair'.

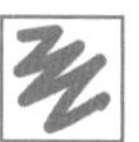 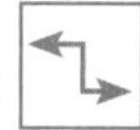 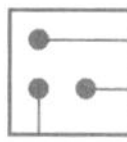

COLOURING, MATCHING AND LABELLING

4. Colour and match the following parts of the neurone on Figure 7.2.

- O Nucleus
- O Terminal boutons
- O Axon hillock
- O Dendrites
- O Myelin sheath

5. Label the parts of the neurone indicated in Figure 7.2

6. Draw an arrow beside the neurone to show the direction of impulse conduction.

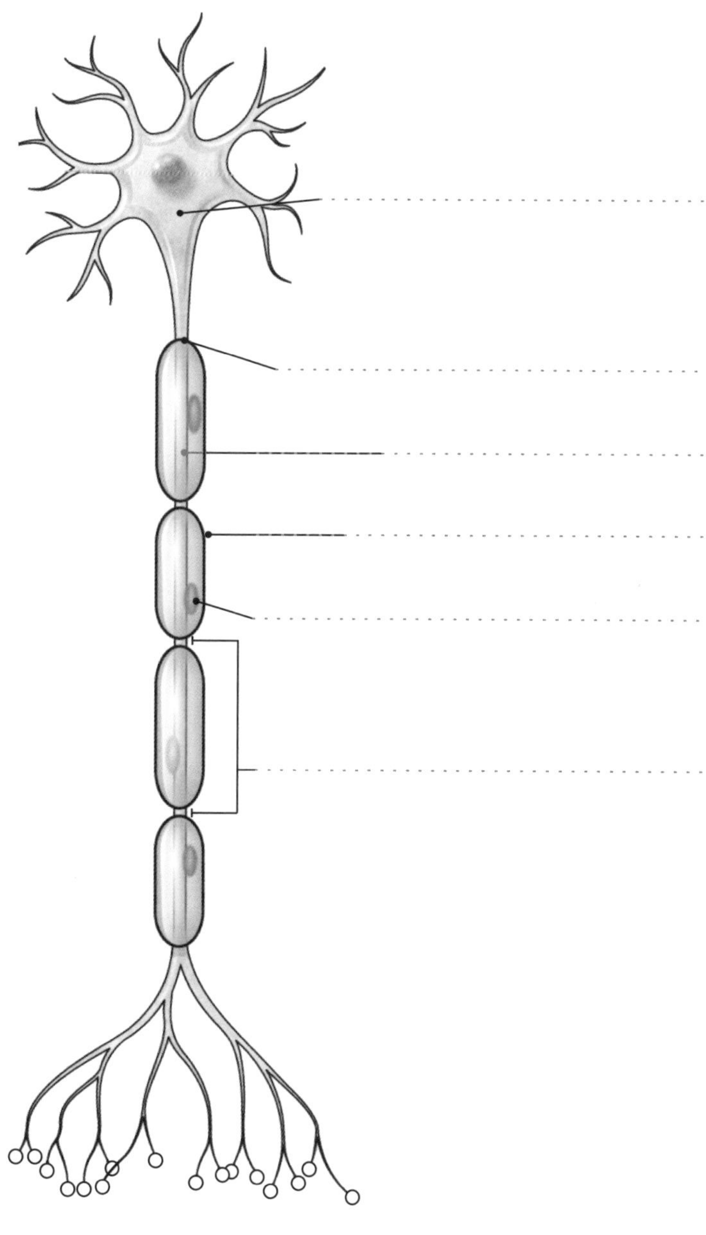

Figure 7.2 The structure of a myelinated neurone

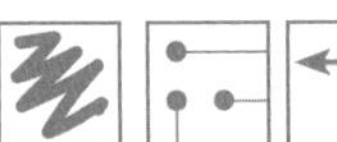

COLOURING, LABELLING AND MATCHING

7. Figure 7.3 illustrates the main parts of a synapse. Colour and match the following:

○ Presynaptic neurone ○ Postsynaptic neurone

8. Label the structures indicated on Figure 7.3.

9. Add arrows showing the direction of impulse transmission in the neurones.

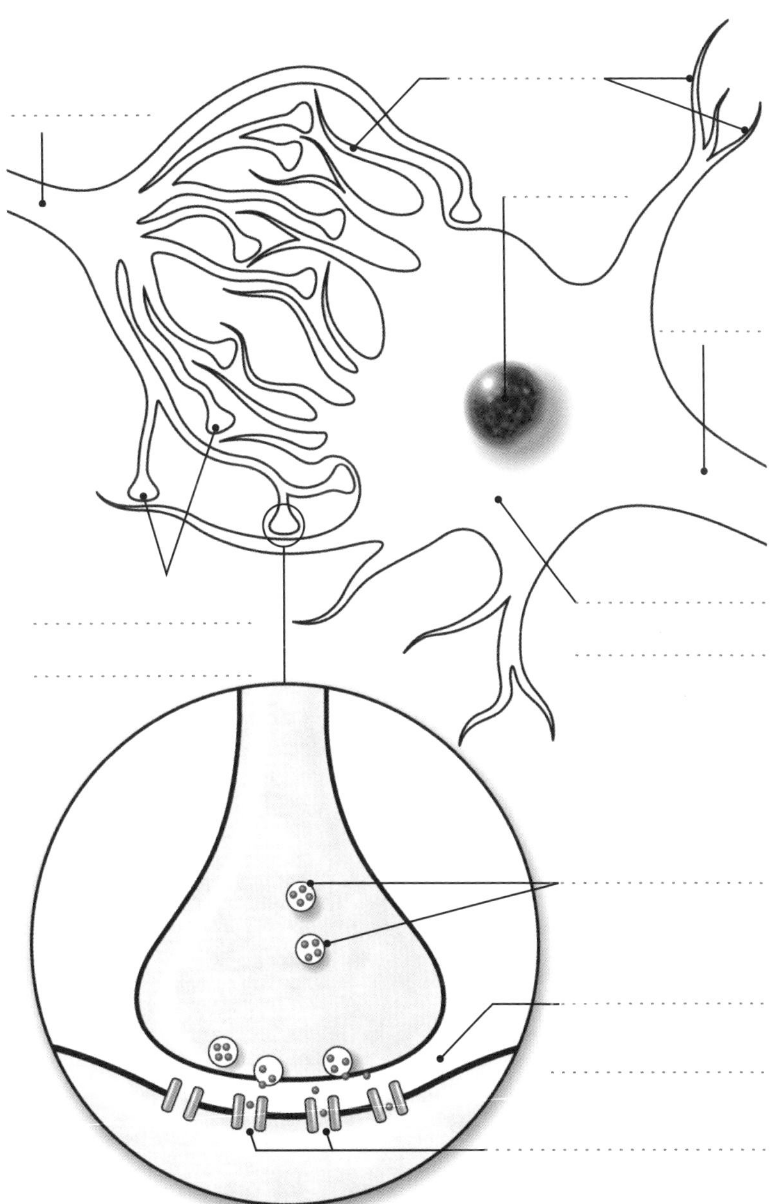

Figure 7.3 Diagram of a synapse

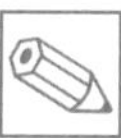

COMPLETION

10. Fill in the blanks in the paragraph below to describe the conduction of nerve impulses.

Transmission of the _______________, or impulse, is due to movement of _______________ across the nerve cell membrane. In the resting state, the nerve cell membrane is _______________ due to differences in the concentrations of ions across the plasma membrane. This means that there is a different electrical charge on each side of the membrane, which is called the resting _______________. At rest, the charge outside the cell is _______________ and inside it is _______________. The principal ions involved are _______________ and _______________. In the resting state, there is a continual tendency for these ions to diffuse down their _______________. During the action potential, sodium ions flood _______________ the neurone, causing _______________. This is followed by _______________, when potassium ions move _______________ the neurone. In myelinated neurones, the insulating properties of the _______________ prevent the movement of ions across the membrane when this is present. In these neurones, impulses pass from one _______________ to the next and transmission is called _______________. In unmyelinated fibres, nerve impulses are conducted by the process called _______________. Impulse conduction is faster when the mechanism of transmission is _______________ than when it is _______________. The diameter of the neurone also affects the rate of impulse conduction – the _______________ the diameter, the faster the conduction.

? MCQs

11. A nerve impulse passes from a presynaptic neurone to the postsynaptic neurone across the: ________
    a. Axon b. Axon hillock c. Neuromuscular junction d. Synapse

12. Neurotransmitters are stored in membrane-bound packages known as: ________
    a. Golgi bodies b. Mitochondria c. Vesicles d. Lysosomes

13. Neurotransmitters cross the gap between the presynaptic neurone and the postsynaptic neurone by: ________
    a. Active transport b. Diffusion c. Pinocytosis d. Phagocytosis

14. Neurotransmitters act on: ________
    a. Any area of the postsynaptic neurone causing depolarisation
    b. Any area of the postsynaptic neurone causing repolarisation
    c. Specific receptors on the postsynaptic neurone causing depolarisation
    d. Specific receptors on the postsynaptic neurone causing repolarisation

15. Myelinated neurones: ________
    a. Are only found in the peripheral nervous system
    b. Have axons that are completely surrounded by the protein myelin
    c. Conduct impulses more rapidly than unmyelinated neurones
    d. Conduct impulses by simple propagation

CENTRAL NERVOUS SYSTEM

POT LUCK

16. This exercise considers characteristics of the different types of non-excitable glial cells found in the central nervous system. For each statement below, identify which key choice it refers to (you may use the key choices more than once):

Key choices:			
Astrocytes	Microglia	Oligodendrocytes	Ependymal cells

    a. The main supporting tissue of the central nervous system is formed by: ____________________
    b. These cells provide protection when they become phagocytic in areas of inflammation: ____________________.
    c. The cells found along the length of myelinated nerve fibres are: ____________________
    d. The star-shaped supporting cells are: ____________________
    e. The lining of the ventricles of the brain and the central canal of the spinal cord is formed by: ____________________
    f. These cells form and maintain myelin: ____________________
    g. Found in large numbers around blood vessels, with their foot processes forming the blood–brain barrier, these cells are: ____________________

17. Outline the function of the blood–brain barrier. ____________________

18. Outline the functions of cerebrospinal fluid (CSF): ____________________

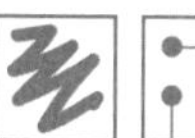
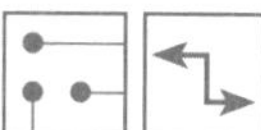

COLOURING, LABELLING AND MATCHING

19. Label the meninges and other structures indicated on Figure 7.4.

20. On Figure 7.4, colour and match the following:

- O Areas where CSF circulates in the brain and spinal cord
- O Venous sinuses
- O Basal ganglia
- O Thalamus
- O Cerebral cortex
- O Cerebellum

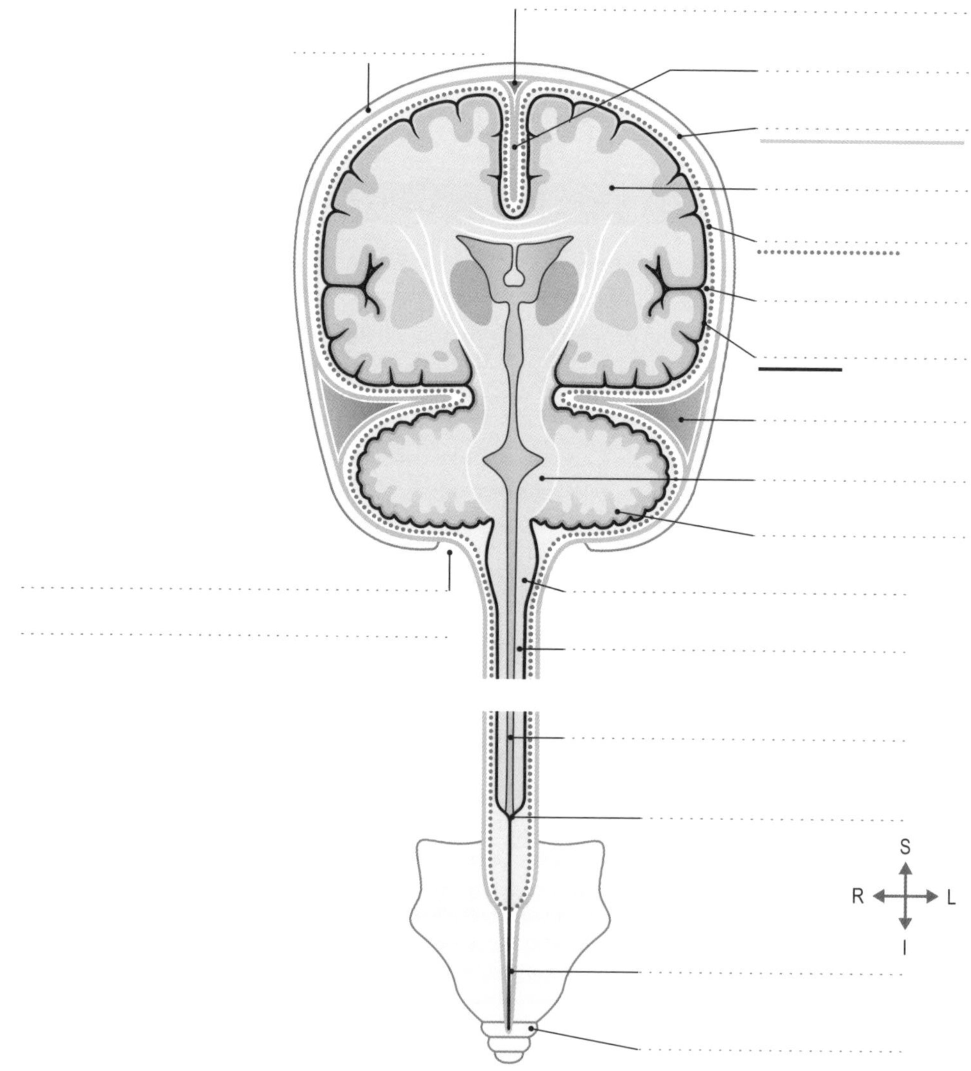

Figure 7.4 The meninges covering the brain and spinal cord

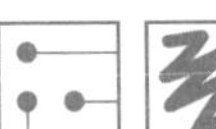

LABELLING AND COLOURING

21. Colour the ventricular system of the brain.

22. Label the components of the ventricular system identified in Figure 7.5.

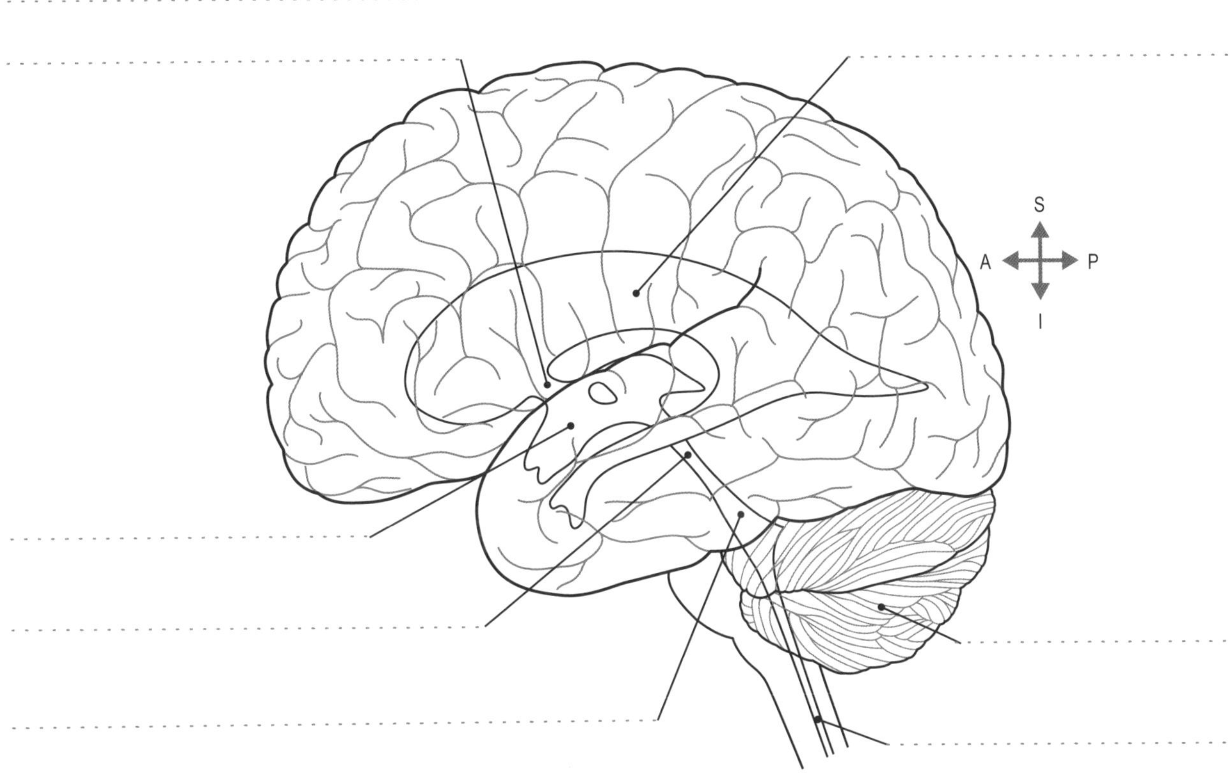

Figure 7.5 The positions of the ventricles in the brain. Viewed from the left side.

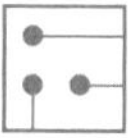 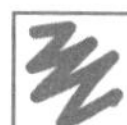 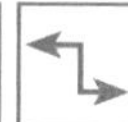

COLOURING, LABELLING AND MATCHING

23. Colour, match and label the corresponding parts of the central nervous system on Figure 7.6:

- O Cerebrum
- O Diencephalon
- O Brain stem
- O Cerebellum
- O Spinal cord

24. Label the other structures shown on Figure 7.6.

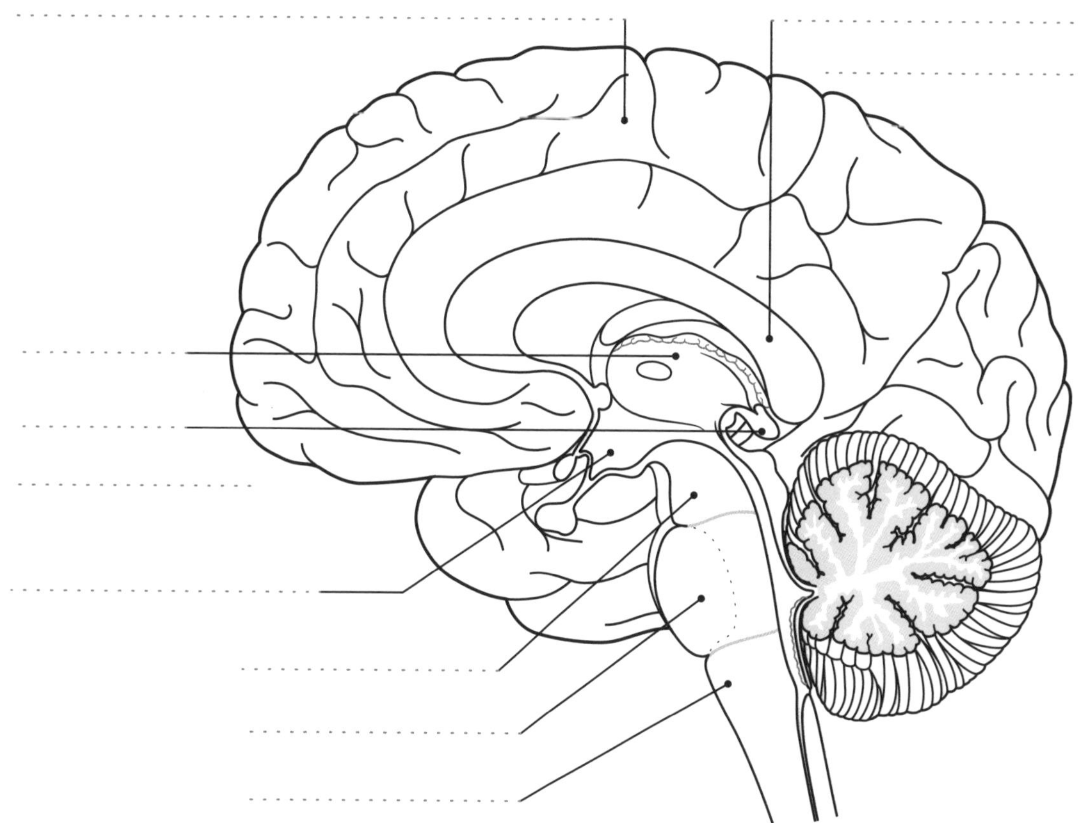

Figure 7.6 The parts of the central nervous system

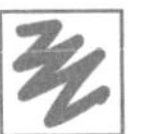 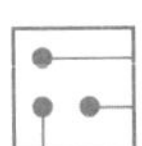 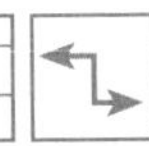

COLOURING, LABELLING AND MATCHING

25. Colour and match the functional areas of the cerebrum listed below with those identified in Figure 7.7:

- O Taste area
- O Somatosensory area
- O Primary motor area
- O Prefrontal area
- O Sensory speech (Wernicke's) area
- O Auditory area
- O Motor speech (Broca's) area
- O Premotor area
- O Visual area

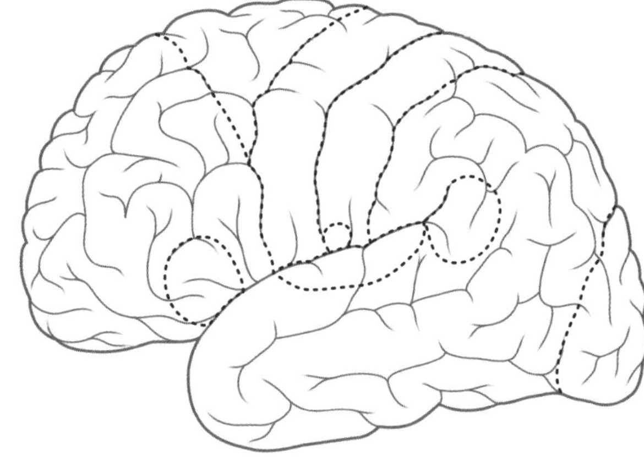

Figure 7.7 The cerebrum showing the functional areas

26. Label the central sulcus

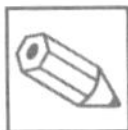

COMPLETION

27. Complete Table 7.1 by ticking the appropriate column(s) for each statement about the meninges.

Table 7.1 Characteristics of the meninges

Characteristic	Dura mater	Arachnoid mater	Pia mater
Consists of two layers of fibrous tissue			
Consists of fine connective tissue			
A delicate serous membrane			
The subdural space lies between these two layers			
Surrounds the venous sinuses			
The subarachnoid space separates these two layers			
Forms the filum terminale			
Cerebrospinal fluid is found in the space between these two layers			
Equivalent to the periosteum of other bones			

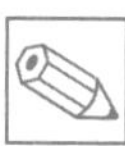

COMPLETION

28. Identify the correct options to describe the structure of the cerebrum.

This is the largest part of the brain and is divided into left and right cerebral **lobes/hemispheres**. Deep inside, the two parts are connected by the **corpus callosum/cerebellum**, which consists of **white/grey** matter. The superficial layer of the cerebrum is known as the **cerebral cortex/cerebellum** and consists of **nerve cell bodies/axons** or **white/grey** matter. The deeper layer consists of **nerve cell bodies/axons** and is **white/grey** in colour. The cerebral cortex has many furrows and folds that vary in depth. The exposed areas are the convolutions or **sulci/gyri** and they are separated by **sulci/gyri**, also known as fissures, which increase the surface area of the cerebrum.

29. The following paragraphs describe aspects of the motor areas of the cerebrum. Cross out the wrong options so that it reads correctly.

The primary motor area lies in the **parietal/temporal/frontal** lobe immediately anterior to the **central/lateral/parieto-occipital** sulcus. The cell bodies are **oval/pyramid-shaped/hexagonal** and stimulation leads to contraction of **smooth/skeletal/cardiac** muscle. Their nerve fibres pass downwards through the **thalamus/internal capsule/hypothalamus** to the **midbrain/cerebellum/medulla**, where they cross to the opposite side and then descend in the spinal cord. These neurones are the upper motor neurones. They synapse with the lower motor neurones in the **spinal cord/medulla/cerebellum**, and lower motor neurones terminate at a **neuromuscular junction/synapse/sensory receptor**. This means that the motor area of the right hemisphere controls skeletal muscle movement on the **left/the right/both** sides(s) of the body.In the motor area of the cerebrum, body areas are represented in **mirror image/the right way up/upside down,** and the proportion of the cerebral cortex that represents a particular part of the body reflects its **size/complexity of movement/distance from the brain**.The motor speech (Broca's) area lies in the **parietal/temporal/frontal** lobe and controls the movements needed for speech. The right hemisphere is dominant in **left-handed/ambidextrous/right-handed** people.

30. Outline the functions of:

a. The reticular activating system ______________________________

____

____

b. The cerebellum ______________________________

____

c. The thalamus ______________________________

____

____

MCQS

31. Which of the following is involved in the secretion of CSF? (Choose all that apply.) _______
    a. Arachnoid villi
    b. Choroid plexuses
    c. Third ventricle
    d. Fourth ventricle

32. CSF circulation is aided by which of the following? (Choose all that apply.) _______
    a. Breathing
    b. Pulsing blood vessels
    c. A pump
    d. Changes in posture

33. CSF normally contains: _______
    a. Glucose, albumin, red blood cells, white blood cells
    b. White blood cells, red blood cells, albumin, globulin
    c. Globulin, red blood cells, glucose, albumin
    d. Albumin, globulin, white blood cells, glucose

34. CSF returns to the blood through the: _______
    a. Foramina in the roof of the fourth ventricle when venous pressure is greater than CSF pressure
    b. Foramina in the roof of the fourth ventricle when CSF pressure is greater than venous pressure
    c. Arachnoid villi when venous pressure is greater than CSF pressure
    d. Arachnoid villi when CSF pressure is greater than venous pressure

35. Normal CSF pressure when lying down is around: _______
    a. 5 cm H_2O
    b. 10 cm H_2O
    c. 15 cm H_2O
    d. 20 cm H_2O

36. Which of the following is not part of the brain stem? _______
    a. Midbrain
    b. Pons
    c. Cerebellum
    d. Medulla

37. The hypothalamus is involved in control of which of the following? (Choose all that apply.) _______
    a. The autonomic nervous system
    b. Body temperature
    c. Blood glucose levels
    d. Thirst and water balance

38. Important masses of grey matter in the cerebrum include which of the following? (Choose all that apply.) _______
    a. Basal ganglia
    b. Pons
    c. Thalamus
    d. Reticular formation

39. The vital centres are found within the: _______
    a. Midbrain
    b. Pons
    c. Cerebellum
    d. Medulla

40. Proprioceptor impulses originate from the: _______
    a. Brain
    b. Skin
    c. Joints
    d. Eyes

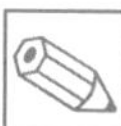 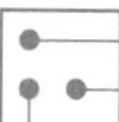

COMPLETION AND LABELLING

41. Label the structures indicated on Figure 7.8.
42. Draw arrows indicating the directions of the nerve impulses in a reflex arc on Figure 7.8.
43. Insert an arrow on Figure 7.8 showing where the knee-jerk reflex is tested.

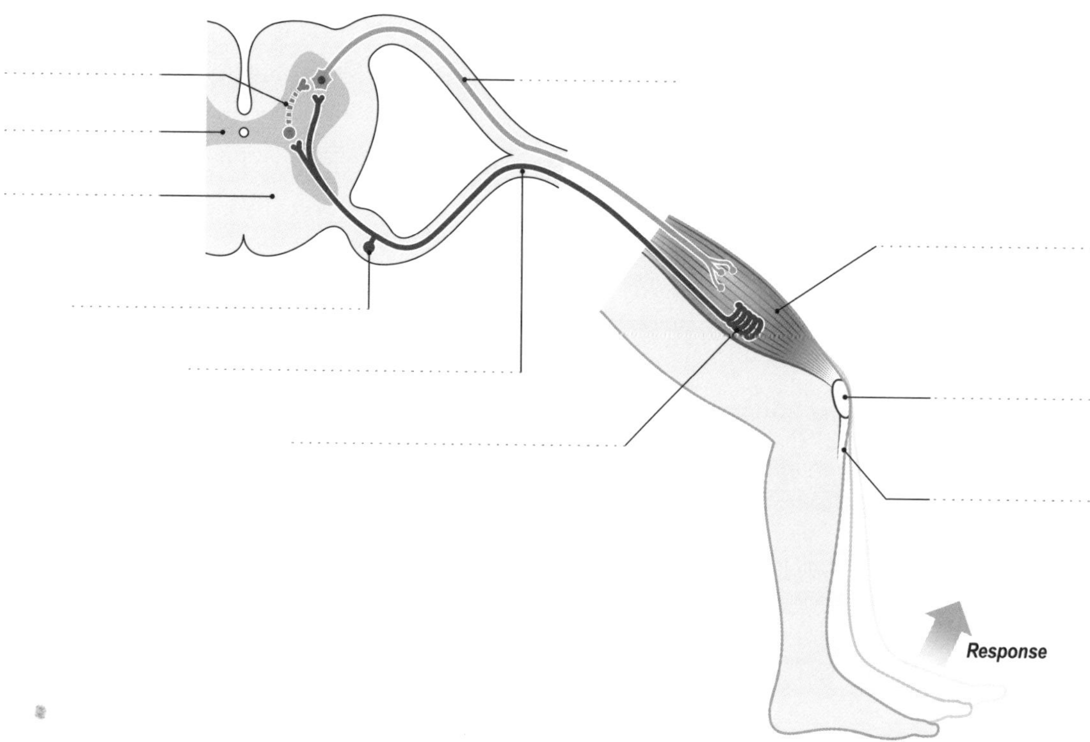

Figure 7.8 The knee-jerk reflex

PERIPHERAL NERVOUS SYSTEM

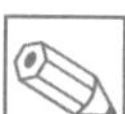

COMPLETION

44. Complete the following paragraph, describing the peripheral nervous system, by filling in the blanks.

Within the peripheral nervous system, there are __________ pairs of spinal nerves and __________ pairs of cranial nerves. These nerves are composed of either __________ nerve fibres conveying afferent impulses to the __________ from __________ organs or __________ nerve fibres that transmit efferent impulses from the __________ to __________ organs. Some nerves, known as __________ nerves, contain both types of fibres.

45. Briefly explain the function of a nerve plexus.

____

____

____

46. Name the nerves that supply the:
    a. Intercostal muscles: ______________________
    b. Diaphragm: ______________________
    c. Hamstrings: ______________________
    d. External anal sphincter: ______________________
    e. External urethral sphincter: ______________________

47. Name the largest nerve in the body: ______________________

LABELLING AND COLOURING

48. Colour the cranial nerves and their associated structures on Figure 7.9.

49. Label the numbered cranial nerves on the right side of Figure 7.9.

50. Identify the structures indicated on the left side of Figure 7.9.

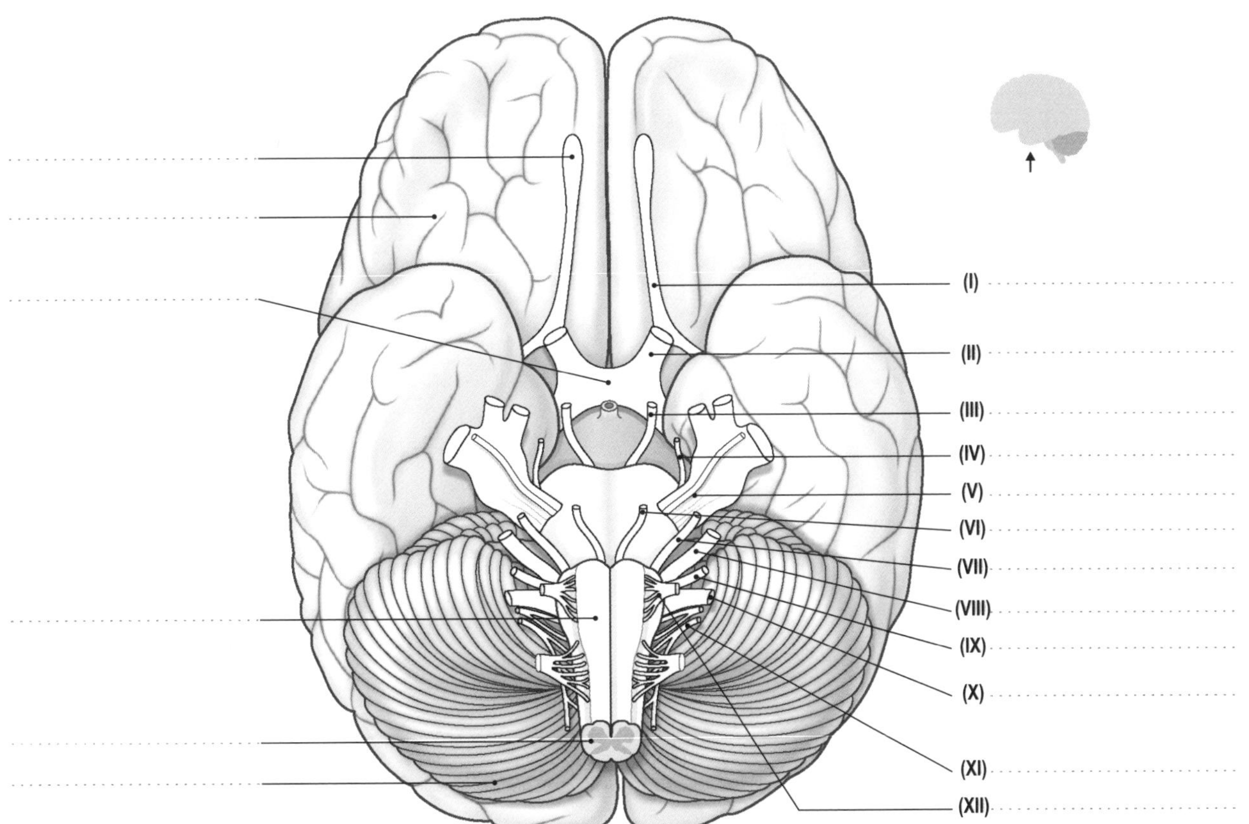

Figure 7.9 The inferior surface of the brain showing the cranial nerves

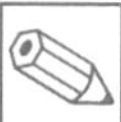 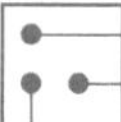 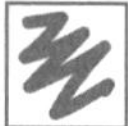 COMPLETION, LABELLING AND COLOURING

51. Draw in lines to represent the postganglionic fibres of the sympathetic nervous system on Figure 7.10.
52. Label the three prevertebral ganglia shown on Figure 7.10.
53. Colour and name the structures supplied by the sympathetic nervous system shown in Figure 7.10.
54. Complete Figure 7.10 to show the effects of sympathetic stimulation by circling the correct options in the right hand column.
55. Describe the principal effects of sympathetic nervous system stimulation that form the fight-or-flight response.

____

____

____

56. Stimulation of the adrenal glands sustains sympathetic nervous system activity. Outline why this occurs.

____

____

____

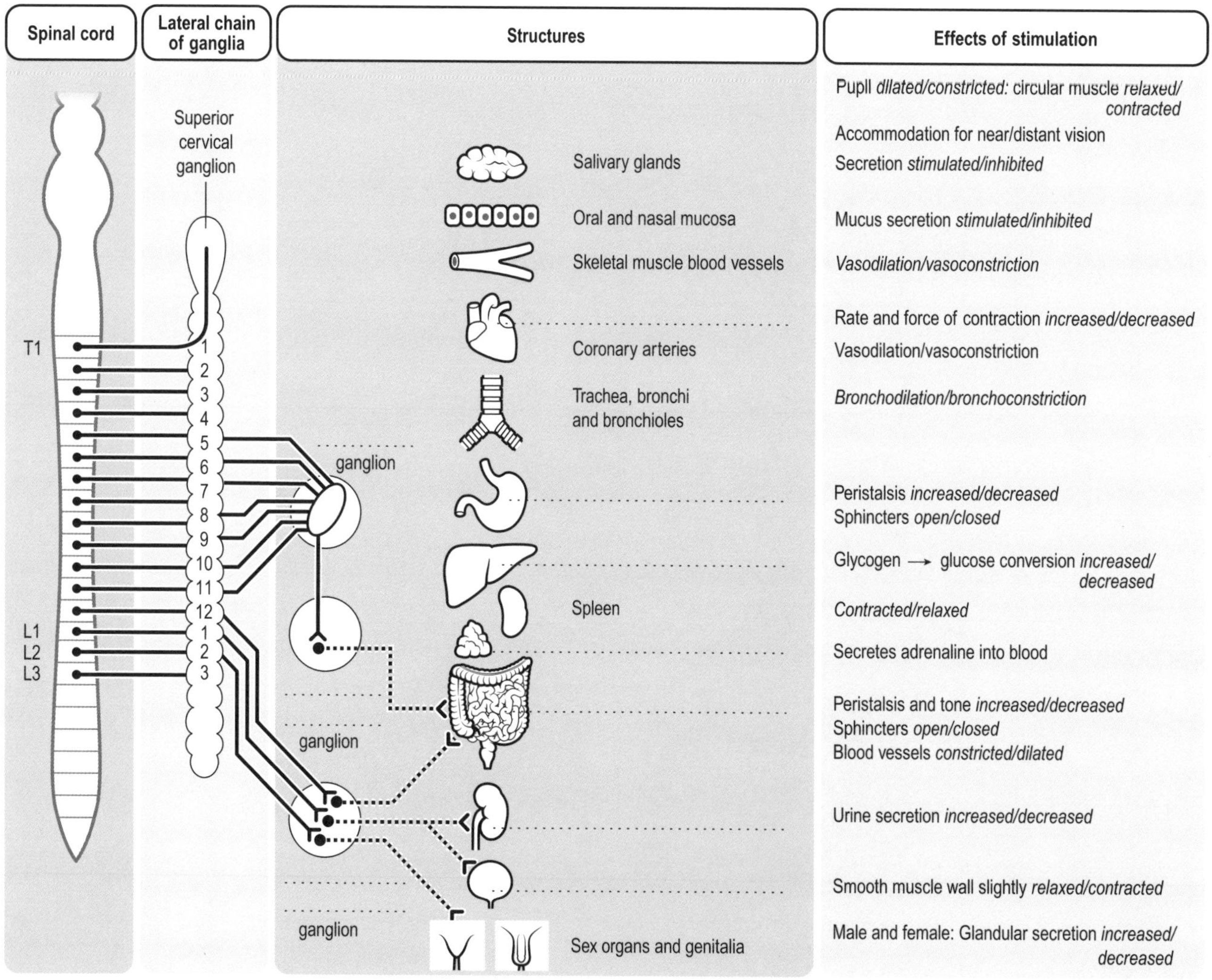

Spinal cord | Lateral chain of ganglia | Structures | Effects of stimulation

Superior cervical ganglion

T1, L1, L2, L3

1, 2, 3, 4, 5, 6, 7, 8, 9, 10, 11, 12, 1, 2, 3

.... ganglion

.... ganglion

.... ganglion

Structures	Effects of stimulation
	Pupil *dilated/constricted:* circular muscle *relaxed/ contracted*
	Accommodation for near/distant vision
Salivary glands	Secretion *stimulated/inhibited*
Oral and nasal mucosa	Mucus secretion *stimulated/inhibited*
Skeletal muscle blood vessels	*Vasodilation/vasoconstriction*
....	Rate and force of contraction *increased/decreased*
Coronary arteries	Vasodilation/vasoconstriction
Trachea, bronchi and bronchioles	*Bronchodilation/bronchoconstriction*
....	Peristalsis *increased/decreased* Sphincters *open/closed*
....	Glycogen → glucose conversion *increased/ decreased*
Spleen	*Contracted/relaxed*
....	Secretes adrenaline into blood
....	Peristalsis and tone *increased/decreased* Sphincters *open/closed* Blood vessels *constricted/dilated*
....	Urine secretion *increased/decreased*
....	Smooth muscle wall slightly *relaxed/contracted*
Sex organs and genitalia	Male and female: Glandular secretion *increased/ decreased*

Figure 7.10 The sympathetic nervous system

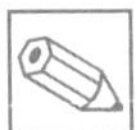

COMPLETION

57. The parasympathetic nervous system acts in a complementary manner to the sympathetic nervous system and their combined activities regulate most involuntary body function. Complete the paragraph below that summarises the main effects of parasympathetic stimulation by crossing out the incorrect options in bold.

    The parasympathetic nervous system **increases/decreases** the heart rate and **increases/decreases** the force of cardiac contraction. In the lungs its effects include mild **bronchoconstriction/bronchodilation** that **increases/decreases** airflow to the alveoli. It **stimulates/inhibits** secretion of saliva and gastric juice. Peristalsis in the digestive tract is **increased/decreased**. This action on the gastrointestinal **smooth/voluntary** muscle **increases/decreases** the rate at which gastrointestinal contents pass along and is facilitated by **relaxation/contraction** of its sphincters. In the liver, storage of glucose is promoted by **increasing/decreasing** its conversion to **glucagon/glycogen**.

? MCQs

58. Which of the following are branches of the trigeminal nerve? (Choose all that apply.) _______
    a. Facial nerve
    b. Ophthalmic nerve
    c. Maxillary nerve
    d. Mandibular nerve

59. The cranial nerves involved in the swallowing and gag reflexes are the: _______
    a. Vagus
    b. Facial
    c. Glossopharyngeal
    d. Abducent

60. The cranial nerves with the most extensive distribution are the: _______
    a. Trigeminal
    b. Vagus
    c. Glossopharyngeal
    d. Facial

61. Which cranial nerves supply the accessory muscles of respiration? _______
    a. Accessory
    b. Abducent
    c. Vagus
    d. Intercostal

8 The special senses

The special senses are those of hearing, balance, sight, smell and taste. For each one, there are specialised sensory receptors located within sensory organs in the head. Incoming information is transmitted to the brain and, together with information from other parts of the brain – for example, the memory – it is integrated, and an effector response ensues. These senses often work together either consciously or subconsciously. Conscious effects include both the taste and smell of foods, which are usually, but not always, associated with enjoyment. At the same time, they subconsciously prepare the digestive system for action. This chapter will help you learn about the special senses.

THE EAR: HEARING AND BALANCE

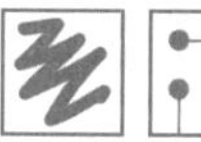
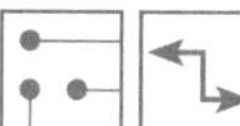

COLOURING, LABELLING AND MATCHING

1. Colour and match the following parts of the ear:

   - O Outer ear
   - O Middle ear
   - O Inner ear

2. Label the structures shown on Figure 8.1.
3. Name the substance secreted by the ceruminous glands in the auditory canal: ____________________

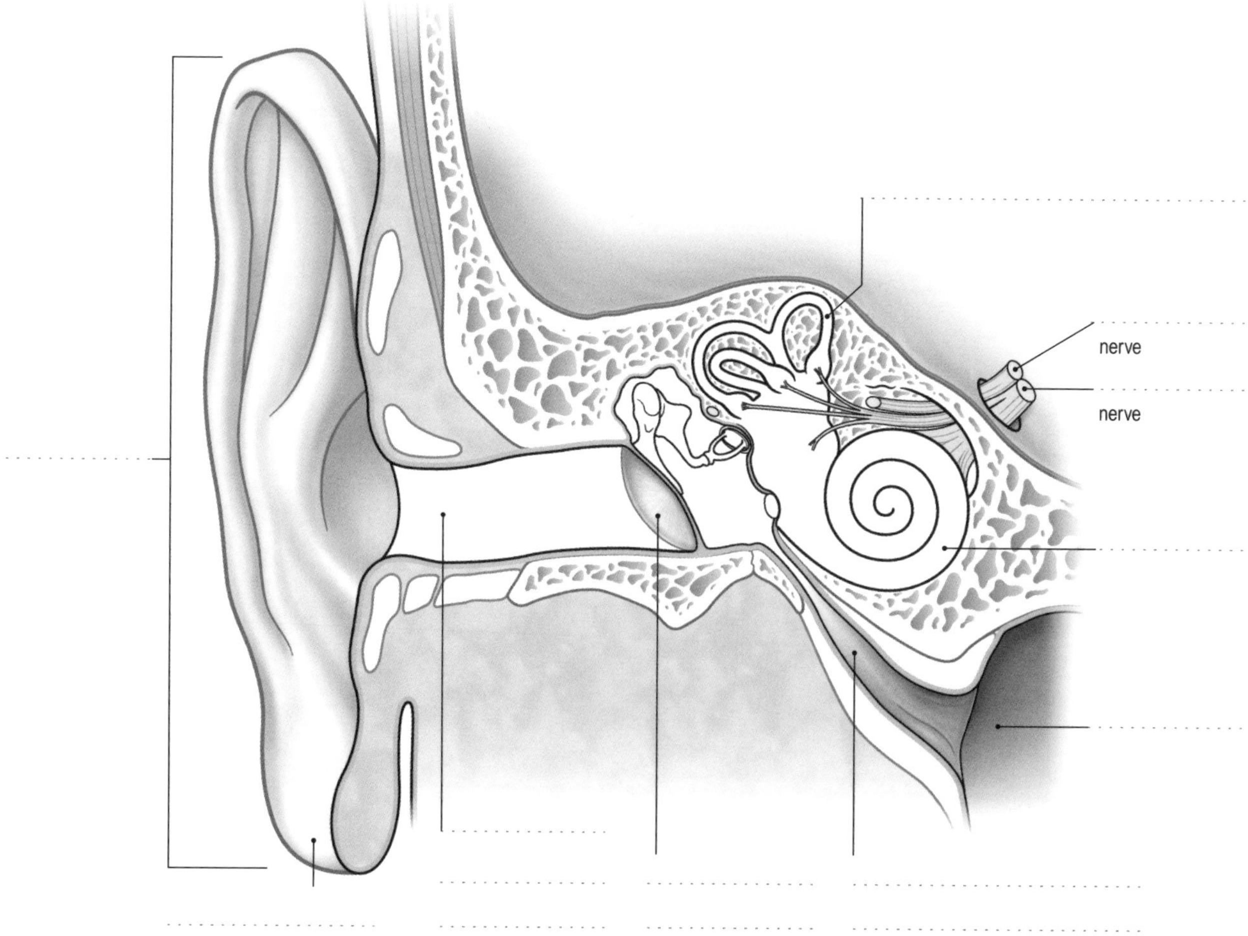

Figure 8.1 Parts of the right ear

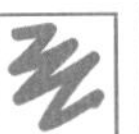 

COLOURING AND MATCHING

4. Colour and match the following parts of the middle ear shown on Figure 8.2:

- O Tympanic cavity
- O Tympanic membrane
- O Oval window
- O Malleus (hammer)
- O Incus (anvil)
- O Stapes (stirrup)
- O Round window

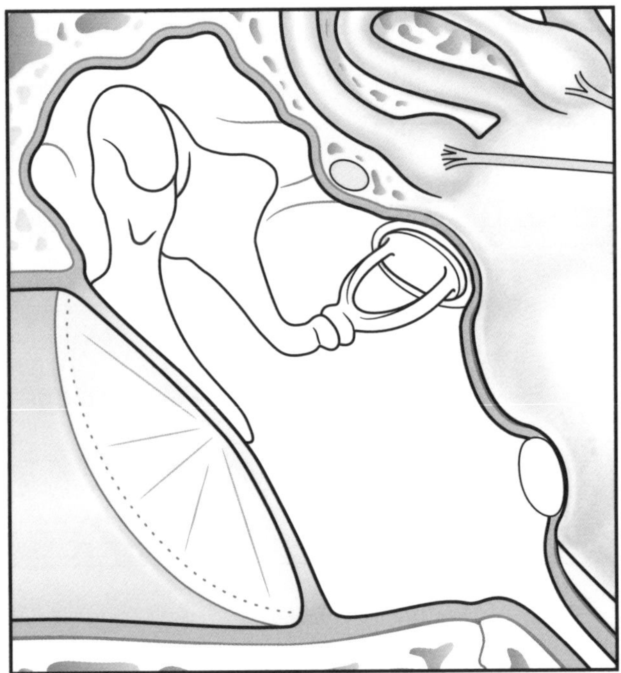

Figure 8.2 The middle ear (right)

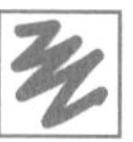
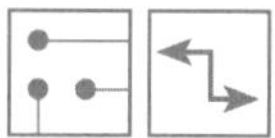

COLOURING, LABELLING AND MATCHING

5. Colour and match the following parts of the inner ear shown on Figure 8.3:

- O Bony labyrinth
- O Membranous labyrinth
- O Temporal bone

6. Label the structures indicated on Figure 8.3.
7. Name the part of the bony labyrinth where the oval and round windows are found: ______________________

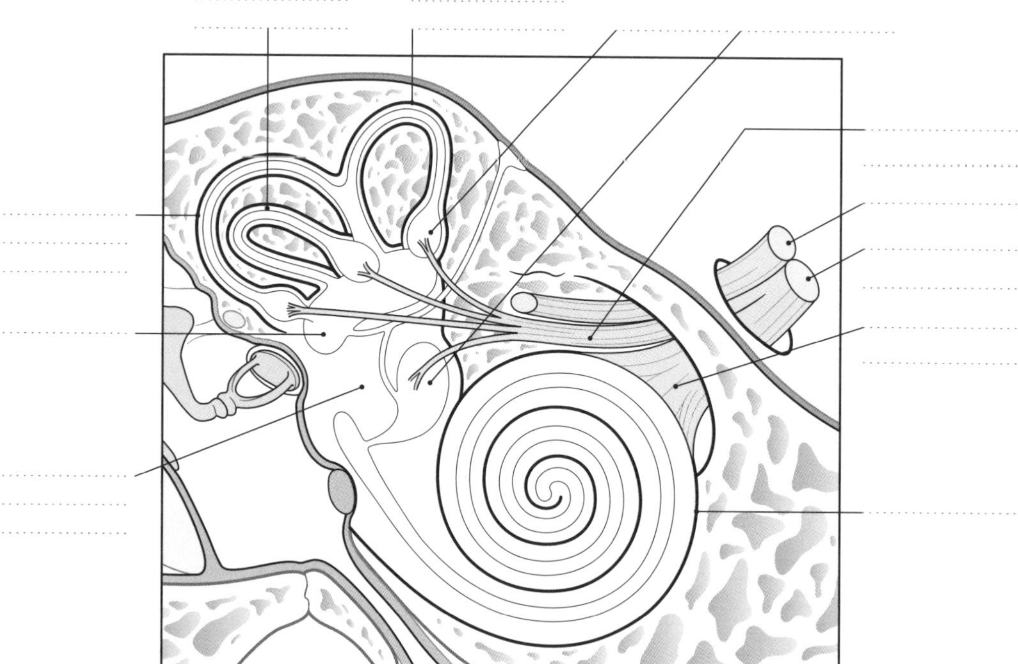

Figure 8.3 The inner ear

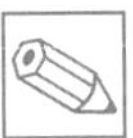

COMPLETION

8. Fill in the blanks to describe the physiology of hearing.

A sound produces ________________ in the air. The auricle ________________ and ________________ them along the ________________ to the ________________. The vibrations are ________________ and ________________ through the middle ear by movement of the ________________ At its medial end, movement of the ________________ in the ________________ window sets up fluid waves in the ________________ of the scala vestibuli. Most of this pressure is transmitted into the ________________, resulting in a corresponding fluid wave in the ________________. This stimulates the auditory receptors in the ________________ cells in the organ of hearing, the ________________. Stimulation of the auditory receptors results in the generation of ________________ that travel to the brain along the ________________ part of the ________________ nerve. The fluid wave is extinguished by vibration of the membrane of the ________________ window.

POT LUCK

9. There are seven errors in the paragraph below. Identify and correct them.

The organs involved with balance are found in the middle ear. They are the three round canals, one in each plane of space, and the vestibule, which comprises two parts, the stapes and the utricle. The canals, like the cochlea, are composed of an outer bony wall and inner membranous ducts. The membranous ducts contain perilymph and are separated from the bony wall by endolymph. They have dilated portions near the vestibule called ampullae containing hair cells with sensory nerve endings between them. Any change in the position of the head causes movement in the endolymph and perilymph. This stimulates the hair cells and nerve impulses are generated. These travel in the vestibular part of the vestibulocochlear nerve to the medulla via the cochlear nucleus. Perception of body position occurs because the cerebrum coordinates impulses from the eyes and proprioceptors in addition to those from the cerebellum.

SIGHT AND THE EYE

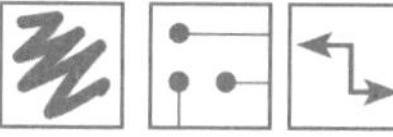

COLOURING, LABELLING AND MATCHING

10. Colour and match the following parts of the eye on Figure 8.4:

O Retina	O Optic nerve	O Cornea	O Lens
O Sclera	O Central retinal artery and vein	O Vitreous chamber	O Choroid

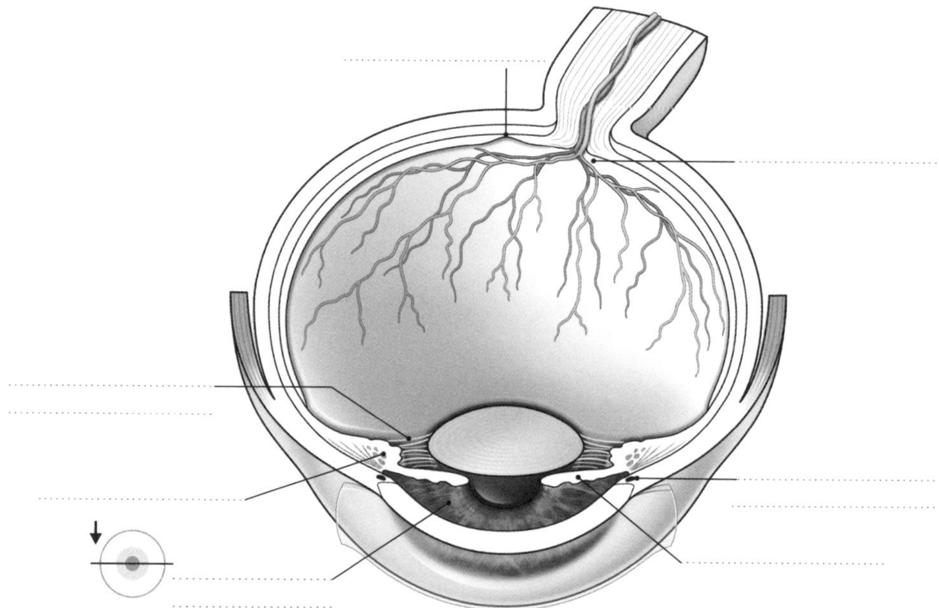

Figure 8.4 A transverse section of the eye

11. Label the structures indicated on Figure 8.4.

12. Name the tissue that lies between the eyeball and orbital cavity to protect the eye:

____

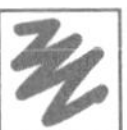
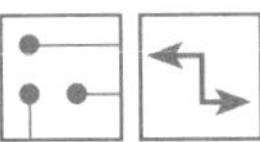

COLOURING, LABELLING AND MATCHING

13. Colour, match and label the following on Figure 8.5:

- O Lacrimal gland
- O Upper and lower eyelids
- O Maxilla
- O Frontal bone
- O Vitreous body
- O Lens
- O Tarsal plate

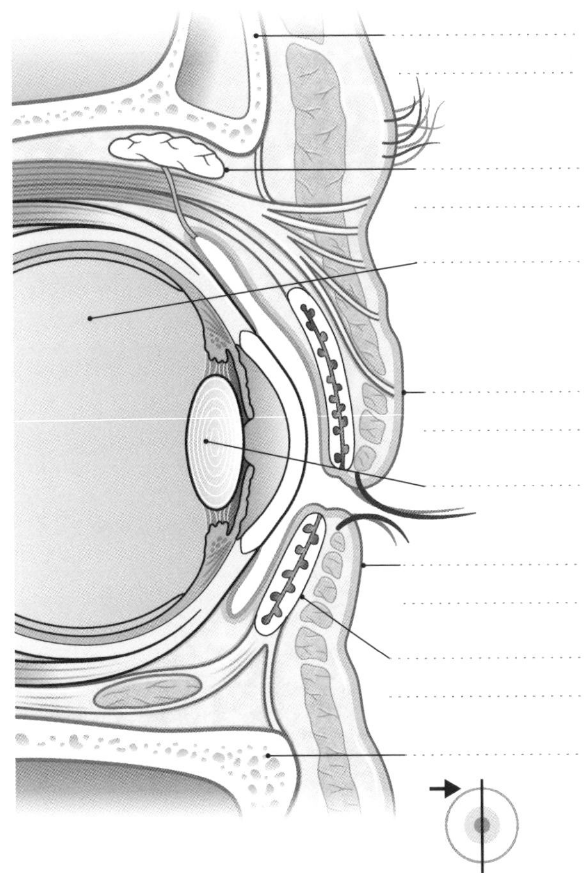

Figure 8.5 A longitudinal section of the eye and its accessory structures

 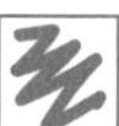

MATCHING AND COLOURING

14. Colour and match the following parts of Figure 8.6A:

- O Iris
- O Lens
- O Vitreous body

15. Label the two structures indicated on Figure 8.6A.
16. Complete Figure 8.6B by drawing in the changes that take place for near vision.
17. At what distance from a viewed object does the eye have to adjust for near vision? ______________________

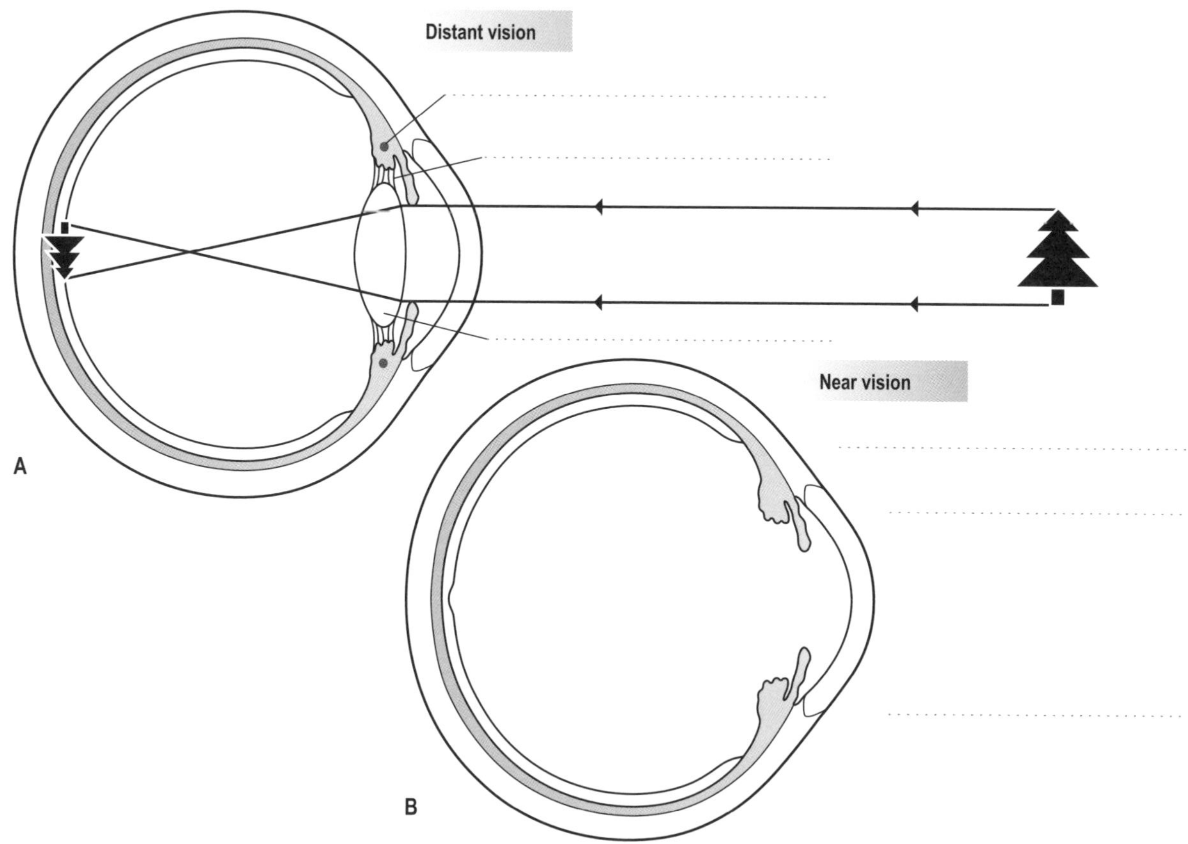

Figure 8.6 Accommodation – action of the ciliary muscle on the shape of the lens. (A) Distant vision. (B) Near vision

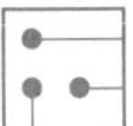

LABELLING

18. Identify the parts of the optic pathways shown in Figure 8.7.

19. Where in the brain is vision perceived?

______________________________.

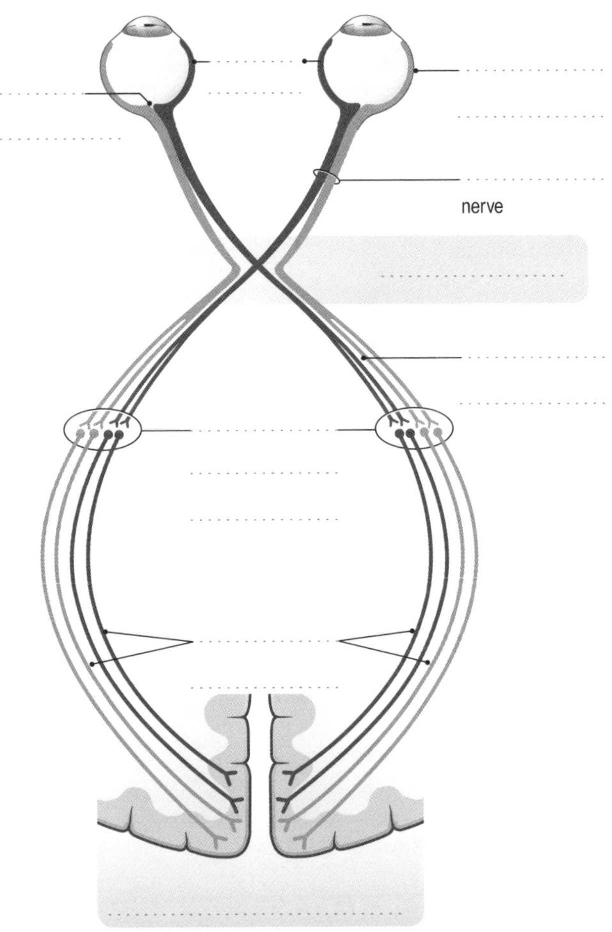

Figure 8.7 The optic nerves and their pathways

COMPLETION

20. Fill in the blanks to describe the interior of the eye.

Internally, the eye is divided into ______ compartments by the iris and the lens: the _________, ___________, and _______________ chambers. The largest is the _____________ chamber, which lies behind the lens and fills the ___________. It contains ___________________, a soft, colourless, transparent substance with a _______________ consistency.

The _______________ chamber lies between the lens and the iris, and the _______________ chamber between the iris and the cornea. These two chambers are filled with another clear substance called __________________________, whose consistency is _______________. This substance is secreted into the _______________ chamber by the ____________________ and drains back into the circulation via the _______________________________ (canal of ____________). Because there is continuous production and drainage, the intraocular pressure remains fairly constant. The structures in the front of the eye, including the cornea and the lens, are supplied with nutrients by the ______________________________.

21. Fill in the blanks to describe the retina.

The retina lines the ____________. Near the centre of the posterior part is the _______________________, or yellow spot. In the centre of the yellow spot is the __________________, which has only one type of light-sensitive receptor, the __________. The area where the optic nerve leaves the retina is the _______________, also known as the __________________.

22. Fill in the blanks to describe the factors that control the amount of light entering the eye.

The amount of light entering the eye is controlled by the _________ of the pupils. In a bright light they are ________________ and in darkness they are __________________. The iris consists of two layers of smooth muscle – contraction of the circular fibres causes ________________ of the pupil, whereas contraction of the radiating fibres causes _______________. The autonomic nervous system controls the size of the pupil – sympathetic stimulation causes _________________, whereas parasympathetic stimulation causes _________________ of the pupil.

POT LUCK

23. Which structures secrete tears?

____

24. List the constituents of tears: ____

____

25. List the four functions of tears: ____

____

26. There are five errors in the paragraph below that describes the sense of smell. Identify and correct them.

All odorous materials give off inert molecules that are carried into the nose in the inhaled air and stimulate the olfactory osmoreceptors. When currents of air are carried to the olfactory tract, the smell receptors are stimulated, setting up impulses in the olfactory nerve endings. These pass through the cribriform plate of the mandible to the olfactory bulb. Nerve fibres that leave the olfactory bulb form the olfactory tract. This passes posteriorly to the olfactory lobe of the cerebellum, where the impulses are interpreted and odour is perceived.

MCQs

27. Light waves travel at the speed of: _______
   a. 300,000 metres per second
   b. 300,000 metres per hour
   c. 300,000 kilometres per second
   d. 300,000 kilometres per hour

28. Light waves of which colour have the shortest wavelength? _______
   a. Red
   b. Yellow
   c. Violet
   d. Blue

29. When light waves pass from a medium of one density to another, they bend. This process is called: _______
   a. Reflection
   b. Radiation
   c. Refraction
   d. Accommodation

30. Which of the following structures is able to change its refractory power? _______
   a. Conjunctiva
   b. Cornea
   c. Lens
   d. Vitreous body

31. Colour vision is discriminated by light-sensitive pigments found in: _______
   a. Visual purple
   b. Rods
   c. Cones
   d. Rods and cones

32. An object appears black when: _______
   a. Light waves of all wavelengths are reflected.
   b. Light waves of all wavelengths are absorbed.
   c. Microwaves are reflected.
   d. Gamma rays are absorbed

33. Which structures in the eye have no blood supply? (Choose all that apply.) _______
   a. Cornea
   b. Iris
   c. Lens
   d. Retina

34. The colour with the longest wavelength in the visible spectrum is: _______
   a. Yellow
   b. Green
   c. Violet
   d. Red

35. In which lobe of the cerebrum is vision perceived? _______
   a. Occipital
   b. Frontal
   c. Temporal
   d. Parietal

DEFINITIONS

Define the following terms:

36. Myopia: ______________________________

____

______________________________.

37. Hyperopia: ______________________________

____

______________________________.

APPLYING WHAT YOU KNOW

38. Insert the commonly used terms that correspond with conditions A and B.

39. In Figure 8.8A, the focal point lies behind the point of focus because the eyeball is too long. In Figure 8.8B, the focal point lies in front of the point of focus because the eyeball is too short. Draw in the correct lenses and their effect on the paths of light rays in Figures 8.8C and D to correct the visual defects in the corresponding figures above.

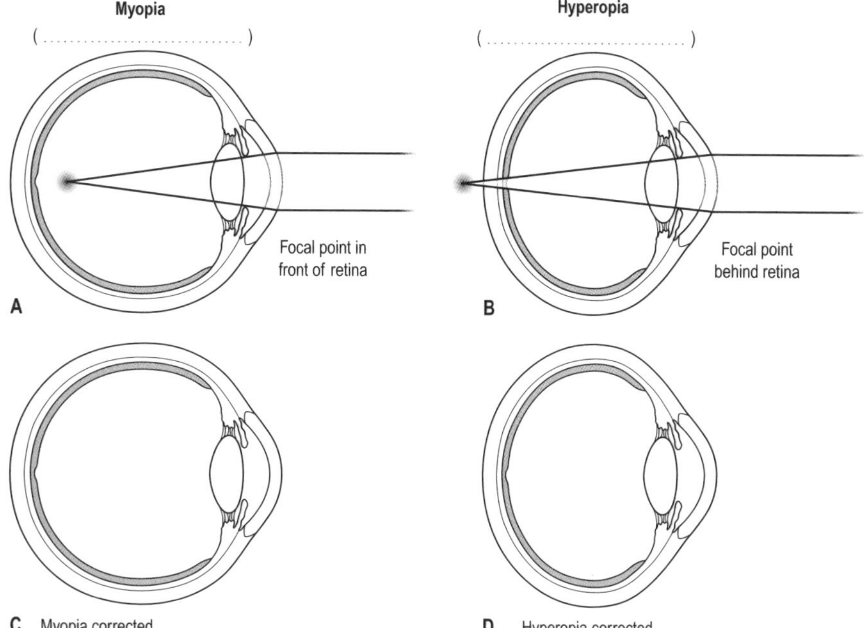

Figure 8.8 (A–D) Common refractive errors of the eye and corrective lenses

9 The endocrine system

The endocrine system consists of ductless glands that secrete hormones. Together with the autonomic nervous system, the endocrine system maintains homeostasis of the internal environment and controls involuntary body functions. This chapter will help you explore the components of the endocrine system and their functions.

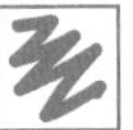
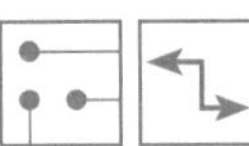

COLOURING, LABELLING AND MATCHING

1. Colour and match the endocrine glands and tissues identified on Figure 9.1:

O Adrenal glands	O Pituitary gland	O Pineal body	O Thyroid gland
O Ovaries (in female)	O Testes (in male)	O Pancreatic islets	O Parathyroid glands

2. Label the endocrine glands and tissues identified on Figure 9.1

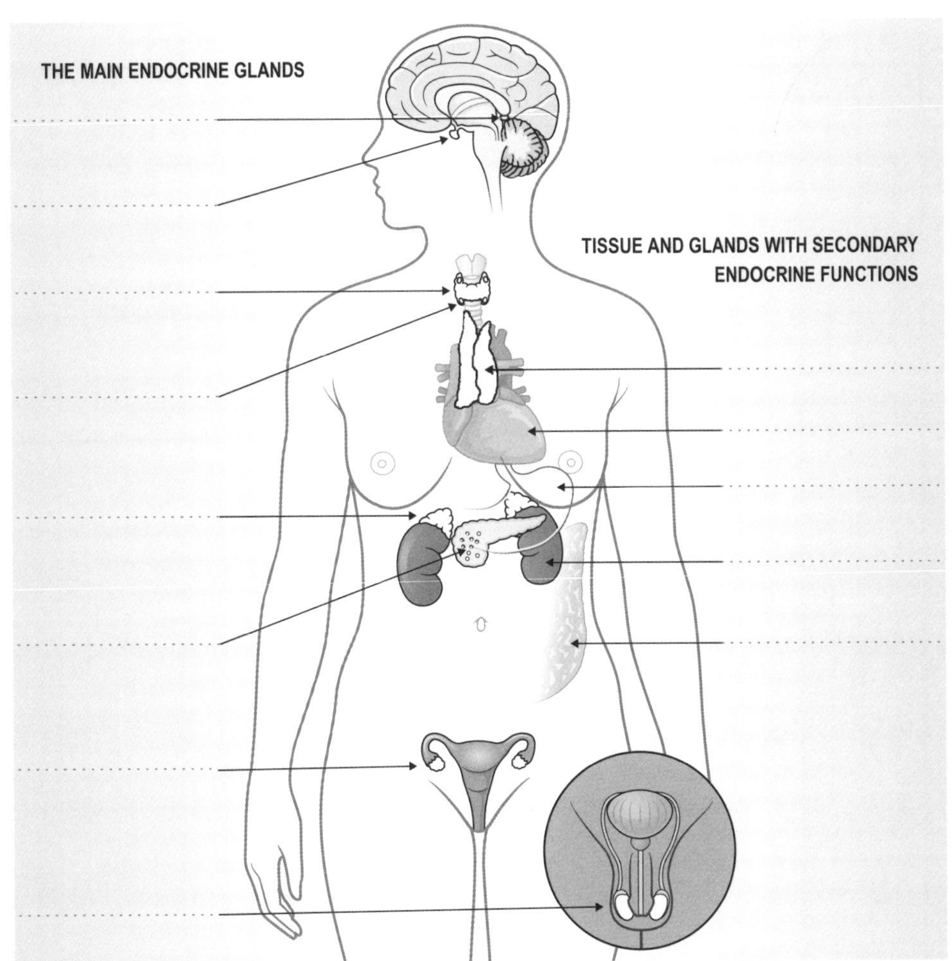

Figure 9.1 Positions of the endocrine glands

3. Match the key choices to the spaces in the paragraph below to provide an overview of hormones.

Key choices:			
Fast	Receptors	Glucagon	Steroids
Target organ/tissue	Water	Thyroid hormones	Secrete
Internal	Bloodstream	Insulin	
Slow	Lipid	Adrenaline	

Hormones are formed by glands or tissues that ______________ them into the ______________ and are transported to their ______________. When a hormone arrives at its site of action, it binds to specific molecular groups on the cell membrane called ______________. Homeostasis of the ______________ environment is maintained partly by the nervous system and partly by the endocrine system. The former is concerned with ______________ changes, whereas those that involve the endocrine system are ______________ and more precise. Chemically, hormones fall into two groups – protein-based and ______________-based. Hormones in the first group are ______________-soluble and include ______________, ______________ and ______________. The latter group includes ______________ and ______________.

COMPLETION AND LABELLING

4. Label the structures identified in Figure 9.2.

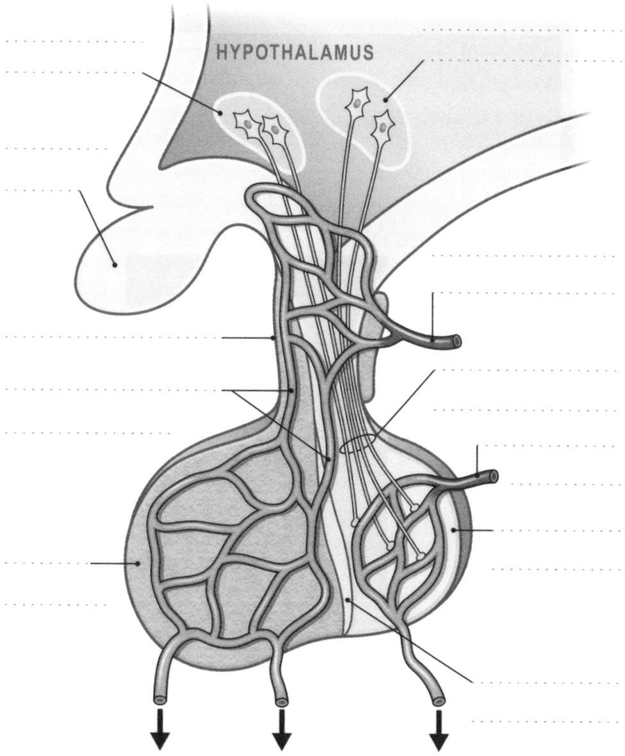

HYPOTHALAMUS

Figure 9.2 The pituitary gland

5. Name the two hormones secreted by the posterior pituitary gland: ______________

____

6. Secretion of which pituitary hormone is through positive feedback? ______________

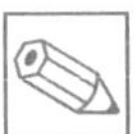

COMPLETION

7. Complete Table 9.1 by inserting the full names and functions of anterior pituitary hormones.

Table 9.1 Summary of the hormones secreted by the anterior pituitary gland

Hormone	Abbreviation	Function
	GH	
	TSH	
	ACTH	
	PRL	
	FSH	Males: Females:
	LH	Males: Females:

8. Outline the effect of a negative feedback control system:

____
____
____
____
____
____

9. Complete the boxes labelled A and B in Figure 9.3.

10. Match the hormones and effects from the key choices with the boxes labelled i, ii, iii and iv in Figure 9.3.

Key choices: Trophic hormones Releasing hormones Lowered Raised

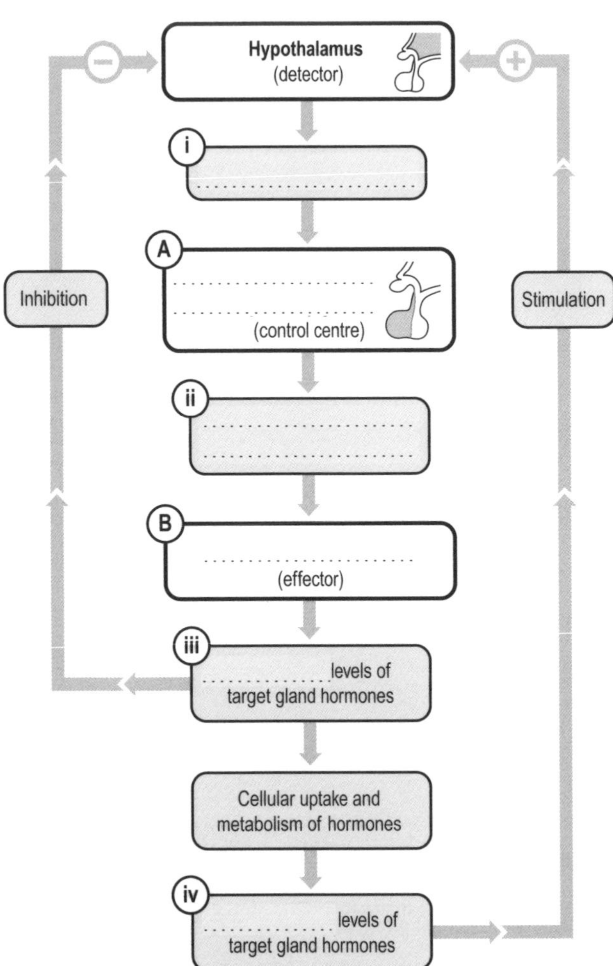

Figure 9.3 Negative feedback regulation of secretion of hormones

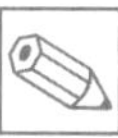

COMPLETION

11. Complete the paragraph below to describe the secretion and effects of antidiuretic hormone (ADH).

An increase in the rate of urine production is called ______________________. ADH is secreted by the ______________________ pituitary gland; its main effect is to ______________________ urine output. It does this by ______________________ the permeability of the ______________________ convoluted tubules and ______________________ ducts in the nephrons to ______________________, thereby increasing its reabsorption from the filtrate. ADH secretion is stimulated by increased ______________________ of the blood, which is detected by ______________________ receptors in the hypothalamus – for example, during ______________________ and ______________________. In more serious situations, ADH also causes ______________________ of smooth muscle, causing ______________________ in small arteries. This has a pressor effect – that is, it increases ______________________ – reflecting the alternative name of this hormone, ______________________.

12. Complete Table 9.2 to summarise the effects of excess and deficiency of T_3 and T_4.

Table 9.2 Effects of abnormal secretion of thyroid hormones

Body function affected	Hypersecretion of T_3 and T_4	Hyposecretion of T_3 and T_4
Metabolic rate		
Weight		
Appetite		
Mental state		
Scalp		
Heart		
Skin		
Faeces		
Eyes		None

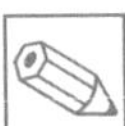

COMPLETION

13. Figure 9.4 summarises the endocrine response to stress. Identify the structures labelled A, B, C and D on Figure 9.4.

14. Insert an arrow in each white box at the bottom of Figure 9.4 to indicate whether the response to stress is to increase or decrease each effect.

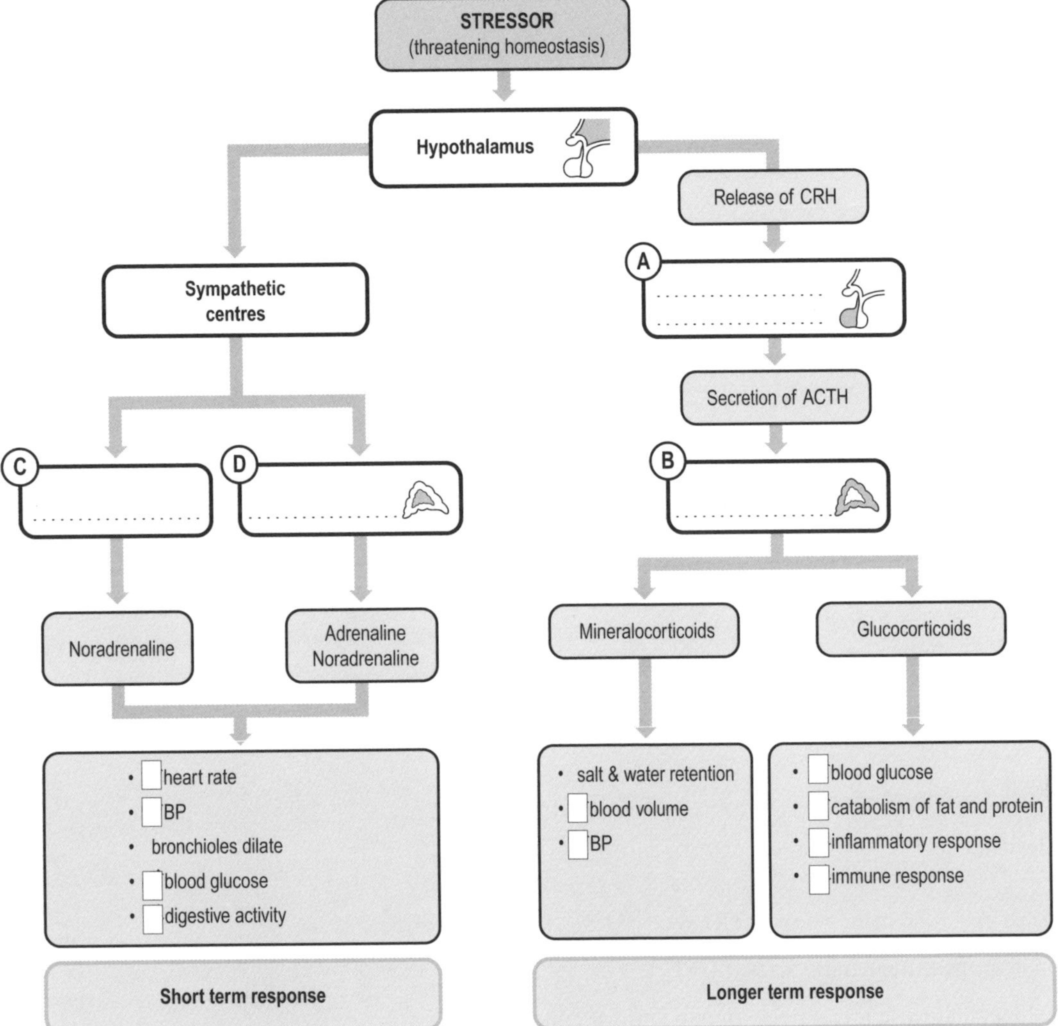

Figure 9.4 Endocrine responses to stress

15. Complete the paragraph below by crossing out the incorrect options.

The adrenal glands are situated on the **upper/lower** pole of each kidney. The outer part of the gland is the **medulla/cortex** and **is/is not** essential for life. The adrenal **cortex/medulla** secretes steroid hormones which are formed from **triglycerides/cholesterol**. There are **two/three** groups of steroid hormones. The main group is the **glucocorticoids/mineralocorticoids.** The adrenal **cortex/medulla** secretes the hormones adrenaline and noradrenaline, which occurs in response to stimulation of the **sympathetic/parasympathetic** nervous system.

POT LUCK

16. Identify whether the following statements related to the thyroid gland are TRUE or FALSE. Circle the correct answer.
    a. The main dietary source of iodine is seafood, which is needed to synthesise the thyroid hormones T_3 and T_4. **(T/F)**
    b. Thyroxine is secreted by the anterior pituitary. **(T/F)**
    c. Thyroid hormones are secreted during fetal life. **(T/F)**
    d. Thyroid hormones are stored in the thyroid follicles until stimulation by thyroid releasing hormone occurs. **(T/F)**
    e. The thyroid gland secretes calcitonin in response to raised blood calcium levels. **(T/F)**

17. Identify the eight mistakes in the paragraph below about the parathyroid glands and correct them.

    There are two parathyroid glands located on each upper pole of the thyroid gland. They secrete parathyroid hormone; blood calcium levels regulate its secretion. When they rise, secretion of PTH is increased and vice versa. The main function of PTH is to decrease the blood calcium level. This is achieved by decreasing the amount of calcium absorbed from the small intestine and reabsorbed from the renal tubules. If these sources do not provide adequate calcium levels, the PTH stimulates osteoblasts (bone destroying cells) and calcium is released into the blood from the parathyroid glands. Normal blood calcium levels are needed for muscle relaxation, blood clotting and nerve impulse transmission.

18. Name the pancreatic cells that secrete these hormones:
    a. Insulin: ___________
    b. Glucagon: ___________
    c. Somatostatin: ___________

19. State whether each statement below is TRUE or FALSE. Circle the correct answer.
    a. Insulin is formed from amino acids. **(T/F)**
    b. Normal blood glucose levels range from 6.1 to 9.9 mmol/L. **(T/F)**
    c. Insulin reduces blood glucose levels. **(T/F)**
    d. Glucagon reduces blood sugar levels. **(T/F)**
    e. Secretion of insulin is stimulated by low blood sugar levels. **(T/F)**
    f. Secretion of insulin is stimulated by gastrin. **(T/F)**
    g. The hypothalamus is involved in secretion of insulin. **(T/F)**
    h. Insulin secretion is decreased by sympathetic stimulation. **(T/F)**

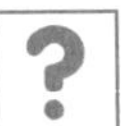

MCQs

20. Levels of which hormones are controlled by negative feedback mechanisms? (Choose all that apply.) _______
    a. Growth hormone
    b. Thyroid-stimulating hormone
    c. Adrenocorticotrophic hormone
    d. Prolactin

21. Which is the most abundant hormone secreted by the anterior pituitary? _______
    a. Growth hormone
    b. Thyroid-stimulating hormone
    c. Adrenocorticotrophic hormone
    d. Prolactin

22. Secretion of which hormone peaks in adolescence? _______
    a. Growth hormone
    b. Thyroid-stimulating hormone
    c. Adrenocorticotrophic hormone
    d. Prolactin

23. Growth hormone stimulates which of the following? (Choose all that apply.) _______
    a. Absorption of calcium
    b. Storage of fats
    c. Division of body cells
    d. Protein synthesis

24. T_3 is also known as: _______
    a. Thyroglobulin
    b. Thyroxine
    c. Triiodothyronine
    d. Thyroid-stimulating hormone

25. Circadian rhythm describes regular fluctuations in hormone secretion during a period of: ______
    a. 12 hours
    b. 24 hours
    c. 7 days
    d. 28 days

26. Which is/are true of prostaglandins? (Choose all that apply.) _______
    a. Cells in the prostate gland
    b. Long-acting substances
    c. Involved in the mediation of fever
    d. Involved in blood clotting

27. The inflammatory process involves which of the following substances? (Choose all that apply.) _______
    a. Histamine
    b. Serotonin
    c. Prostaglandins
    d. Erythropoietin

28. Secretion of which hormone is associated with a circadian rhythm and is highest at night? _______
    a. Prostaglandins
    b. Histamine
    c. Melatonin
    d. Thymosin

29. Which of the following is/are involved in platelet aggregation? (Choose all that apply.) _______
    a. Histamine
    b. Prostaglandins
    c. Serotonin
    d. Secretin

10 The respiratory system

The respiratory system is a collection of tissues and organs whose main collective function is oxygen intake and carbon dioxide elimination. Conventionally, the respiratory system is divided into the upper respiratory tract (those structures not contained within the chest) and the lower respiratory tract (those structures found inside the chest).

STRUCTURES OF THE RESPIRATORY SYSTEM

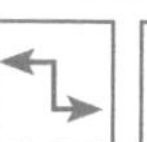
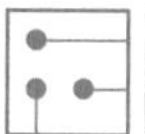
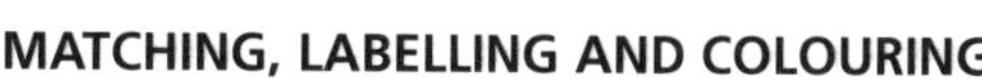

MATCHING, LABELLING AND COLOURING

1. Label the following parts of the respiratory system on Figure 10.1, using the following terms:

Nasal cavity	Parietal pleura	Ribs
Pharynx	Visceral pleura	Space occupied by heart
Epiglottis	Trachea	Cricoid cartilage
Larynx	Left primary bronchus	Thyroid cartilage
Apex of left lung	Right primary bronchus	Right lung
Base of left lung		

2. Colour and match the following:

- ○ Diaphragm
- ○ Pleural cavity
- ○ Clavicles

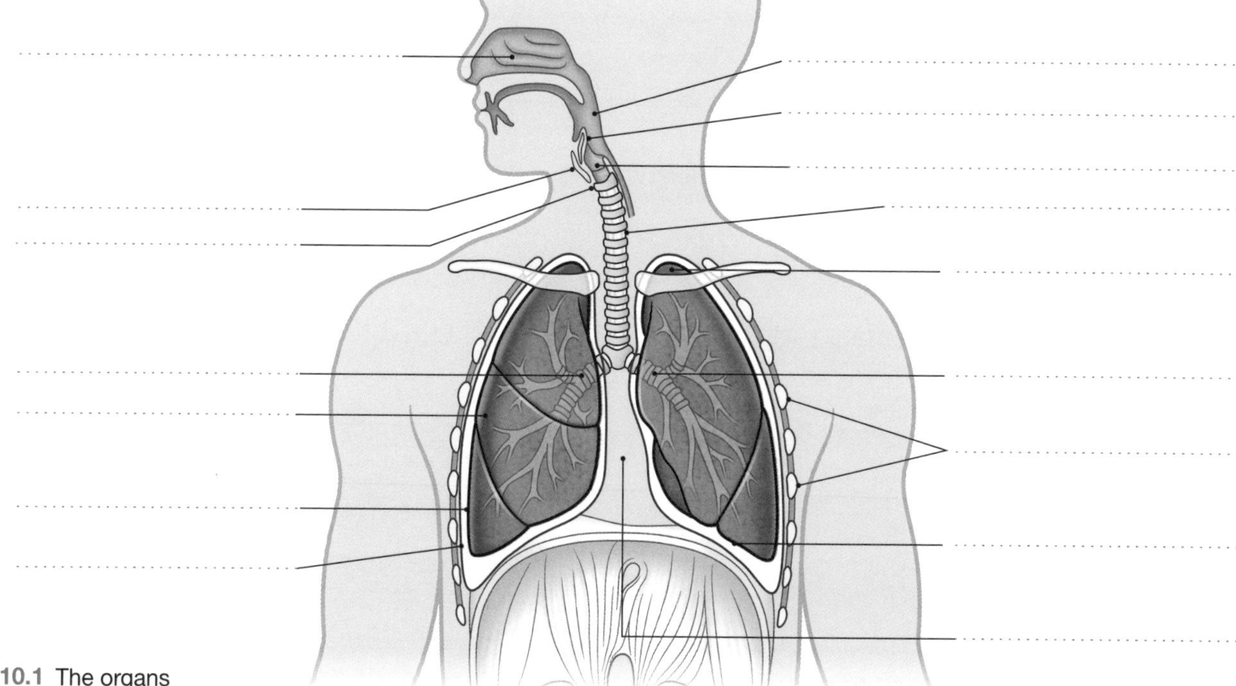

Figure 10.1 The organs of respiration

3. Figure 10.2 shows the lungs and adjacent structures in the thorax. Colour and label the structures indicated.
4. Colour and match the lobes of the lungs.

○ Superior lobe of right lung
○ Middle lobe of right lung
○ Inferior lobe of right lung
○ Superior lobe of left lung
○ Inferior lobe of left lung

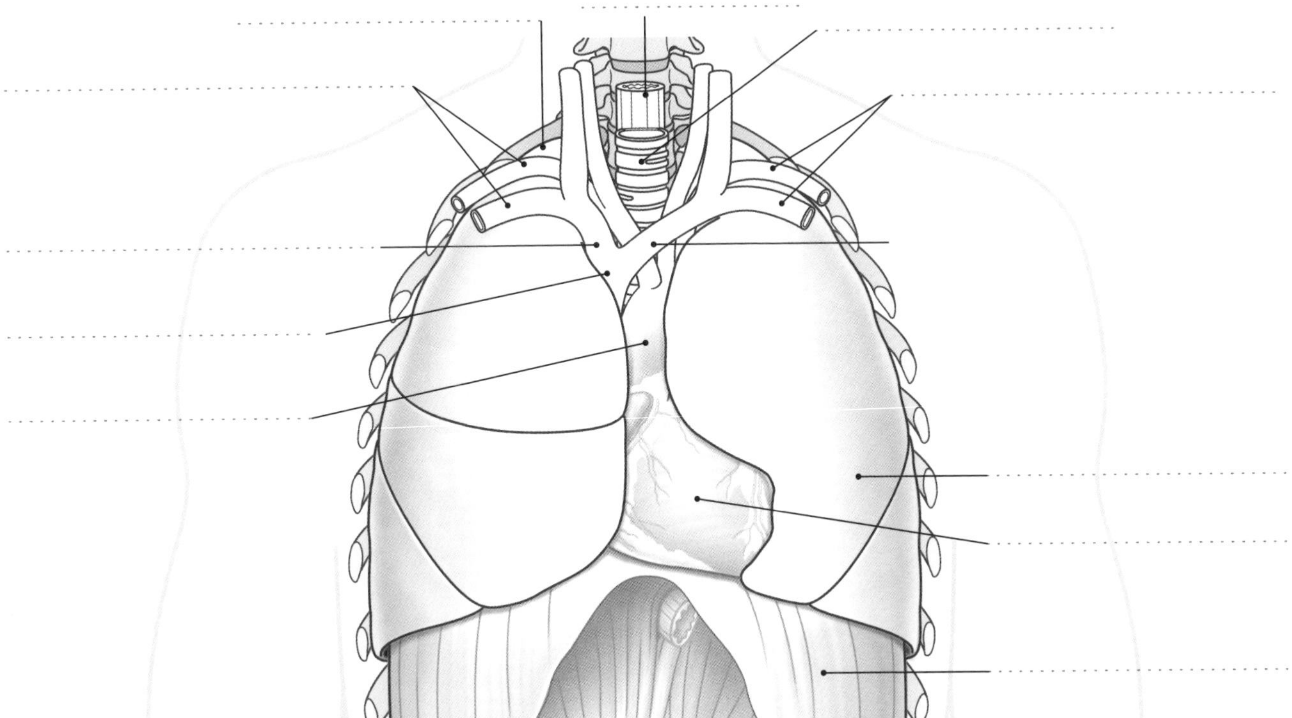

Figure 10.2 Organs associated with the lungs

5. Figure 10.3 shows the relationship of the pleura to the lungs. Label the structures shown.
6. Name the fluid found in the area marked A, and explain its function.

____

____

____

7. The primary bronchus enters the lung at the location marked E on Figure 10.3. What other structures, not shown, enter/leave the lung here?

____

____

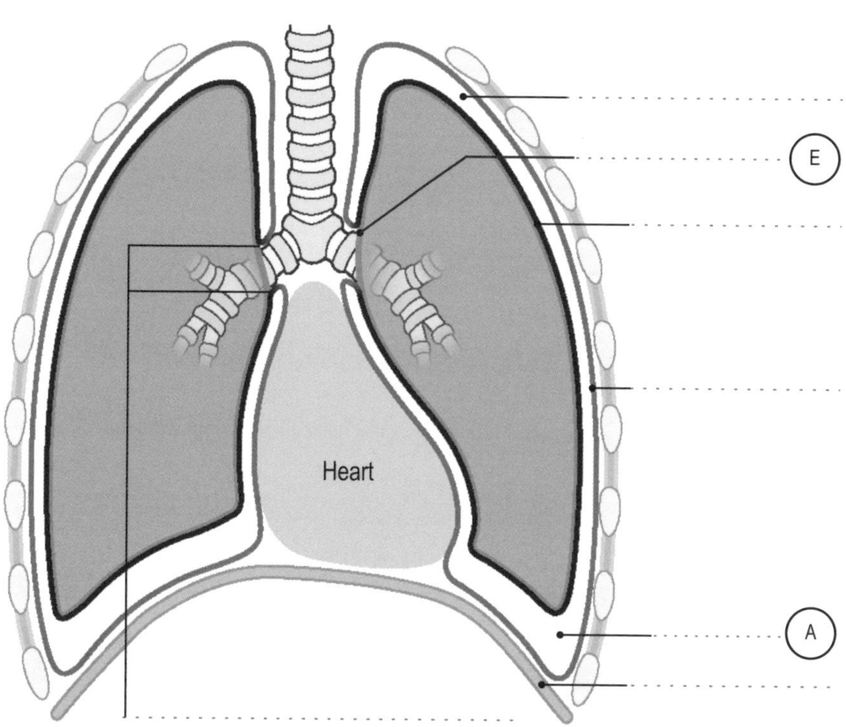

Figure 10.3 Relationship of the pleura to the lungs

8. As the respiratory tree progressively divides, the passageways become narrower and narrower. Label the structures A–J on Figure 10.4.

9. Colour and label the large arrows marked X and Y to show which sections of the respiratory tree are important for air conduction and which are responsible for gas exchange.

○ Air conduction
○ Gas exchange

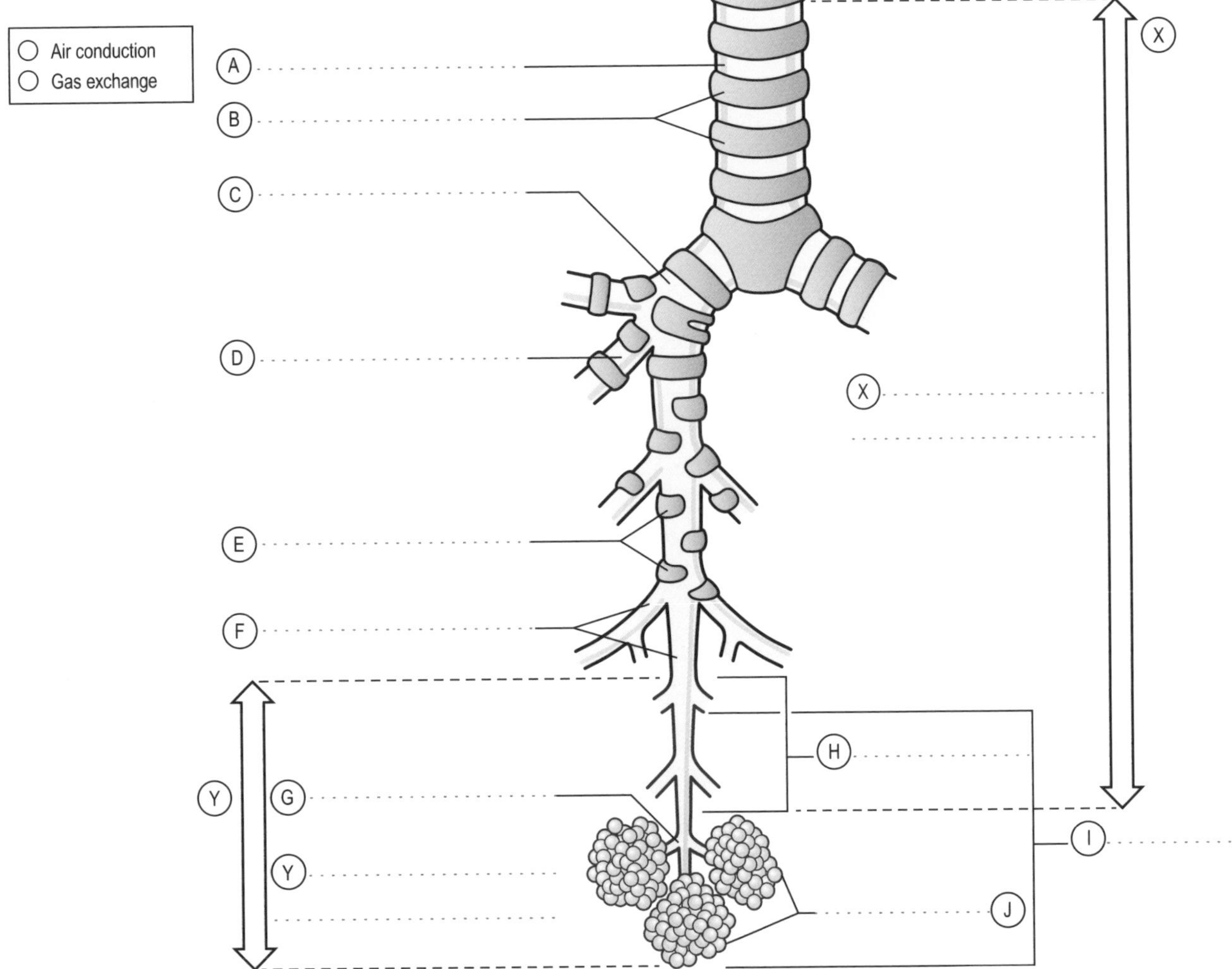

Figure 10.4 Lower respiratory tract

10. Figure 10.5 illustrates a section through an alveolus. Colour, label and match the:

- ○ Alveolar endothelial cells
- ○ Elastic connective tissue
- ○ Blood capillaries

11. Complete the statements below describing cells A and B shown on Figure 10.5.

Cell A is called a _______________ cell and produces a phospholipid fluid called _______________ which lines the alveoli. This fluid reduces alveolar _______________ and keeps the alveoli inflated.

Cell B is involved in protection; it cleans the alveolus by the process of _______________; it is a _______________.

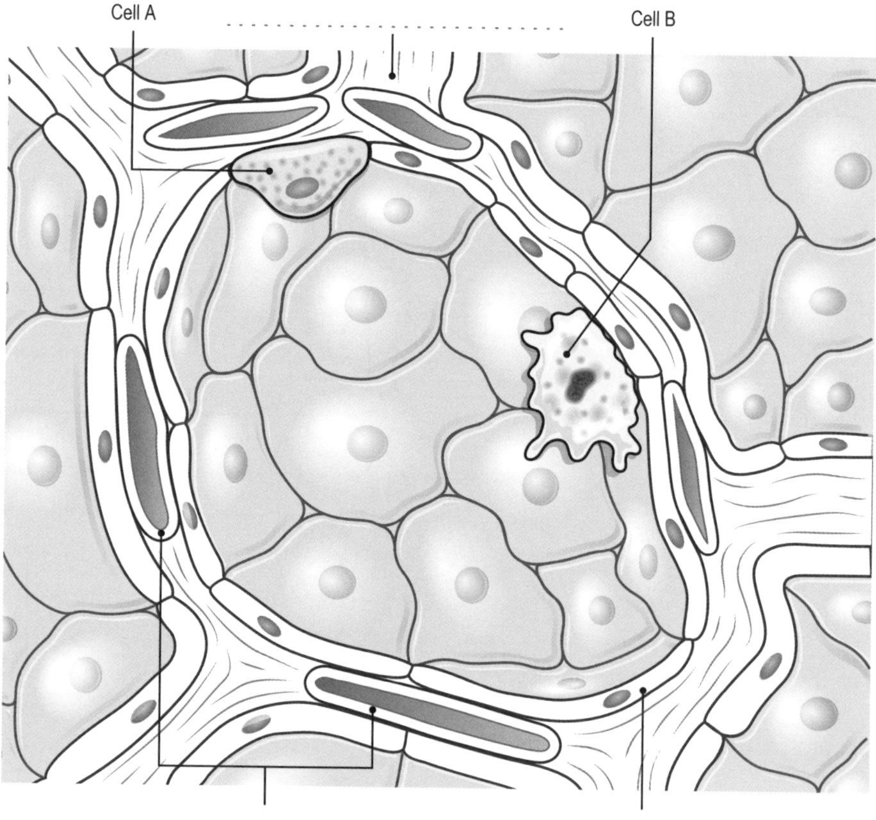

Figure 10.5 Section through an alveolus

MATCHING

12. Match the structures below with their functions.

Functions

a. Produces mucus: ________
b. Contains the vocal cords: ________
c. Opening into the nasal cavity: ________
d. The lid of the larynx, protecting the tracheal opening: ________
e. Air-filled cavity in bone: ________
f. A collection of lymphoid tissue, involved in immunity: ________
g. Links the nasopharynx and middle ear: ________

Structures

Nasopharyngeal tonsil
Epiglottis
Goblet cell
Anterior nares
Larynx
Auditory tube
Sinus

13. For each of the four statements in list A, identify its most appropriate reason from list B. (You won't need all the items in list B.)

List A

a. Mucus is produced in the upper respiratory tract because …

____

____

b. Cilia are present in the upper respiratory tract because …

____

____

c. Cartilage is present in the upper respiratory tract because …

____

____

d. Tracheal cartilages are C-shaped because …

____

____

List B

… the passageway has to be flexible to allow head and neck movement

… the oesophagus is normally collapsed

… the oesophagus needs to expand during swallowing

… mucus needs to be swept away from the lungs

… the tissues need to return to their original shape

… this is an efficient way of removing dust and dirt from inhaled air

… mucus builds up during normal respiration

… the airways have to be kept open at all times

… inspired air must be warmed and humidified

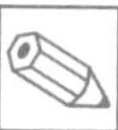

COMPLETION

14. Complete the following paragraph describing the upper respiratory tract by inserting the correct word(s) in the spaces provided.

The right and left nasal cavities are separated by a plate of bone called the ______________, which is formed mainly from two facial bones, the _______ and the ______________. The anterior portion of this plate is made of __________________. The floor of the nasal cavities forms the _______ of the mouth. Anteriorly, it is made from the _________ bone, also called the ___________________. Posteriorly, it is made from __________ muscle, is called the _____________________, and may be seen through the widely open mouth hanging down in the throat; this section is called the ___________. The lateral walls of the nasal cavities are formed partly from the ethmoid bone, which is folded into intricate scroll-like shapes called ____________, and are covered in a very vascular __________ membrane. The main function of the upper respiratory tract is to __________, ____________ and ___________ inspired air.

? POT LUCK

15. In the following paragraph, which describes the lungs, find and correct the eight inaccuracies.

The lungs are identical in shape and size and their lateral surfaces face each other across the space between them. Major structures enter and leave the lung through the lateral surfaces at the area called the pleura. The broad outer surface of the lungs that lies against the ribs is called the medial surface; the surface lying against the diaphragm is the apex, and the lung tip, also called the pyramid, rises above the clavicles. The space between the lungs is called the cardiac notch.

MCQs

16. Which of the following options describing the vocal cords is true? _______
    a. The vocal cords are bands of membrane guarding the entrance to the oesophagus
    b. When the muscles controlling the vocal cords contract, the gap between the cords widens
    c. Speech is produced when air passing into the lungs vibrates the vocal cords
    d. When not in use, the vocal cords lie close together – that is, they are adducted
17. Which of the following is not a function of the larynx? _______
    a. A common passageway for food, air and water
    b. Production of speech
    c. Closing off of the lower respiratory tract by the epiglottis
    d. Sturdy structure keeping the entrance to the trachea open
18. Which of the following statements is true? _______
    a. The larynx is built mainly of smooth muscle
    b. The epiglottis must be closed when speaking
    c. The larynx lies below the oropharynx
    d. The largest pieces of cartilage in the larynx are the arytenoids
19. Which endocrine gland lies very close to the larynx? _______
    a. The pancreas
    b. The thymus gland
    c. The pineal gland
    d. The thyroid gland
20. Snoring is caused by: _______
    a. Adduction of the vocal cords
    b. Mucus accumulation obstructing the upper respiratory tract
    c. Collapse of the pharyngeal walls
    d. Closure of the larynx by the epiglottis
21. The cricoid cartilage: ______
    a. Has its broadest portion posteriorly
    b. Is also called the Adam's apple
    c. Lies superior to the thyroid cartilage
    d. Is linked to the hyoid bone by the cricohyoid cartilage
22. The cough reflex is: _______
    a. A voluntary protective response important in clearing airway obstruction
    b. Initiated by stimulation of sensory nerve endings in the upper airways
    c. Of no use in clearing normal airway mucus
    d. More efficient when the abdominal muscles are relaxed or weak
23. During the cough reflex: _______
    a. Intra-abdominal pressure rises
    b. The glottis is collapsed
    c. The diaphragm moves downwards
    d. There is, initially, a deep expiration
24. Which of the following airways has the smallest diameter? _______
    a. Respiratory bronchiole
    b. Primary bronchus
    c. Trachea
    d. Tertiary bronchus

RESPIRATORY FUNCTION

POT LUCK

25. List two features of the alveolar membrane that increase the efficiency of gas exchange:
    - ______
    - ______

26. List two features of the blood flow through the alveolar capillaries that increase the efficiency of gas exchange:
    - ______
    - ______

27. Decide whether the following statements apply to carbon dioxide, to oxygen, or to both. Complete the list by writing CO_2, O_2 or Both against each in the space provided.

    a. Waste product of metabolism: ______
    b. 23% carried bound to haemoglobin: ______
    c. Raised temperatures increase release from haemoglobin: ______
    d. Mainly carried as bicarbonate ions in the plasma: ______
    e. 98.5% carried bound to haemoglobin: ______
    f. Binds reversibly to haemoglobin: ______
    g. Binding with haemoglobin is tighter in the lungs than in the tissues: ______
    h. 1.5% carried dissolved in plasma: ______
    i. Binding to haemoglobin is tighter in the tissues than in the lungs: ______

COLOURING, MATCHING AND COMPLETION

28. Figure 10.6 shows gas exchange between an alveolus and a lung capillary. What is this process called?

    ______

29. Using different colours for carbon dioxide and oxygen, colour in the arrows to show how each gas moves.
30. Complete the boxes to show the partial pressures of each gas in the arterial capillary, the venous capillary and the alveolus.
31. Colour and match the region on Figure 10.6 that represents the respiratory membrane.

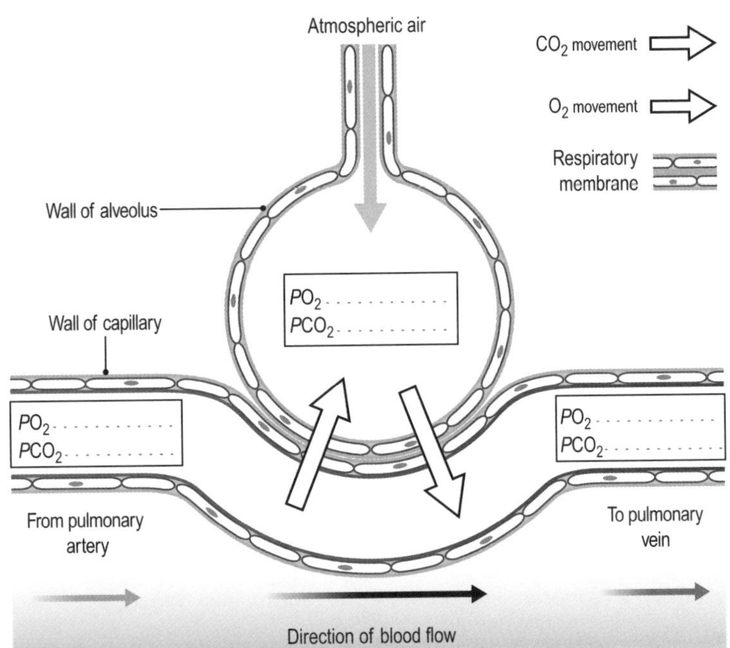

Figure 10.6 Gas exchange between the alveoli and the bloodstream

32. Figure 10.7 shows gas exchange between the bloodstream and tissue cells. What is this process called? ____________________
33. Using different colours for carbon dioxide and oxygen, colour in the arrows to show how each gas moves.
34. Complete the boxes to show the partial pressures of each gas in the arterial capillary, the venous capillary and the tissue cells.

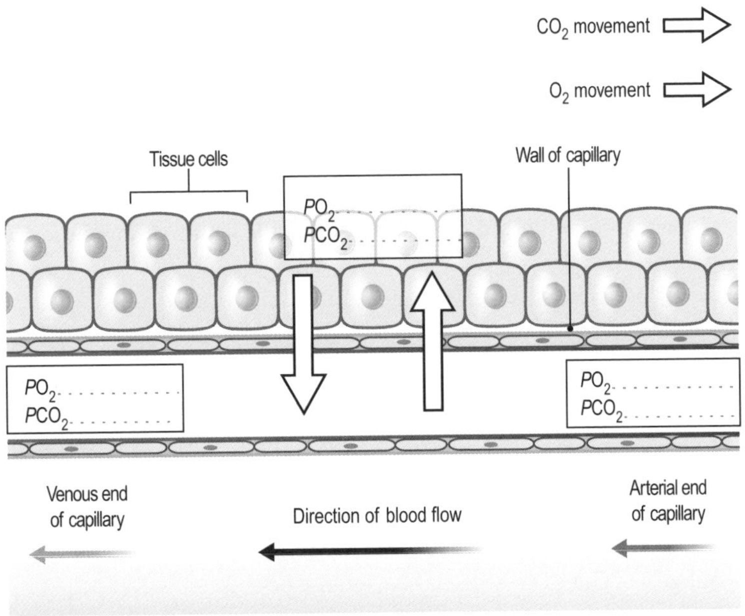

Figure 10.7 Gas exchange between the bloodstream and the tissues

35. The following statements match either to external respiration (ER), internal respiration (IR) or both. Complete the list by writing ER, IR or Both against each in the space provided.
    a. Oxygen and carbon dioxide diffuse in opposite directions across the intervening membrane. ____________________
    b. Takes place across the tissue capillary membranes. ____________________
    c. Takes place across alveolar walls. ____________________
    d. Oxygen diffuses down its concentration gradient. ____________________
    e. Carbon dioxide diffuses into the bloodstream. ____________________
    f. Oxygen diffuses from the bloodstream into the tissues. ____________________

36. The following activity concerns internal respiration. Match the statements in list A with the best reason in list B. (You won't need all the reasons in list B, so choose carefully!)

List A

a. Carbon dioxide diffuses from the body cells into the bloodstream because … ______

b. Tissue levels of oxygen are lower than blood levels because … ______

c. Oxygen diffuses out of the capillary because … ______

d. The arterial end of the capillary is higher in oxygen than the venous end because … ______

List B

…blood flow is slow through the capillary beds
…PO_2 is lower in the tissues than in the bloodstream
…carbon dioxide is continually being produced by the tissues
…PCO_2 is lower in the capillary than in the tissues
…body cells require a constant supply of oxygen
…as the blood flows through the tissues it releases oxygen into the cells
…venous blood is deoxygenated
…body cells are continuously using oxygen

COMPLETION

37. The paragraphs below describe a normal cycle of respiration. Fill in the blanks, using the key choices supplied:

Key choices:

Passive	Increases	Inflate	Upwards
Deflate	Outwards	Muscular effect	Downwards
Inwards	Downwards	Into	Intercostal muscles
Relaxed	Decreases	Contracts	Increases
Relaxes	Intercostal muscles	Out of	Decreases

Just before inspiration commences, the diaphragm is ___________; this occurs in the pause between breaths in normal quiet breathing. Inspiration commences. The rib cage moves ___________ and ___________ owing to contraction of the ______________________. The diaphragm ___________ and moves ___________. This ___________ the volume of the thoracic cavity, and _____________ the pressure. Because of these changes, air moves ________ the lungs, and the lungs _________. Inspiration has taken place.

Unlike inspiration, expiration is usually a __________ process because it requires no ________________. So, following the end of inspiration, the diaphragm _________ and moves back into its resting position. The rib cage moves ___________ and ___________, because the ___________________ have relaxed. This __________ the volume of the thoracic cavity, and so ___________ the pressure within it. Air therefore now moves _________ the lungs, and they _________. There is now a rest period before the next cycle begins.

38. Decide if each stimulus in Table 10.1 increases or decreases respiratory effort, and tick the appropriate column for each.

Table 10.1 Causes of increased or decreased respiratory effort

Stimulus	Increases respiratory effort	Decreases respiratory effort
Fever		
Pain		
Sedative drugs		
Acidification of the cerebrospinal fluid (CSF)		
Sleep		
Exercise		
High blood [H^+]		
Increased alkalinity of the blood		
Increased pH of the CSF		
Hypoxaemia		
Hypercapnia		
Stimulation of the respiratory centre		
Decreased CO_2 excretion		

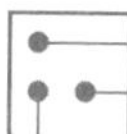

LABELLING

39. Figure 10.8 shows results from a standard spirogram. Complete the list below, identifying each of the standard abbreviations for the main lung volumes and capacities, and use the abbreviations to label Figure 10.8.

a. TV ______________________________

b. VC ______________________________

c. IC ______________________________

d. RV ______________________________

e. IRV ______________________________

f. ERV ______________________________

g. TLC ______________________________

h. FRC ______________________________

40. Using Figure 10.8, complete the following to show how each of the volumes a–f can be calculated from spirometer results.

a. VC = TLC – ___

b. RV = TLC – ___

c. IC = TV + ___

d. VC = TV + ___ + ___

e. ERV = VC – (___ + ___)

f. TLC = TV + ___ + ___ + ___

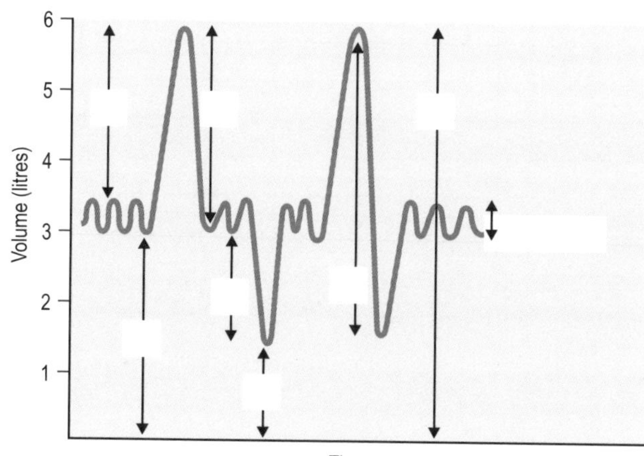

Figure 10.8 Lung volumes and capacities

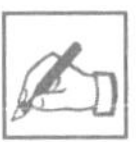

APPLYING WHAT YOU KNOW

41. If the functional residual capacity is 3000 mL, the tidal volume is 500 mL and the total lung capacity is 6000 mL, calculate the inspiratory capacity and the inspiratory reserve volume.

42. If the total lung capacity is 6000 mL and the residual volume is 1200 mL, what is the vital capacity?

43. Calculate the alveolar ventilation for an individual whose tidal volume is 450 mL, anatomical dead space is 160 mL and respiratory rate is 13 breaths/min.

44. Frances is out for a training run. Her pulse is 140 beats/min, the tidal volume is 1200 mL, and her respiratory rate is 20 breaths/min. Of the volumes and capacities labelled in Figure 10.8, which two are relatively fixed and are independent of exercise? Explain your answers.

MCQs

45. Which of the following is true of autonomic innervation of the airways? _______
    a. Sympathetic stimulation causes bronchoconstriction, and parasympathetic stimulation causes bronchodilation
    b. Sympathetic stimulation causes bronchodilation, and parasympathetic stimulation causes bronchoconstriction
    c. Both sympathetic and parasympathetic stimulation cause bronchoconstriction
    d. Both sympathetic and parasympathetic stimulation cause bronchodilation

46. Chemoreceptors that measure pH and relay this information to the respiratory centre to control breathing are found in the (choose all that apply):______
    a. Atria of the heart
    b. Carotid bodies
    c. Surface of the medulla oblongata
    d. Aortic arch

47. A lung that can be stretched easily but that does not return to its original shape is: _______
    a. Elastic but not resistant
    b. Resistant but not compliant
    c. Compliant but not elastic
    d. Elastic but not compliant

48. Compliance is: _______
    a. Stretchability of the lung
    b. Very low in the normal healthy lung
    c. Another term for elasticity
    d. Increased when surfactant levels are low

49. Elasticity is which of the following? (Choose all that apply.) _______
    a. Stretchability of the lung
    b. High in the normal healthy lung
    c. An opposing force to compliance
    d. Important in determining airway resistance

50. Which of the following decreases resistance in the healthy airway? _______
    a. Increased goblet cell activity
    b. Parasympathetic activity
    c. Decreased pleural fluid production
    d. Relaxation of airway smooth muscle

51. Why is there no net movement of nitrogen across the respiratory membrane? _______
    a. Body tissues do not require nitrogen
    b. Nitrogen is not soluble enough to diffuse readily
    c. There is the same amount of nitrogen in the blood as in the alveoli
    d. Nitrogen cannot be transported in the bloodstream

52. In the healthy lung, during quiet breathing: _____
    a. Ventilation and perfusion cannot be adequately matched
    b. Blood flow to all areas of the lung is equal
    c. There is a generalised bronchodilation
    d. Some of the alveoli are collapsed

53. Which of the following are true? (Choose all that apply.) _______
    a. The respiratory centre is located in the brain stem
    b. Accessory muscles of respiration include the diaphragm and the sternocleidomastoid
    c. Stimulation of the vagus nerve supplying aortic chemoreceptors increases the activity of the respiratory centre
    d. Control of breathing is entirely involuntary

54. The Hering–Breuer reflex controls respiration by measuring: _______
    a. Arterial blood pressure
    b. Airway resistance
    c. CO_2 levels in the cerebrospinal fluid
    d. Stretch in the lungs

55. In health, oxygen levels in arterial blood should be in the region of: _______
    a. 13.3 kPa/100 mmHg
    b. 21.4 kPa/160 mmHg
    c. 5.3 kPa/40 mmHg
    d. 10.5 kPa/79 mmHg

11 Introduction to nutrition

All body cells need a supply of nutrients in appropriate quantities, and the ultimate source of these nutrients is the diet. This chapter considers the main groups of nutrients and their roles in body function.

POT LUCK

1. List the main nutrient groups needed for a balanced diet:

- ____________________
- ____________________
- ____________________
- ____________________
- ____________________

2. Calculate the body mass index (BMI) for the following individuals and identify whether the BMI for each person below is underweight, normal, overweight or obese by deleting the incorrect options.

   a. A man who is 1.9 m tall and weighs 60 kg: ____________________. Underweight/normal/overweight/obese

   b. A man who is 1.8 m tall and weighs 90 kg: ____________________. Underweight/normal/overweight/obese

   c. A woman who is 1.6 m tall and weighs 50 kg: ____________________. Underweight/normal/overweight/obese

   d. A woman who is 1.7 m tall and weighs 90 kg: ____________________. Underweight/normal/overweight/obese

3. Outline the main uses of proteins in the body:

- ____________________
- ____________________
- ____________________

4. Define the term essential amino acid. ____________________

5. Outline the main uses of digestible carbohydrates in the body:

- ____________________
- ____________________
- ____________________

6. Which dietary constituent is abbreviated to NSP?____________________

7. List the five main functions of NSP.

- ____________________
- ____________________
- ____________________
- ____________________
- ____________________

8. Name the main dietary sources of NSP ____________________

COMPLETION

9. The following paragraphs discuss the structure and function of the fats. Complete them by filling in the blanks.

Fats are usually divided into two groups; __________ fats are found in foods from animal sources, such as __________, __________ and __________. The second group, the __________ fats, is found in vegetable oils. Certain hormones, such as __________ (e.g. cortisone), are synthesised from the fatty precursor __________, also found in the cell membrane. The same precursor substance is transported in the __________ combined with proteins, forming lipoproteins, such as __________ __________ (LDL). This carries __________ from the __________ to the body cells. Excessive blood LDL levels have a __________ effect on health; LDL is sometimes known as '__________.' Fats in a meal have the direct effect of __________ gastric emptying and __________ the return of a feeling of hunger.

The main use of fat is as a __________ source of __________ and __________. It is stored in __________ tissue in cells called __________. Fats enable absorption, transport and storage of the __________-soluble vitamins _____, _____, _____ and __________. Fats are essential constituents of __________, the outer covering of some nerve fibres that enables rapid transmission of impulses and __________, the oily substance secreted by sebaceous glands in the skin.

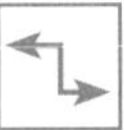

MATCHING

10. Vitamins act as cofactors in a range of important biochemical reactions in the body. Assign to each of the functions in list A the appropriate vitamin from list B. (You may need the items in list B more than once, and you can use more than one vitamin for each function.)

List A

a. Antioxidant: ________________

b. Connective tissue synthesis: ________________

c. Manufacture of visual pigments: ________________

d. Nonessential amino acid synthesis: ________________

e. Cell growth and differentiation, especially fast-growing tissues: ________________

f. Carbohydrate metabolism: ________________

g. Synthesis of clotting factors: ________________

h. DNA synthesis: ________________

i. Amino acid and protein metabolism: ________________

j. Myelin production: ________________

List B

Vitamin A

Vitamin B_1

Vitamin B_2

Vitamin B_6

Vitamin B_{12}

Folate (folic acid)

Pantothenic acid

Biotin

Vitamin E

Vitamin K

Vitamin C

MATCHING

11. Complete Table 11.1 by ticking the appropriate boxes against each of the minerals shown.

Table 11.1 Functions of minerals

Function	Calcium	Phosphate	Sodium	Potassium	Iron	Iodine
Needed for haemoglobin synthesis						
Used in thyroxine manufacture						
Most abundant cation outside the cells						
99% of body stock is found in bones						
Most abundant cation inside the cells						
May be added to table salt						
Vitamin D needed for use						
Involved in muscle contraction						
Used to make high-energy ATP						
Needed for normal blood clotting						
Required for hardening of teeth						
Needed for normal nerve transmission						

MCQS

12. In the UK, it is recommended that the diet includes what proportion of bread, potatoes and other starchy carbohydrates? _____
    a. A quarter
    b. A third
    c. A half
    d. Two thirds

13. Which foods should be eaten sparingly? _____
    a. Beans & pulses
    b. Cucumber and tomatoes
    c. Pasta and porridge
    d. Mayonnaise and crisps.

14. Which of the following is not a recommendation about healthy eating in the UK? _______
    a. Eat unlimited red meat
    b. Eat one portion of oily fish per week
    c. Eat two portions of fish per week
    d. Fruit and vegetables should make up about a third of the diet

15. Vitamin B_{12} is needed for DNA synthesis, and deficiency leads to: _______
    a. Haemolytic anaemia
    b. Iron deficiency anaemia
    c. Megaloblastic anaemia
    d. Pellagra

16. Deficiency of which vitamin causes scurvy? _______
    a. Vitamin B
    b. Vitamin C
    c. Vitamin D
    d. Vitamin E

17. Which of the following are good sources of calcium? (Choose all that apply.) _______
    a. Cheese
    b. Milk
    c. Drinking water
    d. Sardines

18. Which foods have high sodium levels? (Choose all that apply.) _______
    a. Processed foods
    b. Oatmeal
    c. Table salt
    d. Meat

19. Which foods are especially rich in potassium? (Choose all that apply.) _______
    a. Fruit and vegetables
    b. Table salt
    c. Seafood
    d. Meat

20. Which of the foods below are good sources of iron? (Choose all that apply.) _______
    a. Liver
    b. Nuts
    c. Red meat
    d. Green vegetables

12 The digestive system

The digestive system is a varied collection of organs and tissues, which operate together to enable the food we eat and drink to be converted into a suitable form to fuel the activities of the body.

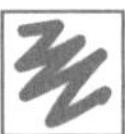 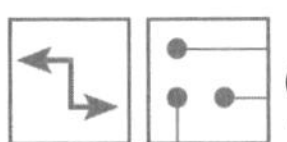

COLOURING, MATCHING AND LABELLING

1. Figure 12.1 shows the digestive system. Colour and match the main parts using the key provided.

○ Rectum	○ Sigmoid colon	○ Small intestine
○ Diaphragm	○ Transverse colon	○ Descending colon
○ Liver	○ Pancreas	○ Duodenum
○ Stomach	○ Oesophagus	○ Appendix
○ Ascending colon	○ Gall bladder	

2. Label the other structures indicated.
3. Highlight the labels identifying the accessory organs of digestion shown on Figure 12.1.

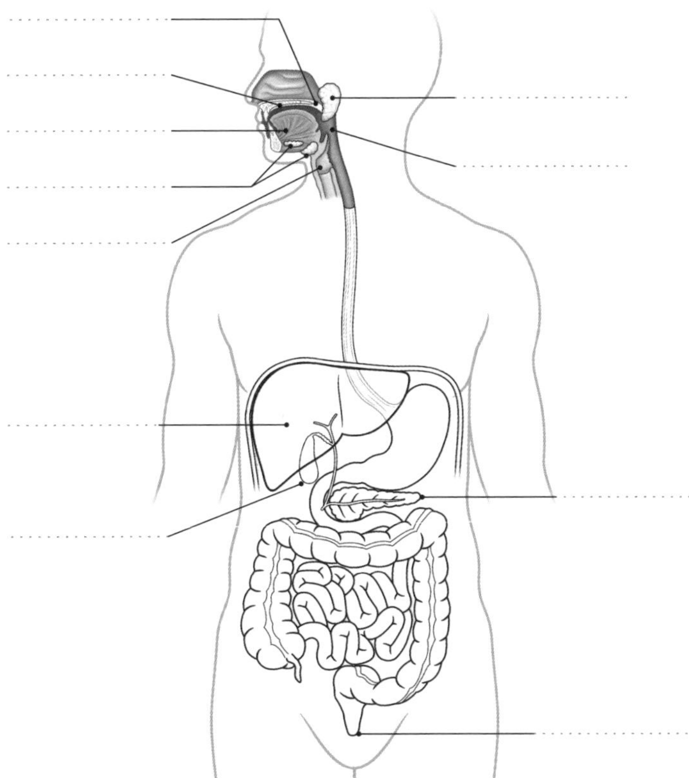

Figure 12.1 The digestive system

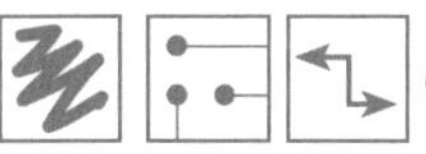

COLOURING, LABELLING AND MATCHING

4. Figure 12.2 shows a section through the wall of the alimentary canal and, although the digestive organs are varied in shape and function, this basic structure is seen in almost all regions. Colour, match and label the nerve plexuses on Figure 12.2.

○ Myenteric plexus	○ Submucosal plexus

5. Label the layers shown on Figure 12.2.

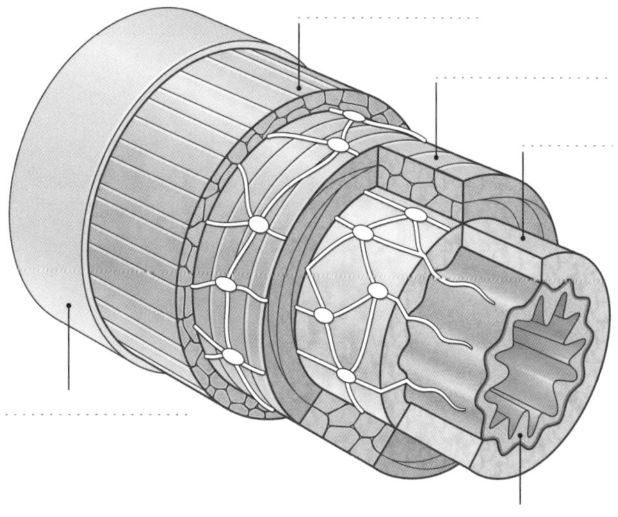

Figure 12.2 General structure of the alimentary canal

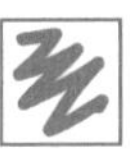 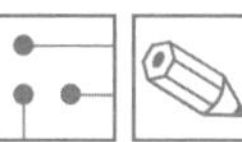

COLOURING, LABELLING AND COMPLETION

6. What type of tissue is shown in Figure 12.3? ______________________________

____

7. Colour and label the two cell types and the product of cell A identified in Figure 12.3.

8. Name two functions of the product of cell A:

- ______________________________
- ______________________________

9. In which regions of the digestive tract is the tissue in Figure 12.3 found?

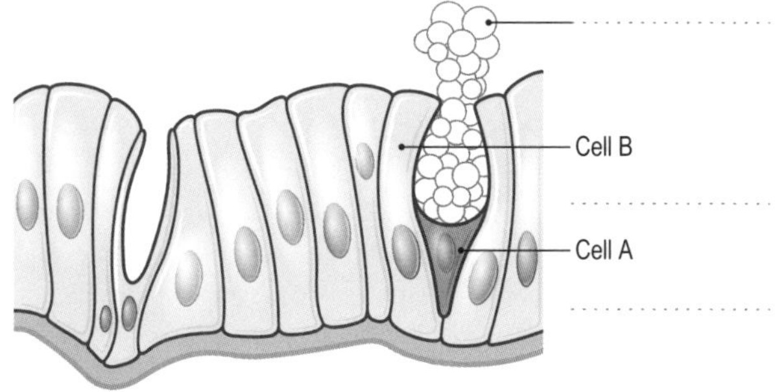

Figure 12.3 Cells of the digestive mucosa

POT LUCK

10. In sequence, list the five processes that take place in the alimentary canal:
    -
    -
    -
    -
    -

11. Distinguish between mechanical breakdown and chemical digestion of food:

12. Define the following terms:

    a. Peristalsis

    b. Sphincter

MCQs

13. Which of the following statements concerning the peritoneum is true? _______
    a. It contains many lymph nodes
    b. It is a large mucous membrane
    c. The uterus is covered only on its posterior surface
    d. The peritoneal cavity is lubricated with lymph

14. The parietal peritoneum: _______
    a. Forms the greater omentum
    b. Covers the pelvic organs
    c. Lines the alimentary canal
    d. Lines the abdominal wall

15. In parts of the alimentary canal that are subjected to considerable wear and tear, the mucous membrane is formed from: _______
    a. Stratified squamous epithelium
    b. Simple squamous epithelium
    c. Columnar epithelium
    d. Transitional epithelium

16. Muscle tissue in the wall of the alimentary canal is: _______
    a. Striated
    b. Voluntary
    c. Smooth
    d. All of these

THE DIGESTIVE SYSTEM AND METABOLISM

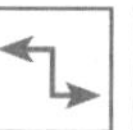 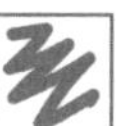

MATCHING AND COLOURING

17. Figure 12.4 shows structures of the mouth. Colour and match the following:

- ○ Teeth
- ○ Lower lip
- ○ Upper lip
- ○ Tongue
- ○ Palatine tonsils
- ○ Soft palate
- ○ Uvula
- ○ Palatopharyngeal arch
- ○ Posterior wall of the pharynx
- ○ Palatoglossal arch

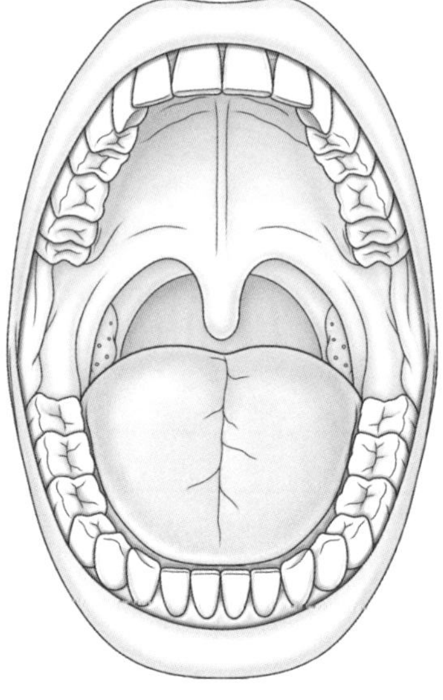

Figure 12.4 Structures of the widely open mouth

COLOURING, MATCHING AND LABELLING

18. Figure 12.5 shows the internal structure of a tooth. Label the structures indicated.
19. Colour and match the following parts on Figure 12.5 and describe the function and main characteristics of each.

- ○ Cementum: ____________________
- ○ Dentine: ____________________
- ○ Enamel: ____________________

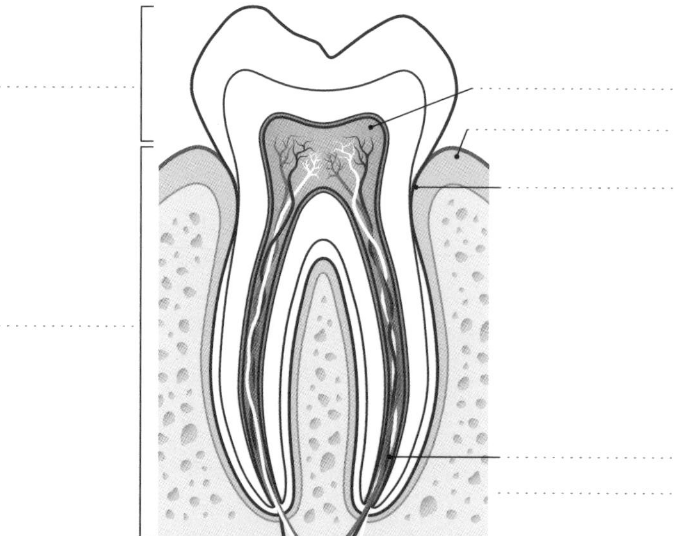

Figure 12.5 A section of a tooth

20. Figure 12.6A shows the stomach and nearby structures. Colour and label the structures indicated.
21. Figure 12.6B shows the main parts of the stomach. Label the structures indicated.
22. Colour and match the following regions of the stomach:

- ○ Body
- ○ Fundus
- ○ Pylorus

23. How many layers of smooth muscle are present in the stomach wall? ____________________
24. Briefly explain why the structure of the stomach wall makes it well suited to its function ____________________

____

____

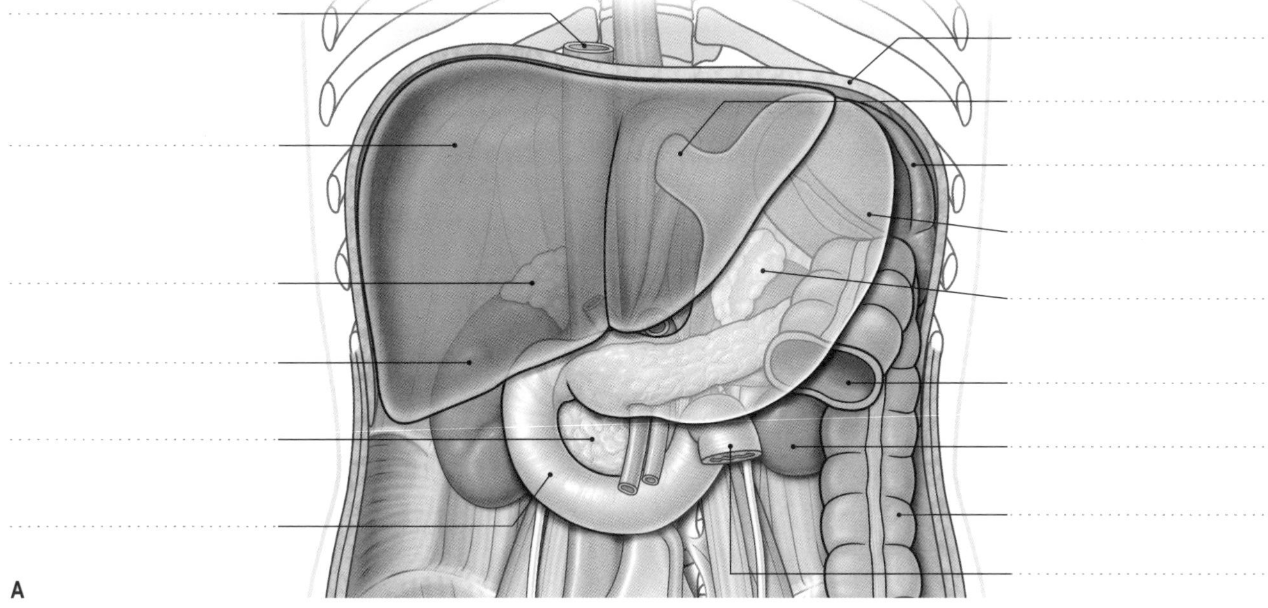

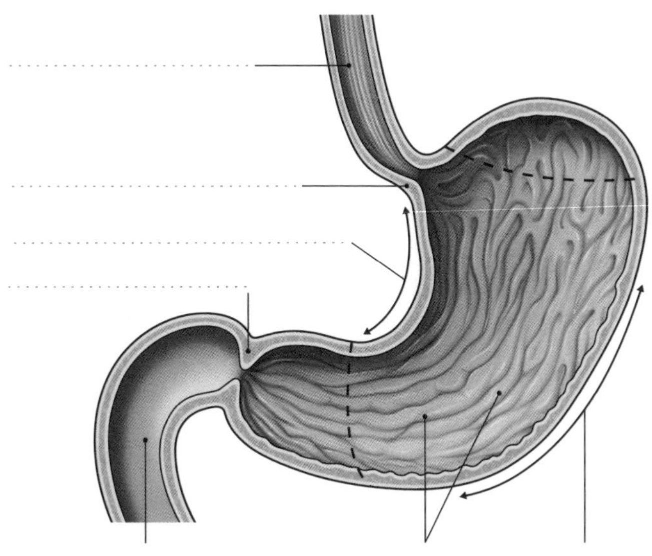

Figure 12.6 A. Stomach and associated structures. B. Longitudinal section of the stomach

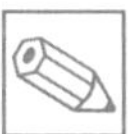
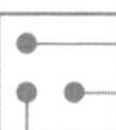

COMPLETION AND LABELLING

25. Figure 12.7 shows two intestinal villi and their specialised modifications that optimise absorption from the gastrointestinal tract.
    a. Label the structures shown.
    b. Colour the arterial supply red, the venous drainage blue and the lymphatic vessels green
    c. The three main nutrients – glucose, amino acids and fatty acids – are represented by different symbols in the key and on the figure. Using the distribution of symbols as a guide, identify which nutrient is represented by the following:

○ ______________________________

● ______________________________

☆ ______________________________

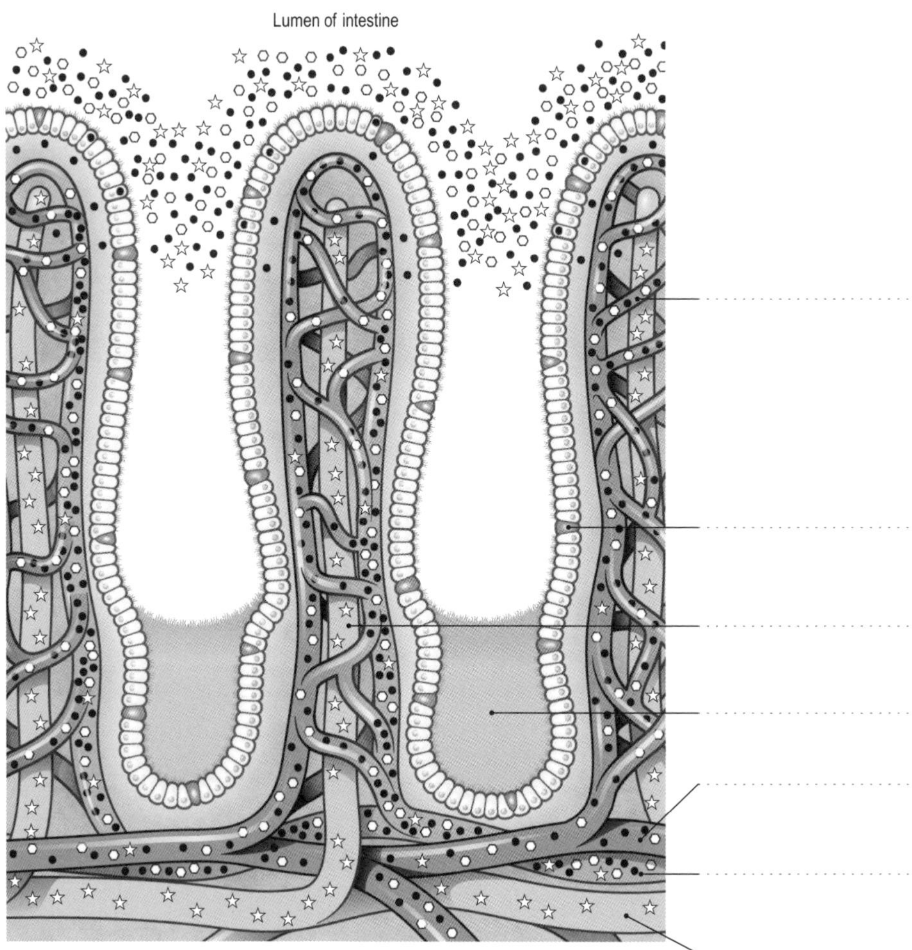

Figure 12.7 The absorption of nutrients into villi

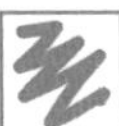 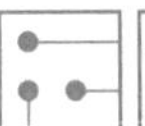 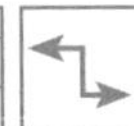

COLOURING, LABELLING AND MATCHING

26. Figure 12.8 shows the pancreas, gall bladder, bile ducts and their connections with the duodenum. Label the structures indicated.

27. Using the key below insert coloured arrows to show the direction of movement of bile in the biliary tract

⟹ Flow from liver to gall bladder

⟹ Flow from gall bladder to duodenum

28. Colour and match the following.

○ Gall bladder
○ Duodenum
○ Pancreas

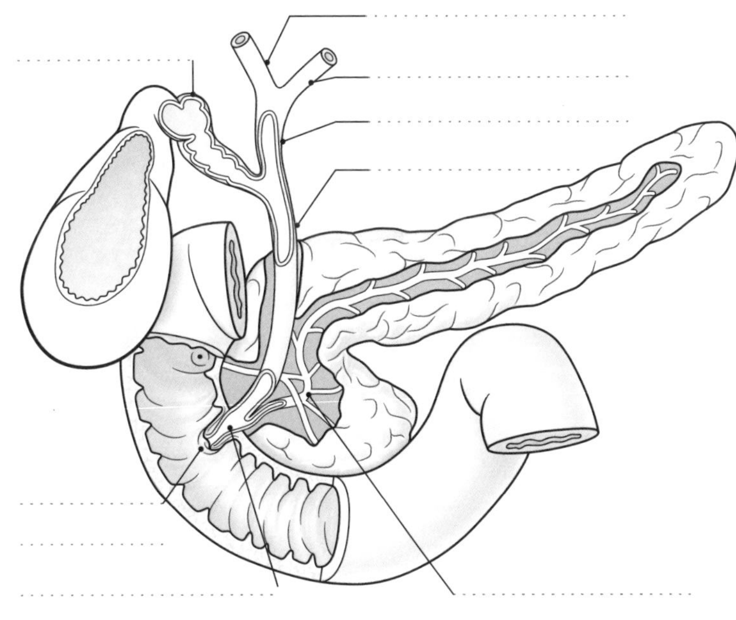

Figure 12.8 The pancreas in relation to the duodenum and biliary tract

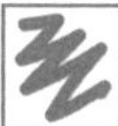 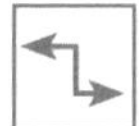

COLOURING AND MATCHING

29. Figure 12.9 shows a magnified transverse section of a liver lobule. Colour and match the following structures:

- ○ Sinusoids
- ○ Hepatic macrophages
- ○ Hepatocytes
- ○ Bile canaliculi.

30. Insert coloured arrows above the labels on Figure 12.9B to indicate the direction of:
    a. Blood flow from the hepatic artery
    b. Blood flow from the hepatic portal vein
    c. Flow of bile to the hepatic duct.

31. The liver is unusual in that it receives both an arterial and a venous blood supply. Explain the significance of this.

____

____.

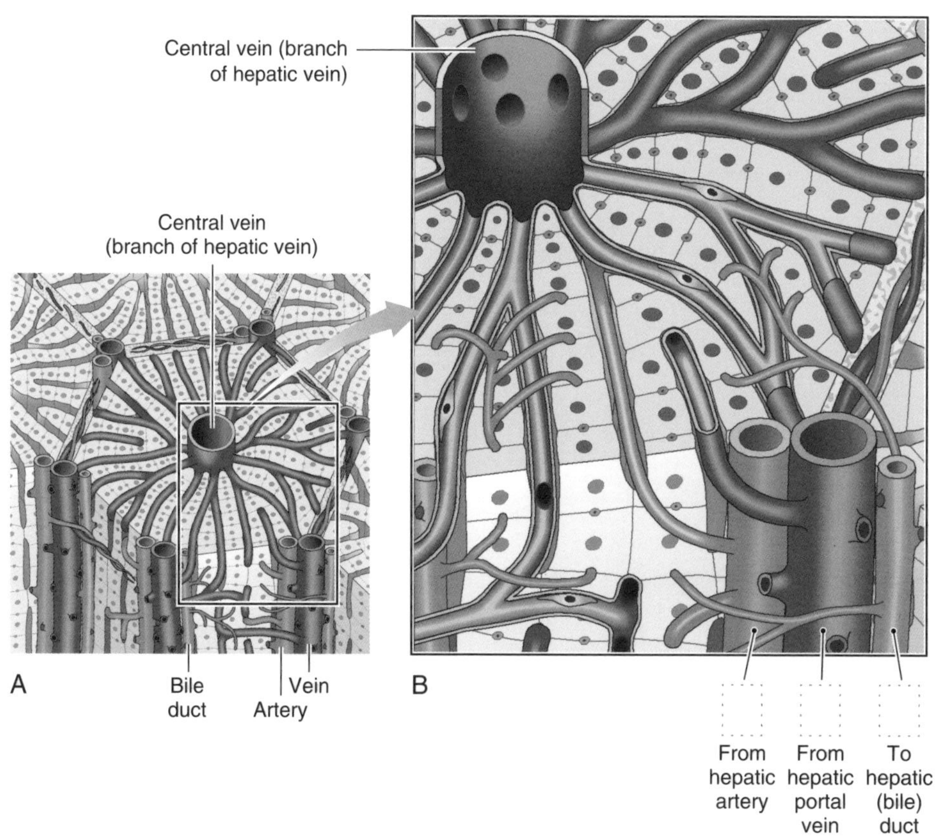

Figure 12.9 A magnified transverse section of a liver lobule

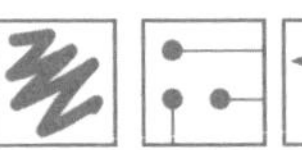

COLOURING, LABELLING AND MATCHING

32. Figure 12.10 shows the biochemical fate of glucose in the cell both in the presence and absence of oxygen. Colour, match and label the arrows to show the three main pathways.

- ○ Glycolysis
- ○ Citric acid (Krebs) cycle
- ○ Oxidative phosphorylation

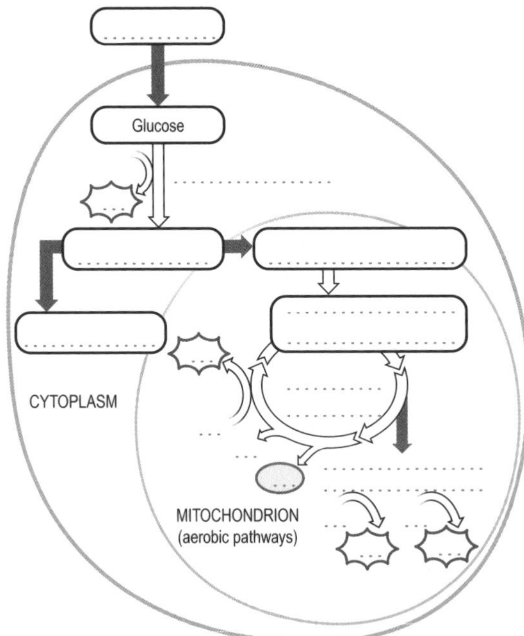

Figure 12.10 Oxidation of glucose

33. Complete the pathways by inserting the correct metabolic intermediates and products in the spaces provided.

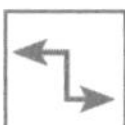
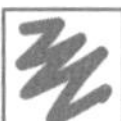

MATCHING AND COLOURING

34. Figure 12.11 summarises the biochemical fates of the main energy sources in the central metabolic pathways, but only the pathways for glucose are complete.
    Using the labels given below, and by inserting arrows appropriately to indicate the conversion of one substance to another, show how proteins and fats also contribute to energy production.

ADP × 4	H_2O
Amino acids	Acetyl coenzyme A
ATP × 4	CO_2
Ketone bodies	Pyruvic acid
Fatty acids	Oxaloacetic acid
Glycerol	

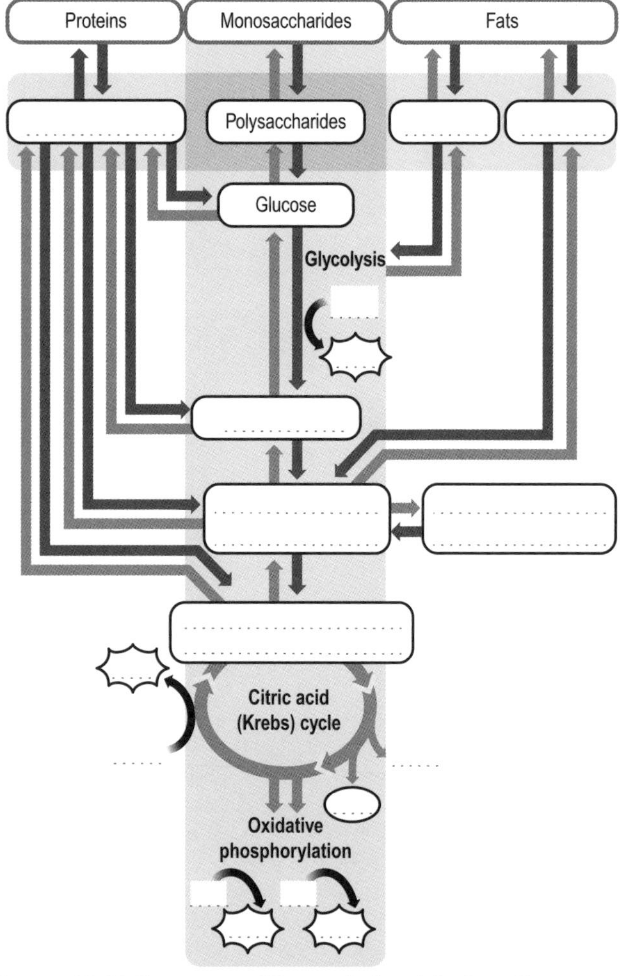

Figure 12.11 Summary of the central metabolic pathways

35. Colour the ATP produced in yellow and the metabolic water in blue.

36. Which substance is essential for the citric acid cycle and oxidative phosphorylation, but is unnecessary for glycolysis? ______________________

POT LUCK

37. List the three stages of swallowing.
    - ______________________
    - ______________________
    - ______________________

38. List A gives some of the important constituents of gastric juice. Match each with the relevant statements in list B. (You might need items in list A more than once.)

List A
Hydrochloric acid
Intrinsic factor
Mucus
Pepsinogens

List B
a. Secreted by parietal cells: ______________________
b. Provides correct pH for stomach enzymes: ______________________
c. Lubricates gastric contents: ______________________
d. Kills ingested bacteria: ______________________
e. Activated to form pepsins: ______________________
f. Secreted by chief cells: ______________________
g. Inactive enzymes: ______________________
h. Required for absorption of vitamin B_{12} in the ileum: ______________________
i. Gives a pH of 1–3 in the stomach: ______________________
j. Secreted by goblet cells: ______________________
k. Precursor for protein digestion: ______________________
l. Stops the action of salivary amylase: ______________________

39. What term describes a soft ball of lubricated food ready for swallowing? ______________________

40. Define the following terms:

    a. Catabolism ______________________

    b. Anabolism ______________________

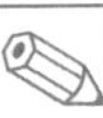

COMPLETION

41. The following paragraphs describe chemical digestion in the small intestine. Complete them by crossing out the incorrect option(s) in bold and leaving the right choice(s).
On a daily basis, the intestine secretes about **1500 mL/2000 mL/2500 mL** of intestinal juices, and its contents are usually acidic, because the pH of the contents coming from the stomach is **acidic/between 7.8 and 8.0/very alkaline to neutralise stomach acid**. In the small intestine, chemical digestion is completed and the end products are absorbed. The main enzyme secreted by the enterocytes is enterokinase, which **breaks down proteins to polypeptides/activates enzymes from the pancreas/neutralises stomach acid and stops the action of pepsin**. However, other enzymes from accessory structures are passed into the **duodenum/jejunum/ileum** as well.
The pancreas secretes **sucrase/amylase/maltase**, which is important in reducing large sugar molecules to **amino acids/glucose/disaccharides**. In addition, pancreatic lipase breaks down fats into **fatty acids and glucose/amino acids and glycerol/fatty acids and glycerol**, which can be absorbed in the intestine. The third major nutrient group, the proteins, are broken down to **amino acids/dipeptides/polypeptides** by pancreatic **trypsin and chymotrypsin/pepsin and trypsin/chymotrypsin and pepsin**. Pancreatic juice is also rich in **chloride/hydrogen/bicarbonate** ions, important in neutralising the acid chyme from the stomach.
Even after the multiple digestive actions of these enzymes, the digested proteins and carbohydrates are still not in a readily absorbable form, and digestion is completed by enzymes made by the **enterocytes/goblet cells/lacteals**. Thus, the final stage of protein digestion produces **glucose/amino acids/dipeptides,** and the final stage of carbohydrate digestion produces **monosaccharides/disaccharides/glycogen**.

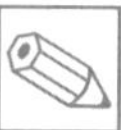

COMPLETION

42. The following paragraphs describe the functions of the liver. Fill in the blanks.

The liver is involved in the metabolism of carbohydrates; it converts glucose to ________________ for storage; the hormone that is important for this is ________________. In the opposite reaction, glucose is released to meet the body's energy needs, and the important hormone for this is ________________. This action of the liver maintains the blood sugar levels within close limits. Other metabolic processes include the formation of waste, including ________________, from the breakdown of protein, and ________________, from the breakdown of nucleic acids. Transamination is the process whereby new ________________ are made from ________________. Proteins are also made here; two important groups of plasma proteins are the ________________ and the ________________.

The liver detoxifies many ingested chemicals, including ________________ and ________________. It also breaks down some of the body's own products, such as ________________. Red blood cells and other cellular material such as microbes are broken down in the ________________ cells. It synthesises vitamin ________________ from ________________, a provitamin found in plants such as carrots, and stores it, along with other vitamins. The liver is also the main storage site of ________________ (essential for haemoglobin synthesis).

The liver makes ________________, which is stored in the gall bladder and facilitates the digestion of ________________. Bile salts are important for ________________ fats in the small intestine, and are themselves reabsorbed from the gut and returned to the liver in the ________________. This is called the ________________ circulation, and helps to conserve the body's store of bile salts. Bilirubin is released when ________________ are broken down (this occurs mainly in the ________________ and the ________________). On its passage through the intestine, it is converted by bacteria to ________________, which is excreted in the faeces; some, however, is reabsorbed and excreted in the urine as ________________. If levels of bilirubin in the blood are high, its yellow colour is seen in the tissues as ________________.

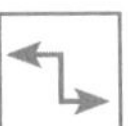

MATCHING

43. The pancreas is both an exocrine and endocrine gland and secretes two types of substances. Complete Table 12.1 using the key choices listed to summarise the characteristics and functions of the pancreas.

Key choices:

Secretions leave via the pancreatic duct
Control of blood sugar levels
Substances are passed directly into blood
Role is in digestion
Synthesis takes place in pancreatic alveoli
Secretion of enzymes
Synthesis takes place in the pancreatic islets
Secretion of glucagon
Secretions include amylase, lipase and proteases
Secretion of hormones
Passes secretions into duodenum
Secretion of insulin

Table 12.1 Functions of the pancreas

Exocrine functions	Endocrine functions

MCQs

44. Which of the following does not form part of the roof of the mouth? _______
    a. The palatine bones
    b. The soft palate
    c. The maxillary bone
    d. The palatine tonsil

45. The uvula is formed from which tissue? _______
    a. Lymphoid
    b. Muscle
    c. Bone
    d. Connective

46. Which of the following statements concerning the tongue is true? _______
    a. It is made of involuntary muscle
    b. Its base is anchored to the hyoid bone
    c. It is the only structure in the mouth possessing nerves for taste
    d. Its role in swallowing is minimal

47. The flow of gastric juice can be stimulated by the thought, sight or smell of food. This is typical of which phase of gastric acid secretion? _______
    a. Cephalic phase
    b. Intestinal phase
    c. Pancreatic phase
    d. Gastric phase

48. Which of the following is not a phase of gastric secretion? _______
    a. Intestinal phase
    b. Biliary phase
    c. Gastric phase
    d. Cephalic phase

49. The stomach is adapted to allow stretching as it fills. This is permitted by: _______
    a. Aggregated lymph follicles
    b. Gastric glands
    c. Villi
    d. Rugae

50. Which of the following meals will remain the longest in the stomach? _______
    a. Mixed salad, low fat yoghurt and an apple
    b. Pasta in a tomato-based sauce
    c. Steak pie and chips
    d. Chicken, mashed potatoes and green beans

51. Why does the pancreas secrete its proteolytic enzymes in an inactive form? _______
    a. To reduce waste
    b. To prevent the active enzymes from digesting the duodenum
    c. To increase the body's control of the digestive processes
    d. To prevent pancreatic damage

52. Which of the following statements concerning control of pancreatic secretion is true? _______
    a. It is regulated by secretin and gastrin, which are made in the duodenum
    b. Secretin and cholecystokinin stimulate pancreatic secretion
    c. The stretching of the duodenal walls when food enters stimulates secretin release
    d. Gastrin is released directly into the pancreas from the enteroendocrine cells that secrete it

53. Which of the following vitamins would be absorbed in reduced amounts if bile were absent from the intestine? (Choose all that apply.) _______
    a. A
    b. B
    c. C
    d. D

54. Which hormone is released when a high-fat meal has been eaten and stimulates contraction of the gall bladder? _______
    a. Bile
    b. Cholecystokinin
    c. Secretin
    d. Gastrin

55. Constipation may arise due to which of the following? (Choose all that apply.) _______
    a. Increased peristalsis in the small intestine
    b. Slow transit along the alimentary canal
    c. Presence of commensal microbes in the large intestine
    d. Postponing the need to defaecate

56. What are the main functions of the colon? (Choose all that apply) _______
    a. Absorption of water
    b. Absorption of nutrients
    c. Absorption of vitamin K produced by commensal bacteria
    d. Regular peristalsis that moves the contents along

57. Which of the following statements concerning defaecation is true? _______
    a. The anal columns allow contraction of the anal canal
    b. The anal sphincters are a continuation of the longitudinal muscle of the colon
    c. The internal anal sphincter is under conscious voluntary control
    d. The desire to defaecate is initiated by the stimulation of stretch receptors in the rectum

58. Which of the following statements concerning faeces is true? _______
    a. The main constituent is fibrous and indigestible material
    b. The bacteria present are dead
    c. They can be runny in diarrhoea
    d. Their brown colour comes from the fatty content

59. The tiny porous blood vessels that allow easy passage of substances between the blood and hepatocytes are: _______
    a. Venules
    b. Arterioles
    c. Capillaries
    d. Sinusoids

60. The vessels in liver lobules that carry bile are the: _______
    a. Capillaries
    b. Canaliculi
    c. Lymphatics
    d. Sinusoids

61. The volume of bile secreted daily is: _______
    a. 200 mL
    b. 800 mL
    c. 500 mL
    d. 300 mL

62. Which section of the biliary tract does bile have to pass through twice? _______
    a. Hepatic duct
    b. Biliary duct
    c. Cystic duct
    d. Common bile duct

63. Which of the following statements concerning the gall bladder is true? _______
    a. Bile is concentrated because water is absorbed through the gall bladder wall
    b. The two layers of muscle in the wall of the gall bladder contract to expel bile
    c. Fatty and acid chyme in the stomach stimulates release of bile
    d. Sympathetic activity in the gall bladder nerve supply stimulates bile release

64. Which of the following concerning the basal metabolic rate (BMR) is true? _______
    a. The individual should not have eaten within 6 hours of the test
    b. The BMR is independent of age or body weight
    c. The BMR reflects the level of energy production needed for only the most vital of body functions
    d. Reduction in food intake increases the BMR and causes loss of body weight

65. Normal blood sugar levels are: _______.
    a. 2–5 mmol/L
    b. 5–8 mmol/L
    c. 8–11 mmol/L
    d. 11–14 mmol/L

66. What normally happens to excess glucose in the body? (Choose all that apply.) _______
    a. It is excreted in the urine
    b. It is converted to fat
    c. It is converted to glucagon
    d. It is stored in liver and skeletal muscle in a polymerised form

67. Gluconeogenesis is an important metabolic process because it is the: _______
    a. Use by body cells of noncarbohydrate sources of energy, such as fats or proteins
    b. Production of glycogen from glucose for energy storage
    c. Conversion of molecules other than carbohydrates to glucose
    d. Production of ATP from energy sources, such as glucose and other carbohydrates

68. Which of the following does not increase the BMR? _______
    a. Resting in a warm room in the postabsorptive state
    b. Ingestion of food
    c. Age
    d. Fever

13 The urinary system

The urinary system has important regulatory and excretory functions that play a vital part in maintaining homeostasis of water and electrolyte concentrations. This chapter will help you understand how this occurs.

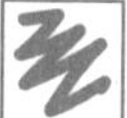 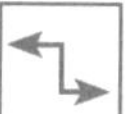 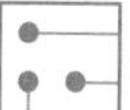

COLOURING, MATCHING AND LABELLING

1. Colour and match the following structures on Figure 13.1:

- O Left kidney
- O Right kidney
- O Bladder
- O Ureters (left and right)
- O Urethra

2. Draw in the left and right adrenal glands on Figure 13.1.
3. Label the remaining structures identified on Figure 13.1.

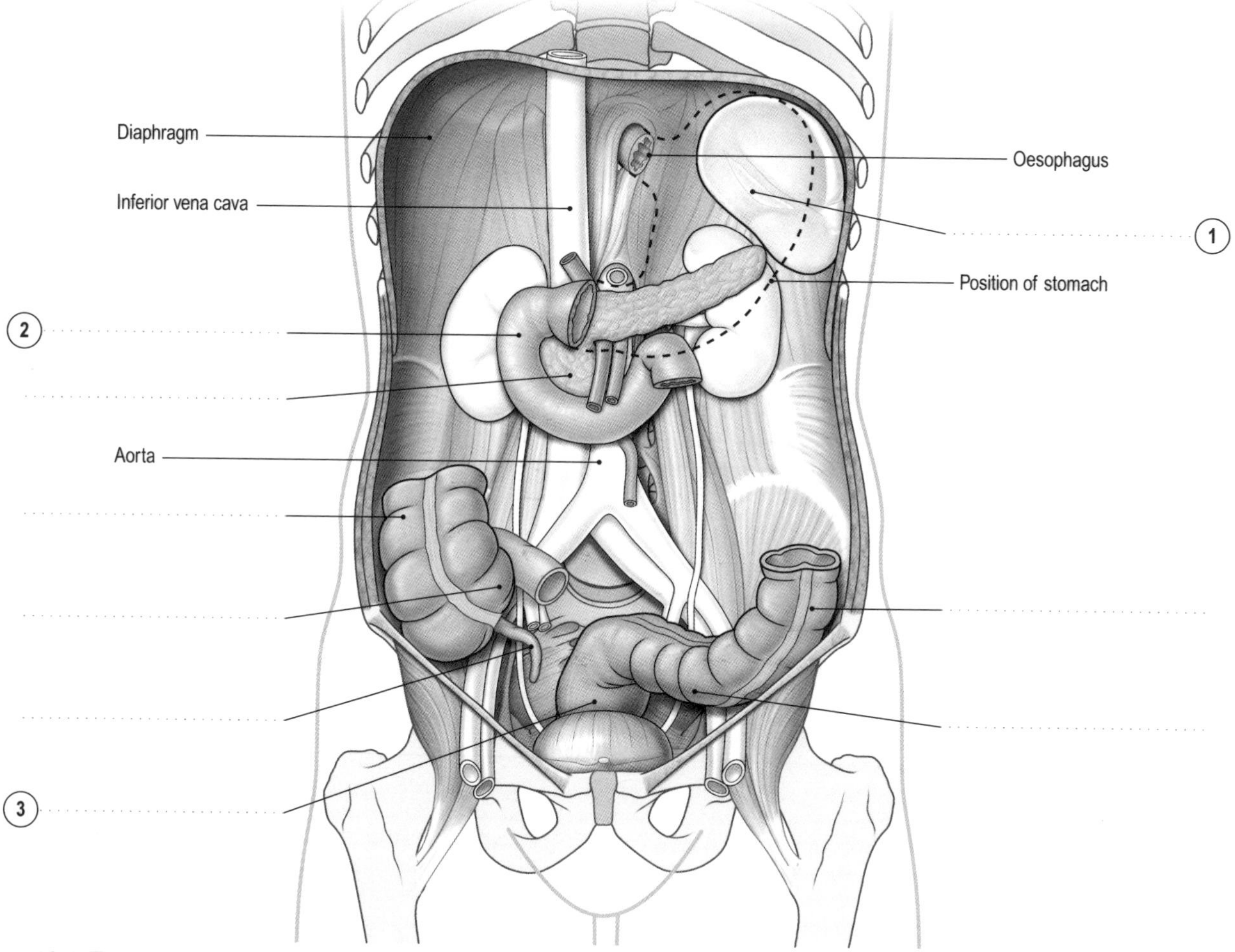

Figure 13.1 The urinary system and associated structures

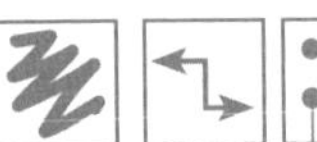

COLORING, MATCHING AND LABELLING

4. Colour, match and label the following parts of the kidney shown on Figure 13.2:

- O Cortex
- O Ureter
- O Pyramids (medulla)
- O Papilla
- O Major calyces
- O Minor calyces
- O Pelvis
- O Capsule

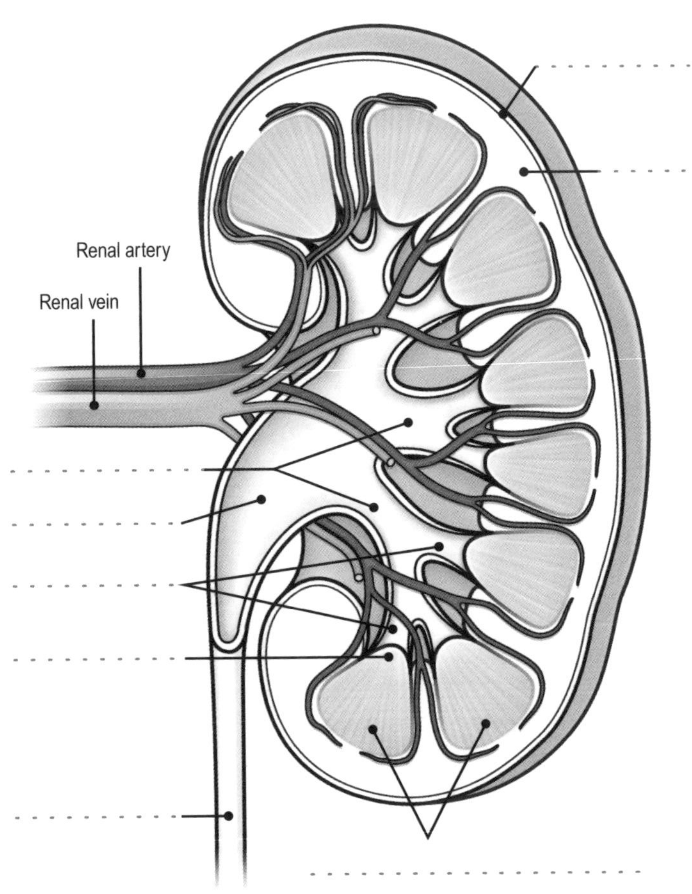

Figure 13.2 A longitudinal section of the kidney

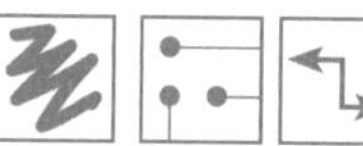

COLOURING, LABELLING AND MATCHING

5. Label the structures identified on Figure 13.3.

6. Colour and match the arrows showing the following:

- ○ Renal medulla
- ○ Renal cortex

7. Insert coloured arrows on Figure 13.3 to indicate:

- ○ Direction of blood flow
- ○ Direction of flow of filtrate

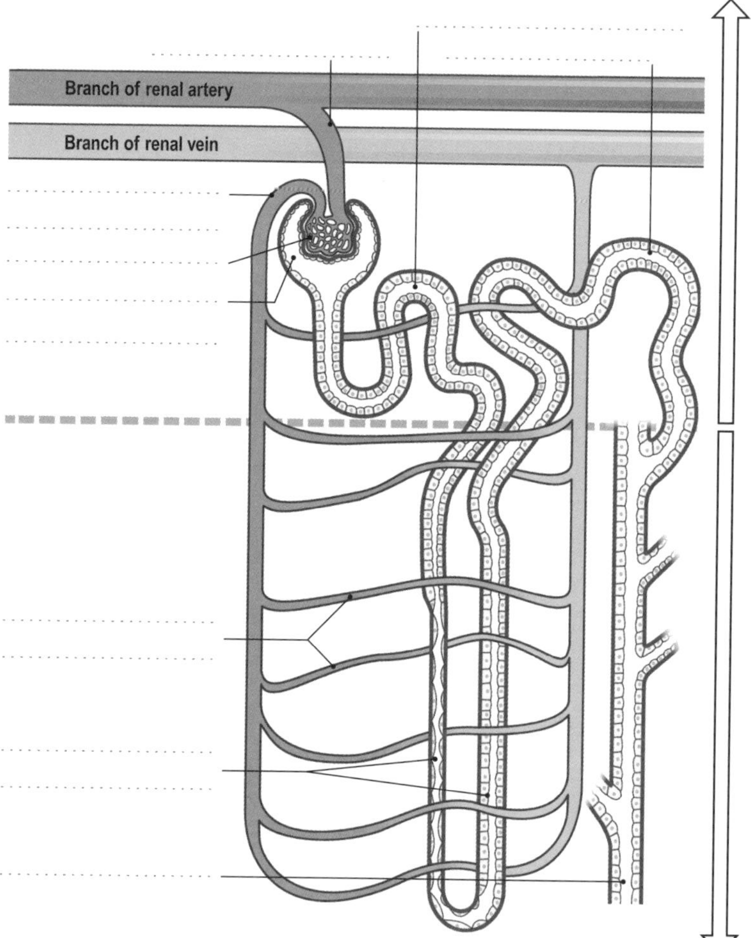

Figure 13.3 A nephron and associated blood vessels

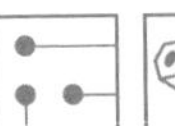

LABELLING AND COMPLETION

8. Label the blood vessels shown on Figure 13.4.
9. Name the three processes involved in the formation of urine at the locations identified on Figure 13.4.

   I. ______________________________

   II. ______________________________

   III. ______________________________

10. Insert three arrows on Figure 13.4 to show the direction of movement of water at locations I, II and III.

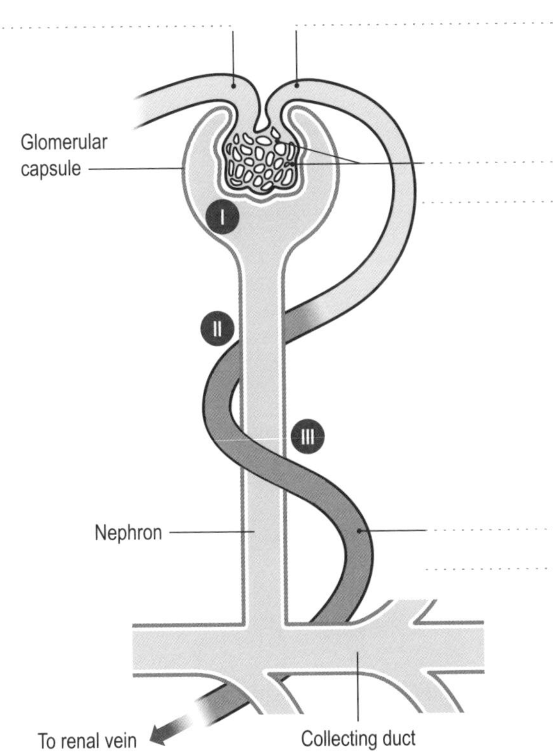

Figure 13.4 Summary of the processes that form urine

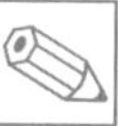

COMPLETION

11. Complete Table 13.1 by identifying which constituents of blood are normally present in the glomerular filtrate and the urine (insert 'normal' or 'abnormal' as appropriate in each column).

Table 13.1 Normal constituents of glomerular filtrate and urine

Constituent of blood	Presence in glomerular filtrate	Presence in urine
Water		
Sodium		
Potassium		
Glucose		
Urea		
Creatinine		
Proteins		
Uric acid		
Red blood cells		
White blood cells		
Platelets		

12. Complete the blanks in the paragraph below to explain the control of water volume in the body.

Water is excreted through the lungs in ____________________, through the skin as ____________________ and via the kidneys as the main constituent of ____________________. Of these three organs, the most important in controlling fluid balance are the ____________________. The minimum urinary output required to excrete the body's waste products is about ____________________ per day. The volume in excess of this is controlled mainly by the hormone ____________________. Sensory nerve cells, called ____________________, detect changes in blood osmotic pressure. When the osmotic pressure increases, the secretion of ADH is ____________________, and ____________________ is reabsorbed by the distal collecting tubules and collecting ducts. These actions result in the osmotic pressure of the blood being ____________________. This is an example of a ____________________ control system.

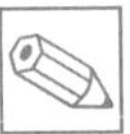

COMPLETION

13. Fill in the blanks in the paragraphs below to describe the structure of the ureters and bladder.

The ureters propel urine from the ____________ to the bladder by the process of ____________. Each ureter is about ____________ long and ____________ in diameter; they are lined with ____________. They enter the bladder at an ____________ angle that prevents ____________ of urine into the ureter as the bladder fills and during ____________.

The bladder acts as a ____________ for urine. When empty, its shape resembles a ____________, and it becomes more ____________ as it fills. The posterior surface is the ____________, and the bladder opens into the urethra at its lowest point, the ____________. The bladder wall consists of three layers. The outer layer is composed of ____________ tissue and contains ____________ and ____________ vessels. The muscular layer is formed by ____________ muscle arranged in ____________ layers. Collectively, this is called the ____________ and, when it ____________, the bladder empties. The inner layer is known as the ____________. Three orifices on the posterior bladder wall form the ____________. The two upper openings are formed when each ____________ enters the bladder; the lower one is the opening of the ____________.

POT LUCK

14. Three of the statements below are false. Identify and correct them using the space provided.
   a. Urea and uric acid are nitrogenous waste products excreted in urine.
   b. The kidneys secrete renin, an important hormone in the control of blood pressure.
   c. The kidneys secrete the hormone erythropoietin, which stimulates the production of red blood cells.
   d. Atrial natriuretic peptide is a hormone secreted by the heart that increases the reabsorption of sodium and water by the proximal convoluted tubules.
   e. Antidiuretic hormone (ADH), secreted by the hypothalamus, stimulates the reabsorption of water from the distal convoluted tubules.

- ____
- ____
- ____

MATCHING

15. Figure 13.5 summarizes the main processes involved in the renin–angiotensin–aldosterone system. Enter the appropriate key choice from the list below into the lettered boxes.

Key choices:
Sodium ____
Potassium ____
Water ____
Increased ____
Volume ____
Vasoconstriction ____
Renin ____
ACE (angiotensin-converting enzyme) ____
Aldosterone ____

16. Add + or − into the circles labelled j, k, l and m in Figure 13.5 to indicate whether the arrows indicate activation or inhibition of the step indicated.

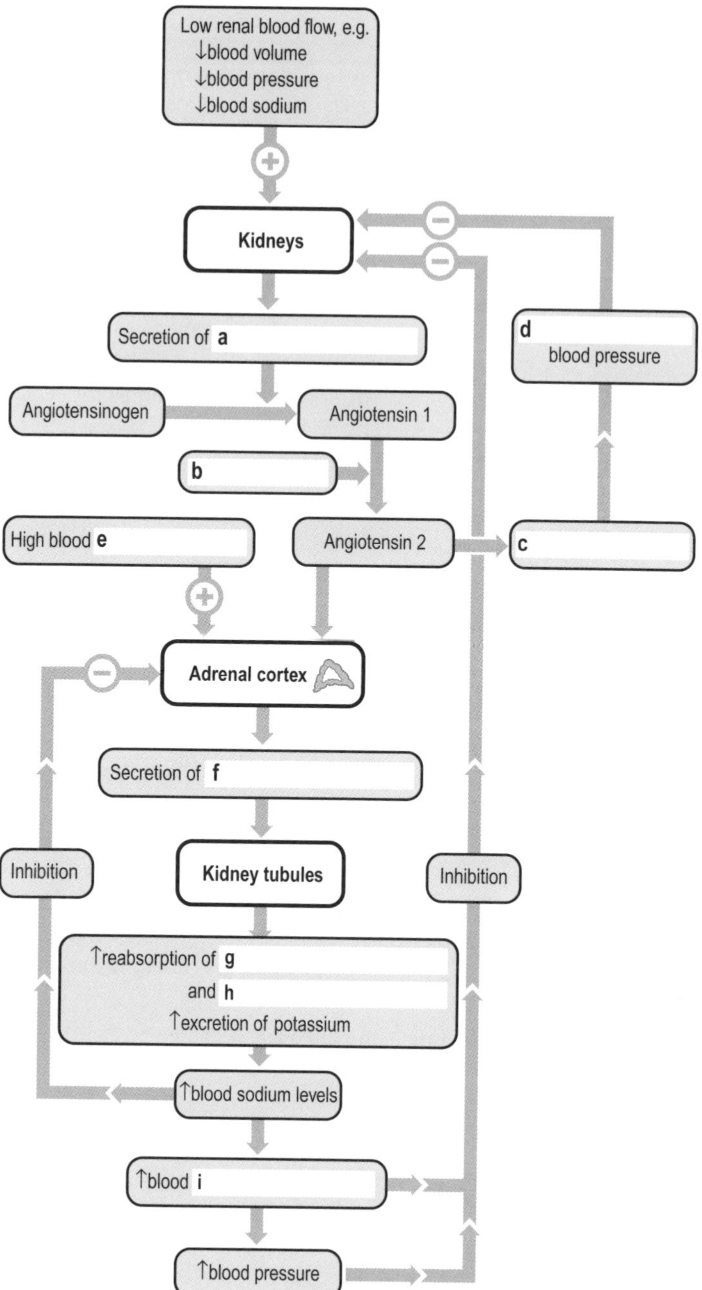

Figure 13.5 Negative feedback regulation of aldosterone secretion

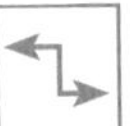

MATCHING

17. Complete the paragraph below, which describes the differences in micturition in infants and adults, with the key choices given.

Key choices:

Brain	Detrusor	Relaxation	Voluntary	Stretching
Contraction	Overridden	Spinal reflex	External	Internal

As the bladder fills and becomes distended, receptors in the wall are stimulated by ________________. In infants, this initiates a ________________, and micturition occurs as nerve impulses to the bladder cause ________________ of the ________________ muscle and ________________ of the ________________ urethral sphincter. When the nervous system is fully developed, the micturition reflex is stimulated, but sensory impulses pass upwards to the ________________. By conscious effort, the reflex can be ________________. In addition to the processes involved in infants, there is ________________ relaxation of the ________________ urethral sphincter.

MCQs

18. The principal effect of aldosterone is to increase the reabsorption of: _______
    a. Potassium
    b. Calcium
    c. Urea
    d. Sodium

19. Renin secretion is stimulated by which of the following? (Choose all that apply.) _______
    a. Low blood potassium level
    b. Low blood sodium level
    c. Low blood volume
    d. Low blood pressure

20. The proportion of glomerular filtrate reabsorbed is about: _______
    a. 1%
    b. 10%
    c. 50%
    d. 99%

21. The glomerular filtration rate (GFR) is normally about: _______
    a. 8 litres per day
    b. 80 litres per day
    c. 180 litres per day
    d. 800 litres per day

22. The kidneys are important in the regulation of: _______
    a. Water balance
    b. Electrolyte balance
    c. pH
    d. All of these

23. The blood vessels and ureters enter or leave the kidneys at the: _______
    a. Hilum
    b. Cortex
    c. Medulla
    d. Capsule

24. The ureters pass through which of the following? (Choose all that apply.) _______
    a. Cranial cavity
    b. Abdominal cavity
    c. Pelvic cavity
    d. Thoracic cavity

25. Peristalsis in the ureters is: _______
    a. An intrinsic property of smooth muscle there
    b. Controlled by the autonomic nervous system
    c. Under voluntary control
    d. Controlled by hormones

26. The urethra extends from the: _______
    a. Kidneys to the external urethral orifice
    b. Trigone to the external urethral orifice
    c. Base of the bladder to the external urethral orifice
    d. Neck of the bladder to the external urethral orifice

27. How many layers of tissue are found in the wall of the urethra? _______
    a. One
    b. Two
    c. Three
    d. Four

28. The internal urethral sphincter is composed of elastic tissue and: _______
    a. Fibrous tissue
    b. Smooth muscle
    c. Skeletal muscle
    d. Cardiac muscle

29. The external urethral sphincter is composed of: _______
    a. Fibrous tissue
    b. Smooth muscle
    c. Skeletal muscle
    d. Cardiac muscle

30. The urethra is which of the following? (Choose all that apply.) _______
    a. Part of the genital tract in males
    b. Part of the genital tract in females
    c. Longer in males than in females
    d. Longer in females than in males

DEFINITIONS

Define the following terms:

31. Polyuria ______________________________

32. Polydipsia ______________________________

33. Ketonuria ______________________________

34. Haematuria ______________________________

35. Anuria ______________________________

14 The skin

The skin completely covers the body and is continuous with the membranes that line the body orifices. This chapter will help you to learn about its structure and functions.

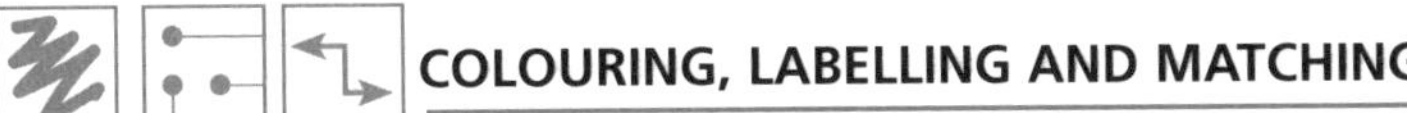

COLOURING, LABELLING AND MATCHING

1. Colour the capillaries on Figure 14.1.
2. Colour and label the structures identified on Figure 14.1.
3. Colour and match the following layers of the skin:

○ Epidermis	○ Dermis	○ Subcutaneous layer

Arterial capillary

Venous capillary

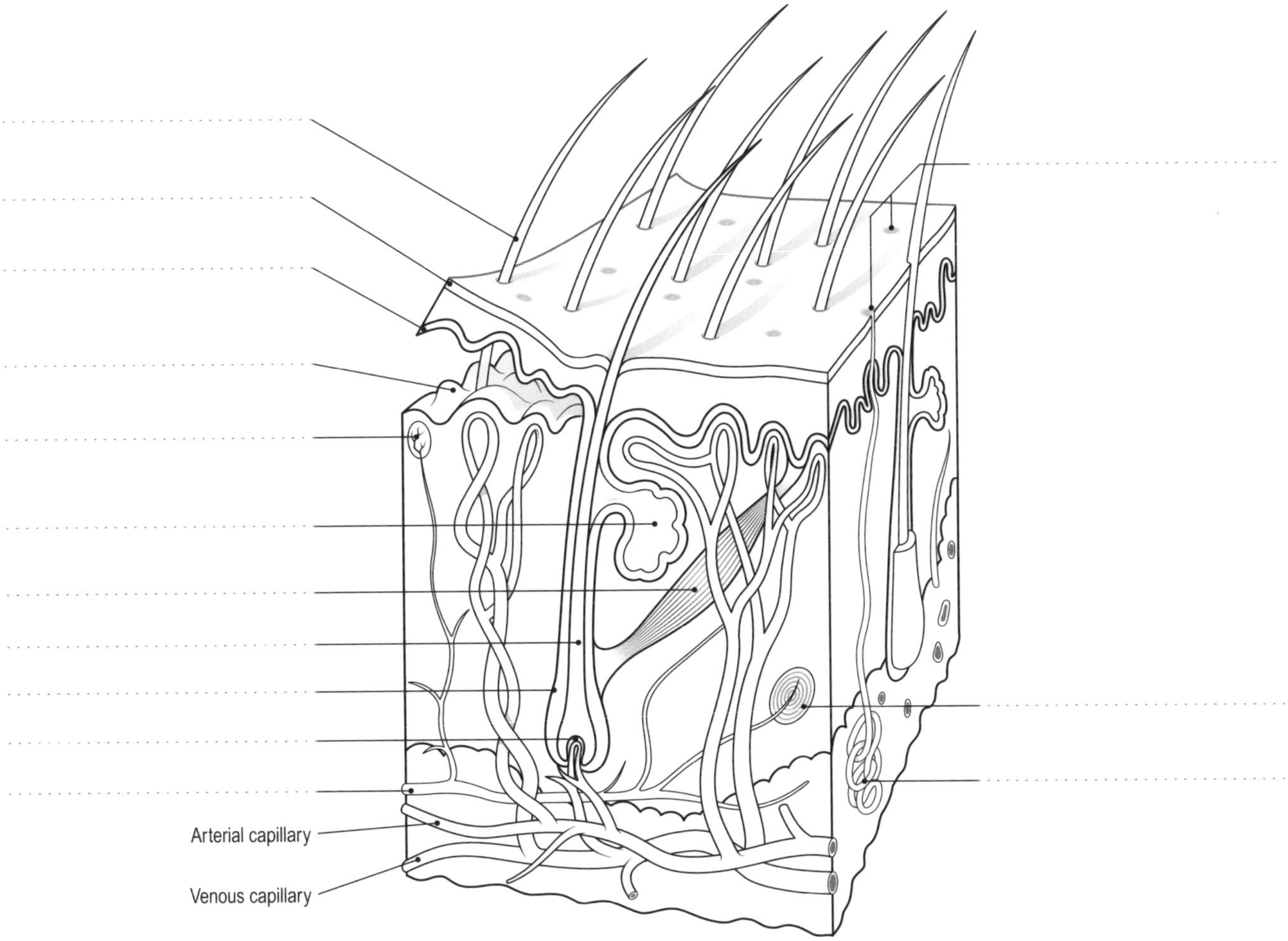

Figure 14.1 The main structures in the skin

POT LUCK

4. State whether each process results in heat loss or heat gain.
   a. Shivering ____________________
   b. Sweating ____________________
   c. Conduction ____________________
   d. Radiation ____________________
   e. Vasodilation ____________________
   f. Vasoconstriction ____________________
   g. Evaporation ____________________
   h. Convection ____________________

MATCHING

5. Match statements a–i with the appropriate correct key choice.

Key choices:
Dendritic cell
Nonspecific defence mechanism
Absorption
Vasodilation
Conduction
Evaporation
Vasoconstriction
Convection
Vitamin D

a. Reduces heat loss from the skin: ____________________
b. Occurs when objects in contact with the skin take up heat: ____________________
c. Results in increased blood flow and is recognised by redness of pale skin: ____________________
d. Formed by conversion of 7-dehydrocholesterol by UV rays in sunlight: ____________________
e. A type of macrophage: ____________________
f. Takes place when heat is used to convert water in sweat to water vapour: ____________________
g. The mechanism whereby a limited number of substances gain entry to the body: ____________________
h. Occurs as cool air replaces warmed air that has risen from the body: ____________________
i. A means of protection against many different potential dangers: ____________________

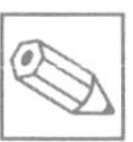

COMPLETION

6. Fill in the blanks to complete the paragraphs describing temperature regulation.

Body temperature is normally maintained around ________________ °C, although it typically ____________ slightly in the evening. The temperature-regulating centre is situated in the ______________ and is responsive to the temperature of circulating ________. When body temperature rises, sweat glands are stimulated by the ______________________. The ________________ centre in the medulla oblongata controls the diameter of small arteries and ______________ and therefore the amount of __________ circulating in the dermis. When body temperature rises, the skin capillaries ____________, and extra blood near the surface increases heat loss by ________________, ________________ and ________________. The skin is warm and pale skin is _______ in colour. When body temperature falls, arteriolar vasoconstriction conserves heat and the skin becomes ____________ and feels cool.

Fever is often the result of ____________. During this process, there is the release of chemicals, also called ____________, from damaged tissue. These chemicals act on the ________________, which releases prostaglandins that reset the temperature thermostat to a _________ temperature. The body responds by activating heat-generating mechanisms, such as ____________ and ______________, until the new temperature is reached. When the thermostat is reset to the normal level, heat loss mechanisms are activated. There is vasodilation and profuse ______________ until the body temperature returns to the normal range again.

? MCQs

7. The healthy epidermis is formed by: _______
   a. One thick layer of columnar epithelium
   b. Several layers of connective tissue
   c. Division of epithelial cells in the basal layer that are pushed upwards
   d. Blood vessels, nerve endings, sebaceous glands and sweat glands

8. Complete regeneration of the epidermis takes about: _______
   a. 1 day
   b. 1 week
   c. 1 month
   d. 2 months

9. Keratin is found in which of the following? (Choose all that apply.) _______
   a. Hair
   b. Nails
   c. Sweat glands
   d. Epidermis

10. The colour of the skin may be affected by: (Choose all that apply) _______
    a. Low oxygen saturation of blood haemoglobin
    b. High levels of bile pigments in the blood
    c. The amount of melanin
    d. Keratinisation of epithelial cells

11. Waterproofing of the skin is provided by: (Choose all that apply) _______
    a. Keratin
    b. Melanin
    c. Sweat
    d. Sebum

12. Bacterial decomposition of secretions from which glands causes the unpleasant odour of stale sweat? _______
    a. Sebaceous glands
    b. Apocrine glands
    c. Eccrine glands
    d. Endocrine glands

WOUND HEALING

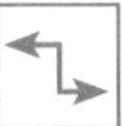 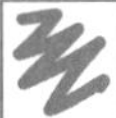

MATCHING AND COLOURING

13. Identify the stages of wound healing shown in Figure 14.2.

14. Match and colour the following on Figure 14.2:

O Fibroblasts	O Platelets	O Scab	O Epidermis
O Phagocytes	O Blood clot	O Capillaries	O Dermis

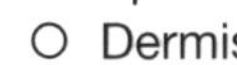

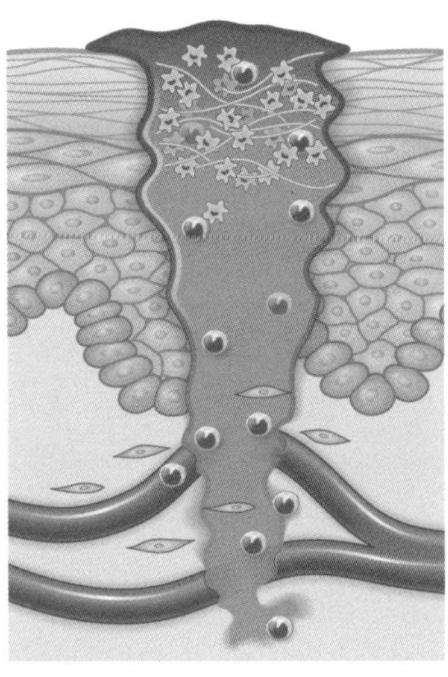 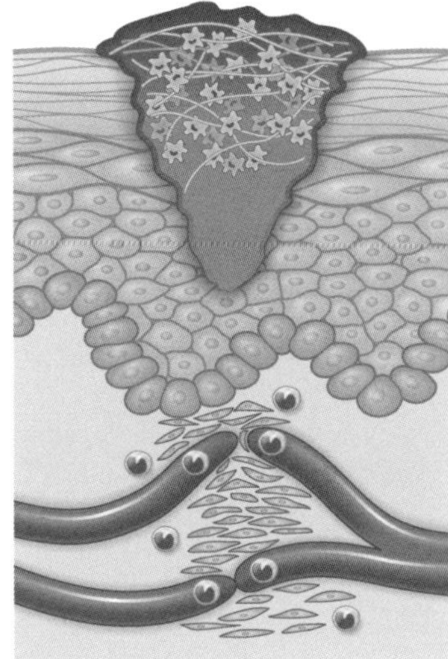 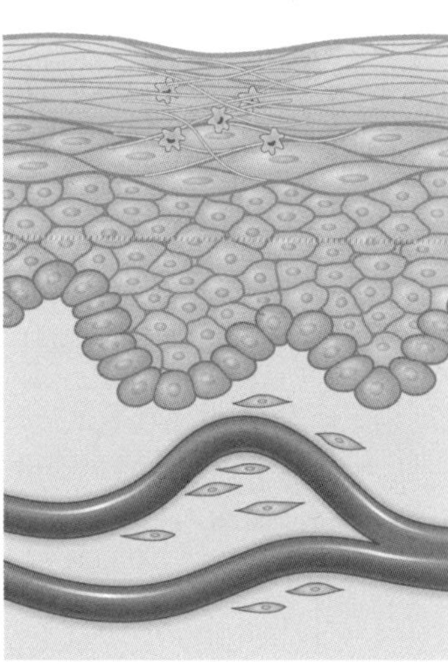

Figure 14.2 Stages in primary wound healing

MATCHING

15. Match the key choices with the statements. Key choices may be used more than once.

Key choices:				
Fibroblasts	Phagocytes	Granulation tissue	Scar tissue	Slouh

a. Blood clot and debris in a wound are removed by: ____________________

b. New collagen fibres are produced by: ____________________

c. Tissue consisting of capillary buds, phagocytes and fibroblasts is called: ____________________

d. Tissue type replaced by fibrous tissue: ____________________

e. Also known as necrotic tissue: ____________________

f. Tissue formed from fibrous tissue: ____________________

g. Cells that travel to a wound in its blood supply: ____________________

15 Resistance and immunity

From life in the womb to the moment of death, an individual is under constant attack from an enormous range of potentially harmful invaders, including bacteria, viruses, parasites and foreign (non-self) cells. The body has therefore developed a wide range of protective measures, both specific and nonspecific, which will be considered in this chapter.

MATCHING

1. Match each of items a to j to either specific (S) or nonspecific (NS) resistance by writing S or NS in the space provided. You may need both for some items.

   a. Targets a range of possible threats ____________

   b. Involves antibody production ____________

   c. Also referred to as immunity ____________

   d. Involves 'memory' ____________

   e. Protects against bacteria ____________

   f. Protects against antigens ____________

   g. An example is skin ____________

   h. Requires lymphocyte activation ____________

   i. Includes body secretions, such as mucus ____________

   j. Effective from birth ____________

2. Match the following statements to each of the five types of antibody listed in the key choices below. You may use more than one antibody type for each statement.

Key choices: IgA, IgD, IgE, IgG, IgM

   a. Involved in allergy _______

   b. Characterises an early immune response _____

   c. Coats epithelia _______

   d. Active against only one particular antigen ____

   e. Produced by plasma cells _______

   f. Powerful activator of complement _______

   g. Expressed on mast cells _______

   h. Expressed on B-cells _______

   i. Found in body fluids like saliva _______

   j. Characterises a mature immune response _____

   k. Largest antibody molecule _______

   l. Found in breast milk _______

   m. Crosses the placenta _______

   n. Neutralises bacterial toxins _______

   o. Most common antibody type _______

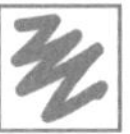
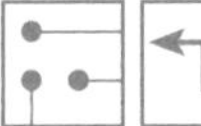

COLOURING, LABELLING AND MATCHING

3. Figure 15.1 summarises the main events of the inflammatory response. Colour and label the free nerve ending and the capillary endothelial cells.

4. Colour, match and label cells A–D.

A ______________________________

B ______________________________

C ______________________________

D ______________________________

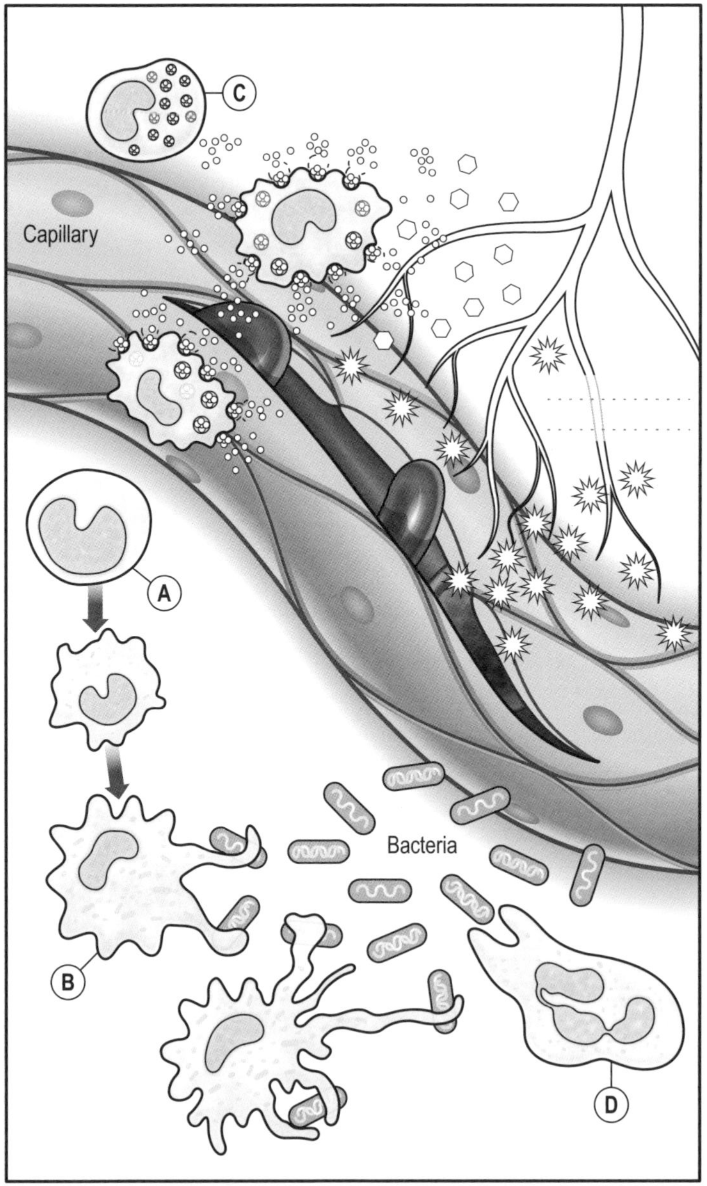

Figure 15.1 The inflammatory response

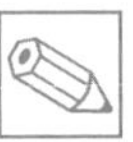

COMPLETION

5. Complete the following paragraph, which describes the functions of cells A–D, using the key choices given. Note that you will not need all the key choices.

Key choices:

Histamine	Monocyte	Microbes	Cell debris	Vasodilation
Diapedesis	Bloodstream	Motile	Smaller	Phagocyte
Phagocyte	Permeable	Lymphocyte	Lymphatic System	Mast Cell
Bradykinin	Neutrophil	Vasoconstriction	Larger	Allergic
Cytotoxic	Viruses	Macrophage	Nonallergic	Active

Cell A, a ______________, travels in the bloodstream and migrates into inflamed tissues. In the tissues, it transforms into cell B, a ______________, which is an active ______________ that engulfs and destroys ______________ and ________________. Cell D is ___________ and more ___________ than cell B and is also an active ______________. It usually travels in the bloodstream and migrates into inflamed tissues by the process called ______________. It is the first inflammatory cell to appear in damaged tissues. Cell C is fixed in body tissues but, in response to cell damage, releases _____________, an important inflammatory mediator associated particularly with _________ inflammation. Capillaries respond to this mediator by becoming more ________________ and widening in diameter, also called __________________.

6. Figure 15.1 shows three different inflammatory mediators. Identify them according to the information given by colouring and matching the symbols in the key.

○ Stored in preformed granules by cell C ____

✲ Causes pain by acting on free nerve endings ____

⬡ Family of mediators made from cell membranes ____

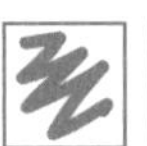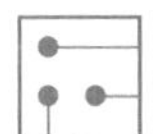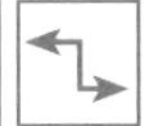

COLOURING, LABELLING AND MATCHING

7. Activation of T-cells is an important element of the immune response. Figure 15.2 shows how the production of the different types of T-cell occurs in response to antigen challenge. Colour and match the different types of cell and outline briefly the function of each in T-cell activation using the key below.

O Macrophage

Function: ______________________________

O T-cell, unspecialised

Function: ______________________________

O Cytotoxic T-cell

Function: ______________________________

O Helper T-cell

Function: ______________________________

O Memory T-cell

Function: ______________________________

O Regulatory T-cell

Function: ______________________________

8. Label the remaining items indicated in Figure 15.2.

9. Colour the receptors for antigen on all cells that you see. What is significant about these receptors when compared between cell types?

____

____

____

10. The process of proliferation and differentiation shown in the centre of the diagram is also called what?

____

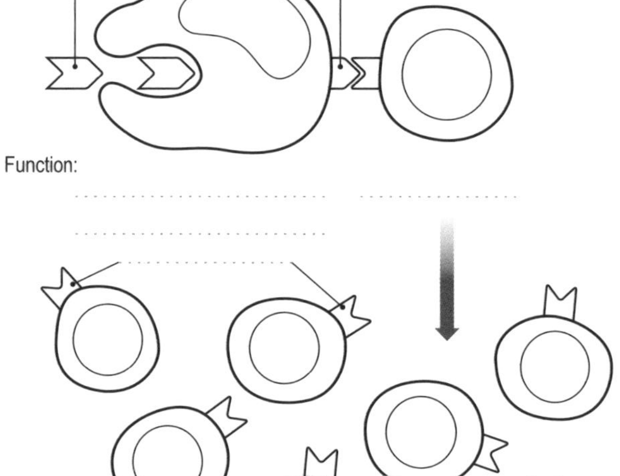

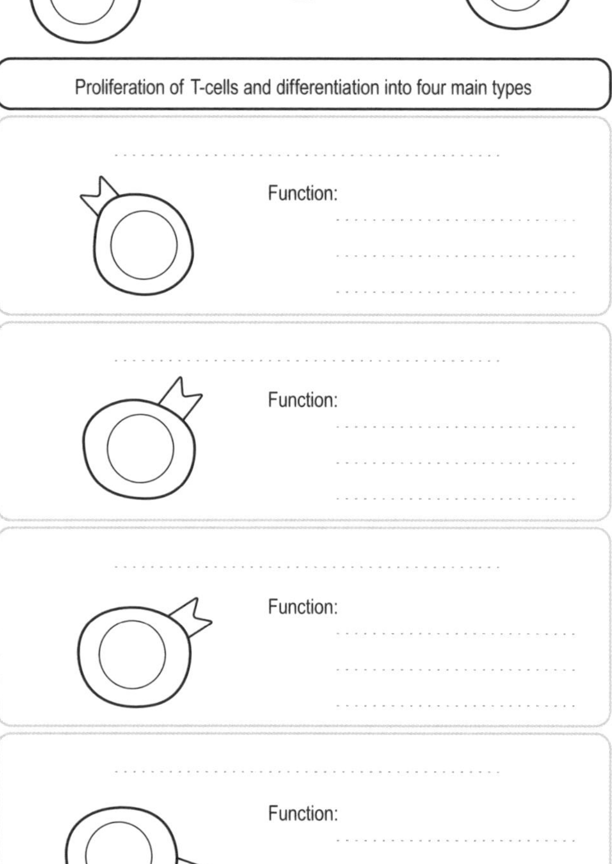

Figure 15.2 The T-cell response to antigen challenge

POT LUCK

11. List the five main signs of the inflammatory response:

- ____
- ____
- ____
- ____
- ____

COMPLETION

12. Table 15.1 presents information about a number of important inflammatory mediators. Complete the table by filling in the blanks.

Table 15.1 Summary of some important inflammatory mediators

Substance	Made by	Trigger for release	Main actions
Histamine			
	Platelets, mast cells and basophils; neurotransmitter in central nervous system		
	Synthesised as required from cell membranes		
			Anticoagulant, maintaining blood supply to an inflamed area
Bradykinin			

13. Table 15.2 lists various characteristics of the two main populations of lymphocyte. Complete the table.

Table 15.2 Lymphocyte characteristics

Characteristic	T-cell	B-cell
Shape of nucleus		
Site of manufacture		
Site of post-manufacture processing		
Nature of immunity involved		
Specific or nonspecific defence		
Production of antibodies		
Processing regulated by thymosin		

14. Complete the paragraph below, which relates to the nature of immunity, by crossing out the incorrect options in bold. Only one of each set is correct.

When the body is exposed to an antigen for the first time, the immune response can be measured as blood antibody levels after about **4 hours/2 days/7 days/3 weeks**; this is the **innate/antibody/acquired/primary** response. The main antibody type here is **IgA/IgD/IgE/IgG/IgM**. Antibody levels fall thereafter and do not rise again unless there is a further exposure to the same antigen, which stimulates a **secondary/delayed/natural/cooperative** response. This is different to the primary response in that it is **faster/less powerful/nonspecific/double-peaked** and is characterised by high levels of **IgA/IgD/IgE/IgG/IgM**. Immunity to an antigen depends on the production of a population of **memory/immune/killer/surveillance** cells.

Immunity is not constant throughout life. Unborn babies are vulnerable to infections because **maternal antibodies do not cross the placenta/they do not make their own antibodies/pregnancy increases the risk of infection/they do not produce white blood cells**. In older age, the immune system can become less efficient. One significant difference in the ageing immune system is **increased incidence of less specific antibodies/more aggressive natural killer cells/enlargement of the thymus/higher levels of autoantibodies**. Additionally, cancer, more common in later years of life, is usually associated with **reduced function of suppressor cells/less efficient immunological surveillance/plasma cell mutations/increased incidence of infections**.

15. Immunity may be acquired in different ways, and the nature of the immunity may vary. Complete Table 15.3 by ticking the appropriate boxes relevant to each of the four listed types of immunity.

Table 15.3 The four types of acquired immunity

Characteristic	Active natural	Active artificial	Passive natural	Passive artificial
An example is a baby's consumption of antibodies in its mother's milk				
Long-lived protection				
Involves production of memory cells				
An example is vaccination				
Short-lived protection				
An example is infusion of antibodies				
Involves production of antibodies by the individual				
An example is a child catching chickenpox at school				
Specific				

? MCQs

16. Complement is which of the following? (Choose all that apply.) _______
    a. A system of about 20 antibodies found in the blood and body fluids
    b. Active against bacteria
    c. An effective attractant for white blood cells
    d. Produced by virally infected cells

17. Which of the following induces resistance to viral infection? _______
    a. Interleukin
    b. Complement
    c. Interferon
    d. Lysozyme

18. Which of the following is involved in specific defence? _______
    a. Antibody
    b. Interferon
    c. Interleukin
    d. Histamine

19. Which of the following binds to and perforates bacterial cell walls? _______
    a. Interferon
    b. Histamine
    c. Lysozyme
    d. Complement

20. The inflammatory response: _______
    a. Is triggered by any form of tissue damage
    b. Is only activated in the presence of infection
    c. Is associated with defensive memory
    d. Adapts depending on the type of invading organism present

21. Which of the following is **not** an action of complement? _______
    a. Damages bacterial cell walls
    b. Vasodilation
    c. Coats bacteria, increasing phagocytosis
    d. Chemoattraction

22. Increased blood flow to an inflamed area is due to: _______
    a. Attraction of large numbers of white blood cells into the region
    b. Loss of plasma proteins from the bloodstream
    c. Dilation of blood vessels supplying the area
    d. Increased vascular permeability, caused by histamine

23. The term meaning pus-forming is: _______
    a. Suppurative
    b. Pyrexial
    c. Pustular
    d. Pyogenic

24. Chemotaxis is which of the following? _______
    a. Movement of white blood cells out of the bloodstream into the tissues
    b. Attraction of white blood cells to an area of inflammation
    c. Stimulated by substances released from white blood cells
    d. Seen only in the early stages of an acute inflammatory response

25. An inflamed area swells because of which of the following? (Choose all that apply.) _______
    a. Blood supply to the area increases
    b. Blood vessels in the region become more permeable
    c. There is loss of plasma proteins from the bloodstream
    d. Hydrostatic pressure in local blood vessels increases

26. Raised temperature, both local and systemic, is beneficial in the inflammatory response because it does which of the following? (Choose all that apply.) ___________
    a. Enhances phagocytosis
    b. Increases chemotaxis
    c. Decreases bacterial viability
    d. Increases production of prostaglandins and other inflammatory mediators

27. Which plasma protein leaks into the tissues and forms an insoluble barrier around an infected area? ______
    a. Thromboplastin
    b. Fibrinogen
    c. Plasmin
    d. Albumin

28. Which mediator resets the internal thermostat in the hypothalamus in infection, leading to fever? _________
    a. Prostaglandin E_2
    b. Bradykinin
    c. Interferon
    d. Interleukin 1

29. Which type of white blood cell predominates in chronic inflammation? _______
    a. Lymphocytes
    b. Macrophages
    c. Neutrophils
    d. Eosinophils

30. Immunological surveillance is: ______
    a. Mediated by macrophages
    b. Ineffective against virally infected cells
    c. An essential part of the acute inflammatory response
    d. Important in the detection of mutated body cells

31. Which of the following cell types is longest-lived? _______
    a. Macrophage
    b. Cytotoxic T-cell
    c. Helper T-cell
    d. Memory T-cell

32. Which of the following cell types is active against different types of antigen (i.e., it is not specific)? _______
    a. Macrophage
    b. Cytotoxic T-cell
    c. Helper T-cell
    d. Memory T-cell

33. How long do plasma cells live? _______
    a. The individual's lifetime
    b. 1 year or more
    c. 1 month
    d. No more than a day

34. Immunological tolerance is mediated by: _______
    a. Cytotoxic T-cells
    b. Memory T-cells
    c. Regulatory T-cells
    d. Helper T-cells

16 The musculoskeletal system

The musculoskeletal system consists of the bones of the skeleton, their joints and the skeletal (voluntary) muscles that move the body. This chapter will help you understand the structure and function of each component of the musculoskeletal system.

THE SKELETON AND ITS JOINTS

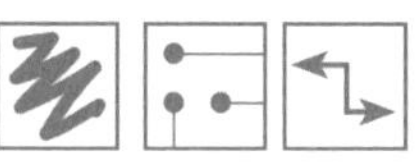

COLOURING, LABELLING AND MATCHING

1. Colour and match the following parts of the long bone in Figure 16.1.

- ○ Periosteum
- ○ Compact bone
- ○ Spongy bone
- ○ Medullary canal
- ○ Nutrient artery
- ○ Articular (hyaline) cartilage
- ○ Epiphyseal line

2. Label the areas of the long bone in Figure 16.1 using the bracketed boxes.
3. In adults, which part of the long bone contains red bone marrow? ______

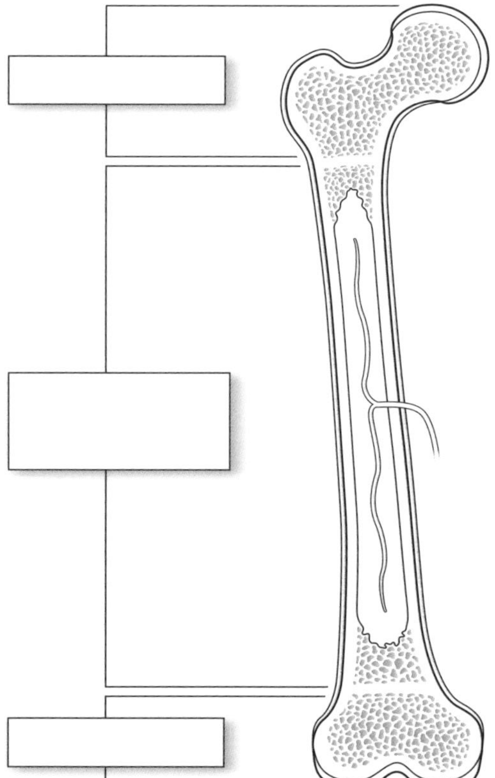

Figure 16.1 Typical features of a long bone

4. Colour and match the following parts of the skeleton in Figure 16.2:

○ Costal cartilages	○ Sacrum and coccyx	○ Metacarpals (hand)
○ Manubrium of sternum	○ Vertebrae	○ Phalanges (hand)
○ Body of sternum	○ Manubrium of sternum	○ Tarsals
○ Xiphoid process of sternum	○ Body of sternum	○ Metatarsals (feet)
○ Intervertebral discs	○ Carpals	○ Phalanges (feet)

5. Label all bones indicated on Figure 16.2.

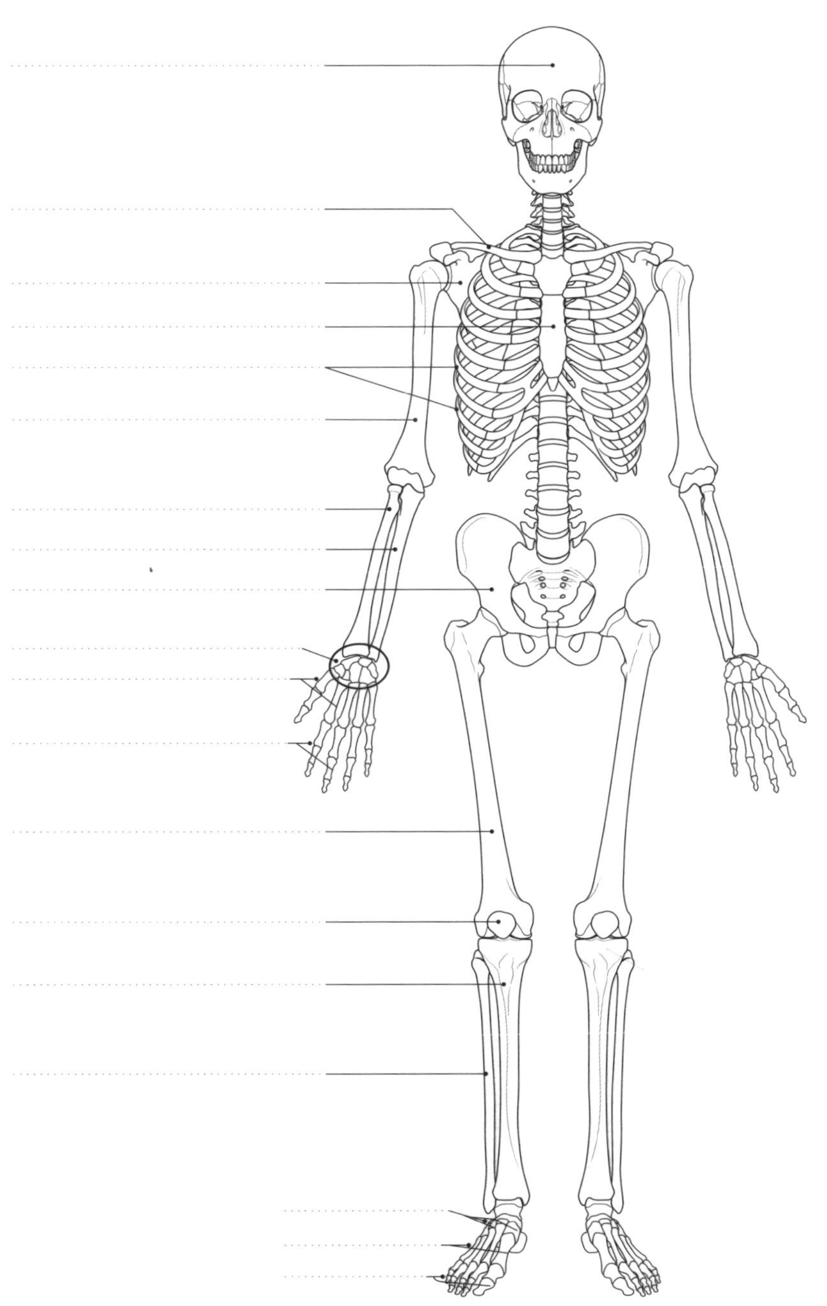

Figure 16.2 The skeleton, anterior view

6. Colour and match the following skull bones shown on Figure 16.3:

○ Ethmoid bone	○ Nasal bone
○ Frontal bone	○ Parietal bone
○ Lacrimal bone	○ Sphenoid bone
○ Occipital bone	○ Temporal bone
○ Maxilla	○ Zygomatic bone
○ Mandible	

7. Label the sutures indicated on Figure 16.3.

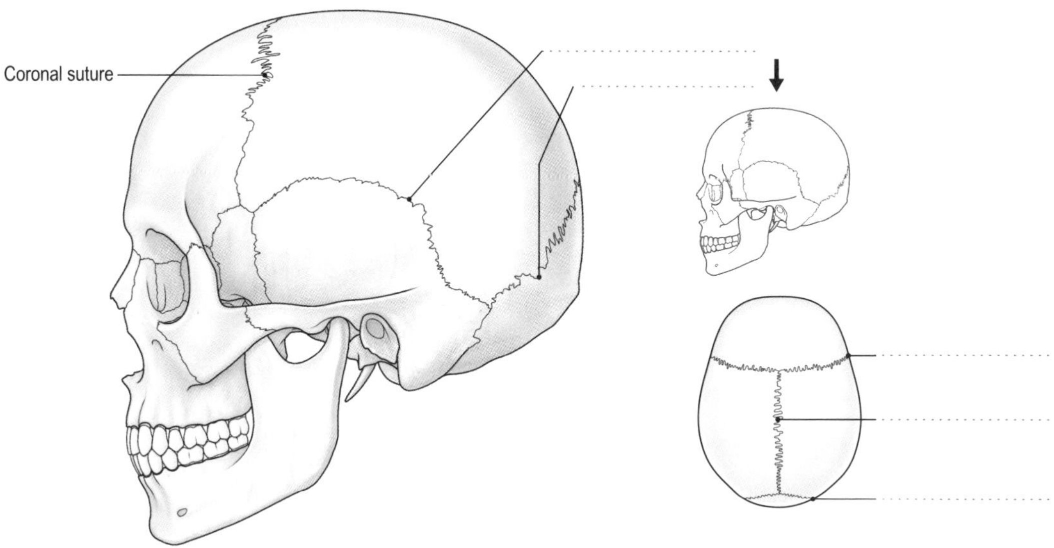

Figure 16.3 The bones and sutures of the skull. (A) Lateral view. (B) Viewed from above.

8. Figure 16.4 shows a lumbar vertebra, which displays the main features of a typical vertebra. Match and label the parts shown.

9. Which structure passes through the part labelled as C?

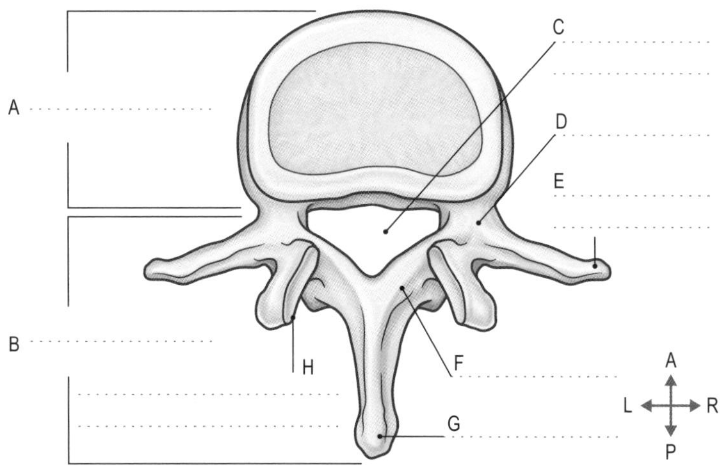

Figure 16.4 A lumbar vertebra, showing features of a typical vertebra, viewed from above

10. Match and label the parts of the humerus on Figure 16.5 using the terms listed below.

Parts of the humerus:	Coronoid fossa
Head	Deltoid tuberosity
Neck	Lateral supracondylar ridge
Shaft	Medial supracondylar ridge
Greater tubercle	Lateral epicondyle
Lesser tubercle	Medial epicondyle
Bicipital groove	Trochlea
Capitulum	

11. On Figure 16.5, colour and match the areas that articulate with the:

- ○ Glenoid cavity of scapula
- ○ Ulna
- ○ Radius

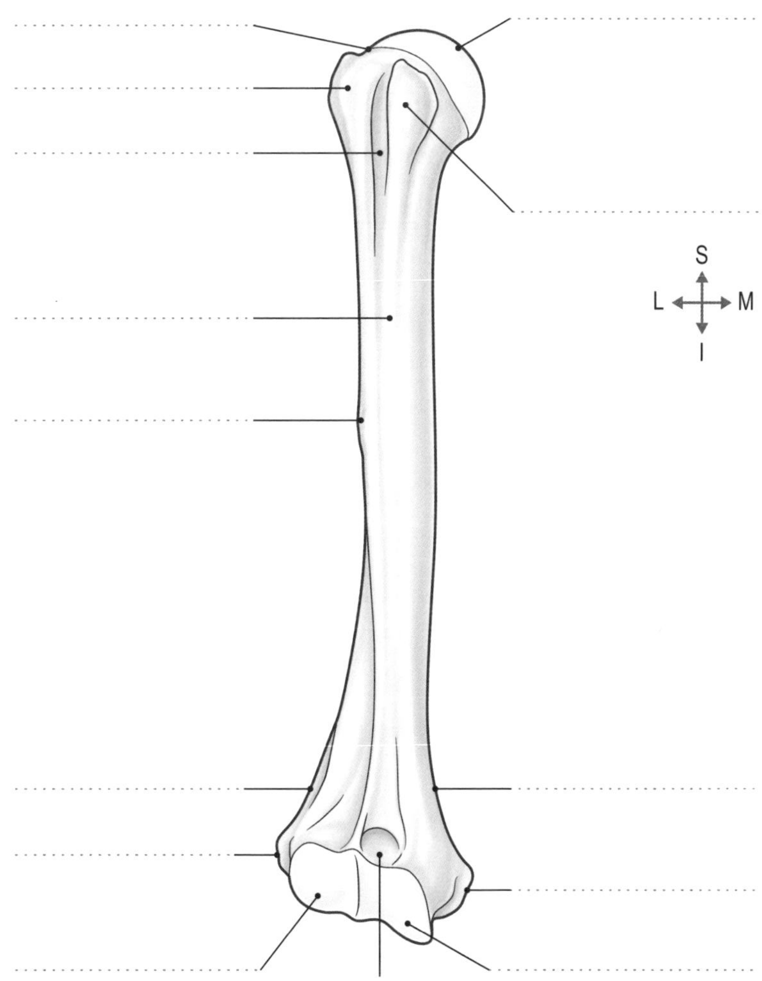

Figure 16.5 The right humerus, anterior view

12. Figure 16.6 shows the bones of the wrist and hand. Colour and match the following bones:

- ○ Carpal bones
- ○ Metacarpal bones
- ○ Proximal phalanges
- ○ Middle phalanges
- ○ Distal phalanges

13. Label the bones of the wrist (the carpal bones) shown on Figure 16.6.

14. On Figure 16.6, circle and label two examples of the following joints:

- ○ Carpal joints
- ○ Carpometacarpal joints
- ○ Metacarpophalangeal joints
- ○ Interphalangeal joints

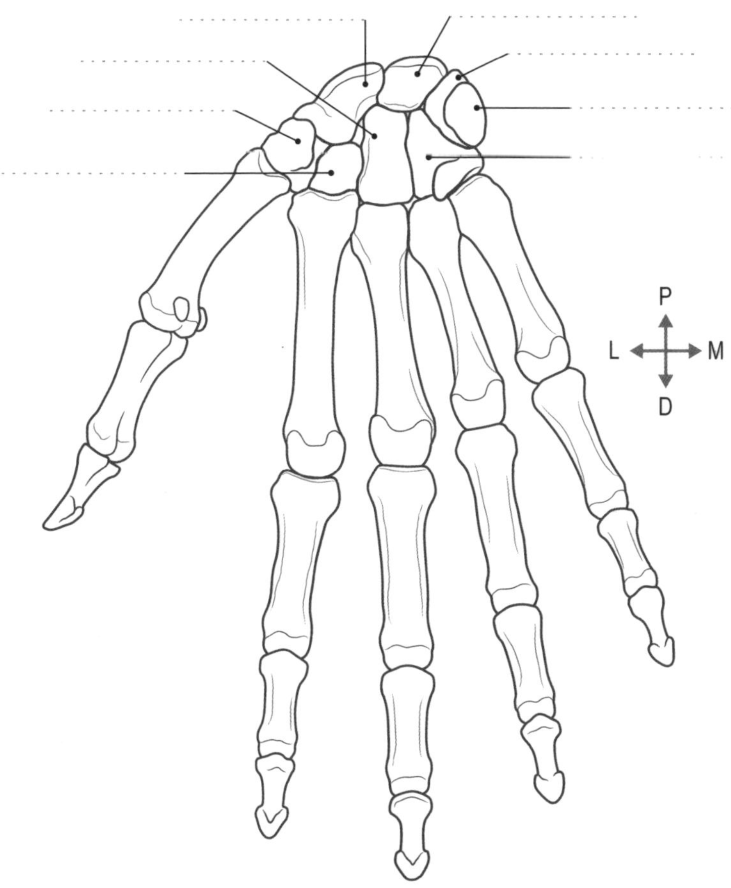

Figure 16.6 The bones and joints of the right wrist, hand and fingers, anterior view

15. On Figure 16.7, colour and match the following parts of the femur:

- ○ Neck
- ○ Head
- ○ Shaft
- ○ Site of articulation with pelvis
- ○ Sites of articulation with tibia

16. Label the landmarks of the femur indicated on Figure 16.7.

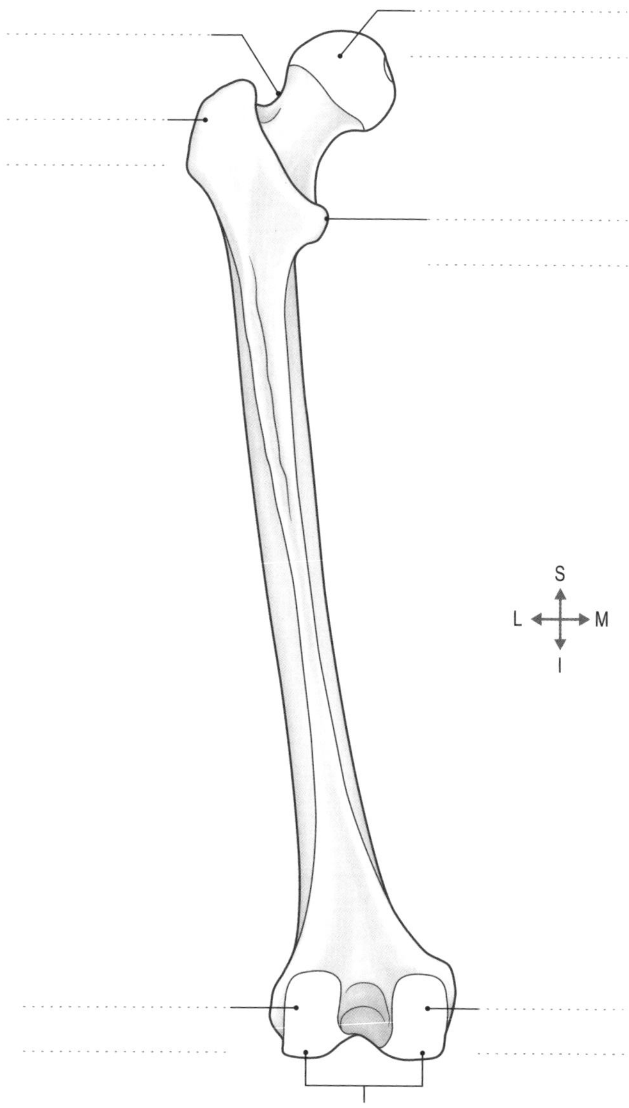

Figure 16.7 The left femur, posterior view

17. On Figure 16.8, colour and match the following parts of the foot:

- ○ Tarsal bones
- ○ Metatarsal bones
- ○ Phalanges

18. Label the individual tarsal bones of the foot shown on Figure 16.8.

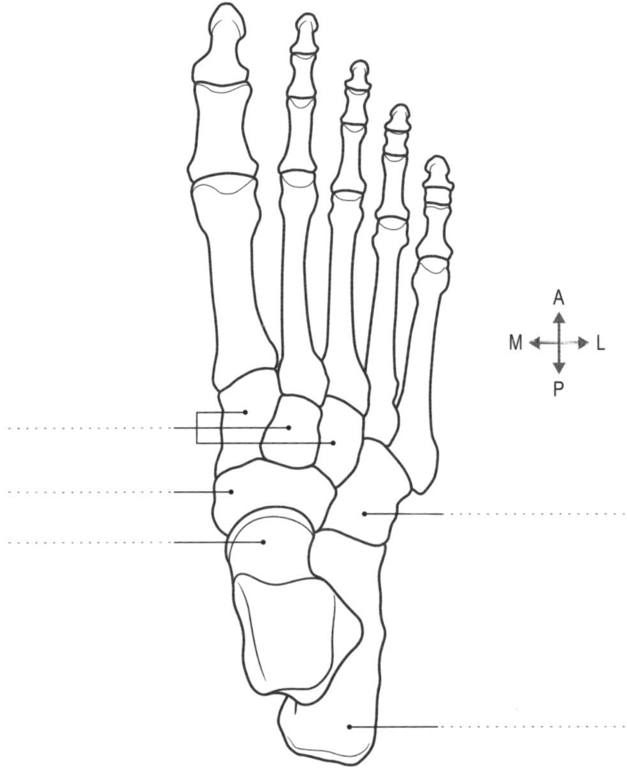

Figure 16.8 The bones of the right foot, viewed from above

COMPLETION

19. Give an example of each type of bone:

a. Long ______________________________

b. Short ______________________________

c. Irregular ______________________________

d. Flat ______________________________

e. Sesamoid ______________________________

20. Fill in the blanks to complete the description of sinuses and fontanelles of the skull.

Sinuses contain ________ and are found in the ____________, ____________, ____________ and ______________ bones. They all communicate with the __________________ and are lined with __________________. Their functions are to give ____________ to the voice and____________ the bones of the face and cranium. Fontanelles are distinct _______________ areas of the skull in infants and are present until _______________ is complete and the skull bones fuse. The largest are the ___________ fontanelle, present until ________ months, and the ____________ fontanelle, which usually closes over by _______ months of age. Their presence allows for moulding of the baby's _________ during childbirth.

21. Insert the characteristics of different types of fractures in Table 16.1.

Table 16.1 Types of fractures

Type of fracture	Characteristics
Simple	
Compound	
Pathological	

22. List four factors that delay the healing of fractures:

- ____
- ____
- ____
- ____

POT LUCK

23. The following statements relate to cells found in skeletal tissue. Four are false. Identify the inaccurate statements and correct them.
    a. Cells that produce cartilage are called chondroblasts. Cartilage is an important constituent of osteoid.
    b. Osteoblasts build new bone. When they mature, they become osteocytes.
    c. Bone is broken down by osteocytes. Healthy bone is constantly subject to the process of breakdown and rebuilding.
    d. Osteoclasts are found mainly under the periosteum and line the medullary canal. These are the smallest of all bone cells.
    e. Bone tissue is constantly monitored by its osteocyte population, which is responsible for depositing the essential minerals iron, calcium and phosphate in the matrix.
    f. The two main cell types in maintaining the correct composition and density of bone are the osteoclasts and osteoblasts. Excessive osteoclast activity leads to lighter, weaker bone tissue.

- ____________________
- ____________________
- ____________________
- ____________________

24. Give the terms that define each of the bony landmarks described below.

    a. A hollow or depression ____________________
    b. A ridge of bone separating two surfaces ____________________
    c. A large rough bony projection for muscle and ligament attachment ____________________
    d. A small hole through a bone ____________________
    e. A smooth rounded projection for making a joint ____________________
    f. A tube-shaped cavity in bone ____________________
    g. An immovable joint between skull bones ____________________
    h. A narrow slit in bone ____________________
    i. A sharp bony ridge (two terms for this) ____________________
    j. A small flat surface for making a joint ____________________
    k. A hollow cavity within a bone ____________________

25. Figure 16.9 shows a number of bony features and surface landmarks identifiable on the anterior view of the skeleton. Complete the figure by labelling all structures indicated.

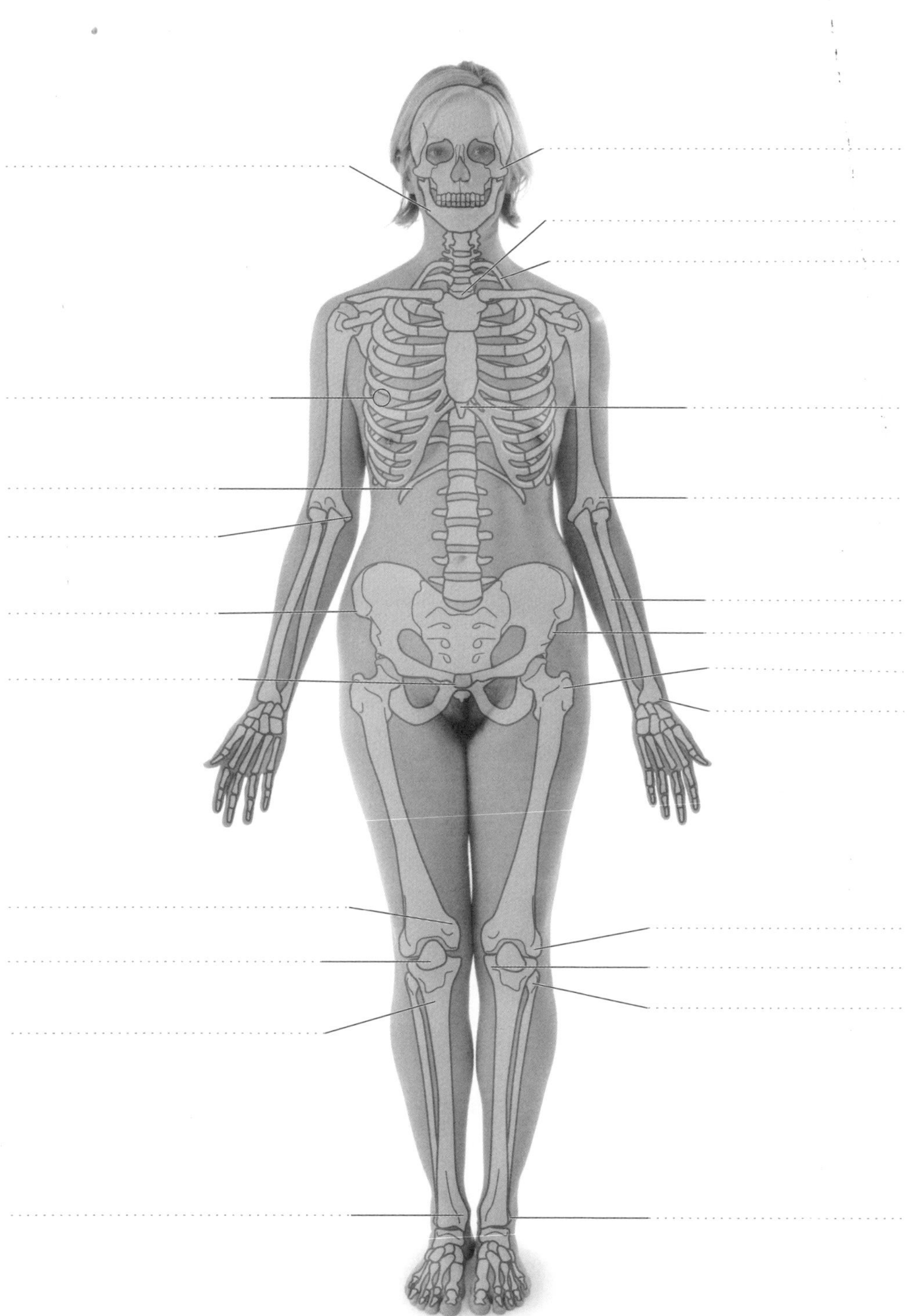

Figure 16.9 The skeleton, anterior view, showing some important bony features and surface landmarks. Modified from Patton K, et al: Brief Atlas of the Human Body Adapted International Edition, 2019, Elsevier.

MATCHING

26. Match the key choices with the statements in Table 16.2 to identify key characteristics of bone.

Table 16.2 Characteristics of bone

Structure	Characteristic
	Looks like a honeycomb to the naked eye
	Haversian system
	Cancellous bone
	Compact bone
	Form the framework of spongy bone
	Remains of old osteons
	Tiny cavities between lamellae containing osteocytes
	Found mainly in spaces within spongy bone
	Develop from membrane models
	Develop from tendon models
	Develop from cartilage models

Key choices:
Sesamoid bones
Flat bones
Long bones
Lacunae
Osteon
Red bone marrow
Trabeculae
Interstitial lamellae
Spongy bone
Spongy bone
Cortical bone

27. List A contains the main hormones that regulate bone growth and development. Match each key choice to the appropriate hormone by writing its letter in the appropriate space in list A. You may use the key choices more than once.

List A
Oestrogen ______
Testosterone ______
Parathyroid hormone
Calcitonin ______
Growth hormone ______
Thyroxine, triiodothyronine

Key choices:

a. Promotes closure of the epiphyseal plate
b. Lack in childhood causes dwarfism
c. Increases calcium deposition in bone
d. Increases calcium loss from bone
e. Promotes bone growth
f. Maintains bone structure in adulthood
g. Essential for normal bone development in infancy and childhood
h. Excess in childhood causes gigantism
i. Excessive quantities predispose to bone thinning

28. Match the key choices listed with the statements about the vertebral column below:

Key choices:	Transverse foramen
Odontoid process	Nucleus pulposus
Intervertebral disc	Atlas
Spinous process	Coccyx
Sacrum	Annulus fibrosus
Axis	Body
Thoracic vertebrae	

a. Consists of four fused vertebrae: ______________________________

b. Part of a cervical vertebra containing the vertebral artery: ______________________________

c. Vertebrae that articulate with ribs: ______________________________

d. First cervical vertebra: ______________________________

e. Second cervical vertebra: ______________________________

f. Articulates with the ilium to form the sacroiliac joints ______________________________

g. Acts as the body of the atlas: ______________________________

h. Region that articulates with the intervertebral discs: ______________________________

i. Separates the bodies of adjacent vertebrae: ______________________________

j. The outer part of the intervertebral disc: ______________________________

k. The central core of the intervertebral disc: ______________________________

l. Bony knob of vertebra felt through skin overlying spine: ______________________________

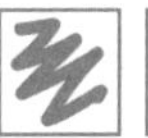 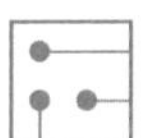 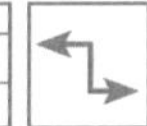

COLOURING, LABELLING AND MATCHING

29. Colour and label the following parts of a typical synovial joint on Figure 16.10:

- ○ Bone
- ○ Joint capsule
- ○ Synovial membrane
- ○ Articular cartilage
- ○ Synovial cavity

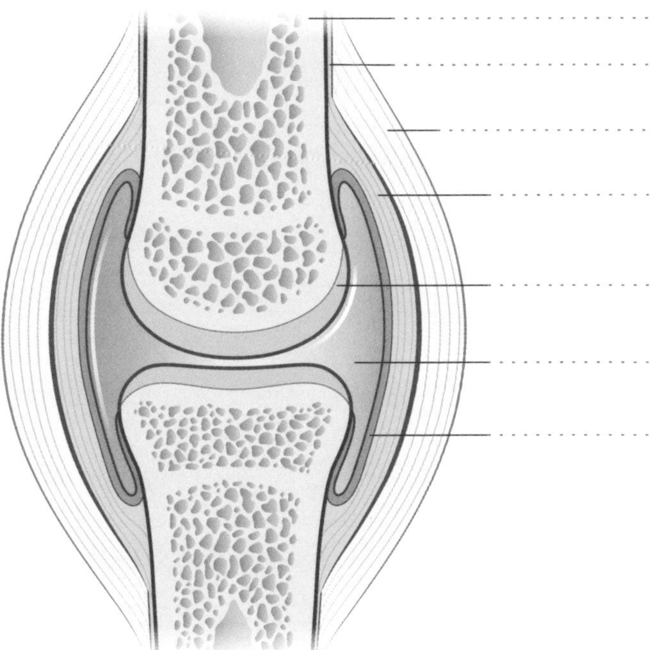

Figure 16.10 The basic structure of a synovial joint

30. Of which type of tissue is synovial membrane made? ______________________________

31. What is the function of articular cartilage? ______________________________

32. Figure 16.11 shows the hip joint. Colour and match the structural features listed below.

- ○ Capsular ligaments forming the joint sleeve
- ○ Synovial membrane
- ○ Articular cartilage
- ○ Synovial cavity containing synovial fluid
- ○ Femur
- ○ Pelvic bone
- ○ Ligament of the head of femur

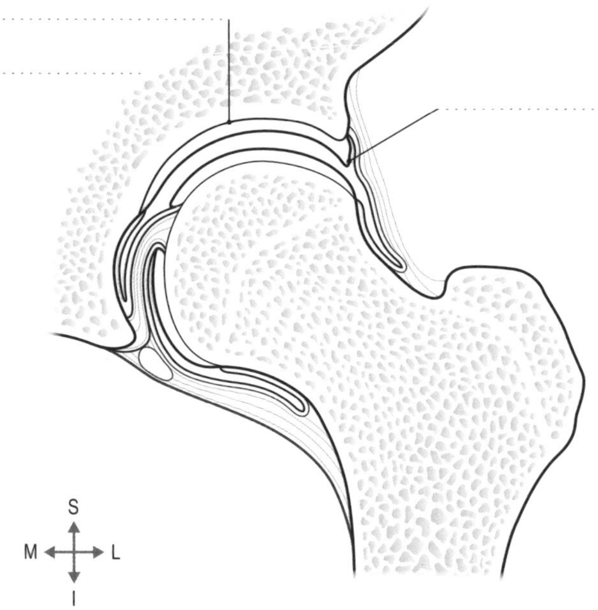

Figure 16.11 The hip joint, anterior view

33. On Figure 16.11, label the acetabulum of the pelvic bone and the acetabular labrum.

34. On Figure 16.11, name and label the area of the joint that most commonly fractures in a hip fracture.

35. What type of synovial joint is the hip joint? ______________________________

36. Colour and match the following structures of the knee joint on Figure 16.12, and label the remaining structures indicated:

○ Articular cartilage	○ Synovial membrane
○ Cruciate ligaments	○ Semilunar cartilages
○ Femur	○ Tibia
○ Fibula	○ Prepatellar bursa
○ Patella	

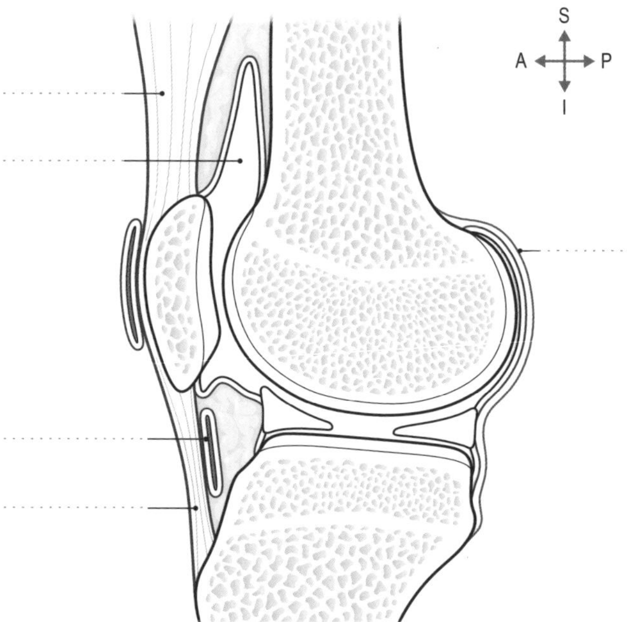

Figure 16.12 The knee joint, viewed from the side

37. Match the key choices to define the movements listed below.

Key choices:	Flexion
Abduction	Inversion
Adduction	Pronation
Circumduction	Rotation
Eversion	Supination
Extension	

a. Bending, usually forwards: ____________________

b. Straightening or bending backwards: ____________________

c. Movement away from the midline of the body: ____________________

d. Movement towards the midline of the body: ____________________

e. Movement of a limb or digit so that it forms a cone in space: ____________

f. Movement round the long axis of a bone: ____________________

g. Turning the palm of the hand down: ____________________

h. Turning the palm of the hand up: ____________________

i. Turning the sole of the foot inwards: ____________________

j. Turning the sole of the foot outwards: ____________________

COMPLETION

38. Complete Table 16.3 by identifying each named joint as synovial, fibrous or cartilaginous, and deciding if it is an immovable, slightly movable or freely movable joint.

Table 16.3 Joints and movements

Joint	Type of joint: Synovial, fibrous or cartilaginous?	Movement at joint: immovable, slightly movable or freely movable?
Suture		
Tooth in jaw		
Shoulder joint		
Symphysis pubis		
Knee joint		
Interosseous membrane		
Hip joint		
Joint between phalanges		
Intervertebral discs		

? POT LUCK

39. List three functions of synovial fluid:

- ____
____
- ____
____
- ____
____

40. State the function of the following extracapsular structures:

a. Ligaments: ____
____

b. Muscles or their tendons: ____
____

41. What is the function of bursae in a joint? ____
____

MCQs

42. The term given to a mass of clotted blood that forms around broken ends of bone is: ______
    a. Haematoma
    b. Haematuria
    c. Haemophilus
    d. Haemostasis

43. The callus that forms around a healing bone is: ______
    a. Granulation tissue
    b. New bone
    c. A dense collection of phagocytes
    d. Produced by osteoclasts

44. The role of macrophages in bone healing is to: ______
    a. Reduce the inflammatory response
    b. Recanalise the repaired bone
    c. Regulate osteoblast activity
    d. Remove dead wound debris

45. New bone that repairs a fracture is synthesised by: ______
    a. Osteoblasts
    b. Osteoclasts
    c. Osteons
    d. Osteocytes

46. In compact bone tissue, osteocytes live in tiny pockets called: ______
    a. Lamellae
    b. Bursae
    c. Lacunae
    d. Canaliculi

47. What is an osteon? ______
    a. A mature bone cell
    b. A cylindrical unit of bone tissue
    c. A channel in bone allowing bone cells to communicate with each other
    d. A plate or pillar of bone found in spongy bone

48. How many thoracic vertebrae are present in the normal spine? ______
    a. 5
    b. 7
    c. 9
    d. 12

49. The nerves running along the grooves on the underside of each rib are called the: ______
    a. Phrenic nerves
    b. Intercostal nerves
    c. Thoracic nerves
    d. Transverse nerves

50. The trochlea of the humerus fits into which structure on the ulna to form the elbow joint? ______
    a. The coronoid process
    b. The styloid process
    c. The ulnar tuberosity
    d. The olecranon process

51. What is the function of the glenoid cavity? ______
    a. With the head of the humerus, it forms the shoulder joint
    b. With the head of the femur, it forms the hip joint
    c. With the occipital bone of the skull, it forms the upper joint of the vertebral column
    d. With the head of the tibia, it forms part of the knee joint

52. Which bones form the hip bone (choose all that apply)? ______
    a. Ilium
    b. Pubis
    c. Ischium
    d. Sacrum

53. The interosseous membrane of the leg: ______
    a. Is a fibrous protective layer around both tibia and fibula
    b. Forms the distal tibiofibular joint
    c. Binds the femur to the tibia and stabilises the knee joint
    d. Holds the shafts of the tibia and fibula close together

MUSCLE

54. Name the three types of muscle tissue.

- ______________________________
- ______________________________
- ______________________________

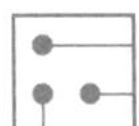 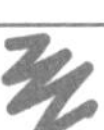

LABELLING AND COLOURING

55. Figure 16.13 shows the levels of structure within skeletal muscle, from the gross structure of an individual muscle attached to a bone down to the contractile filaments within individual muscle cells. Colour and label the structures shown on Figure 16.13.

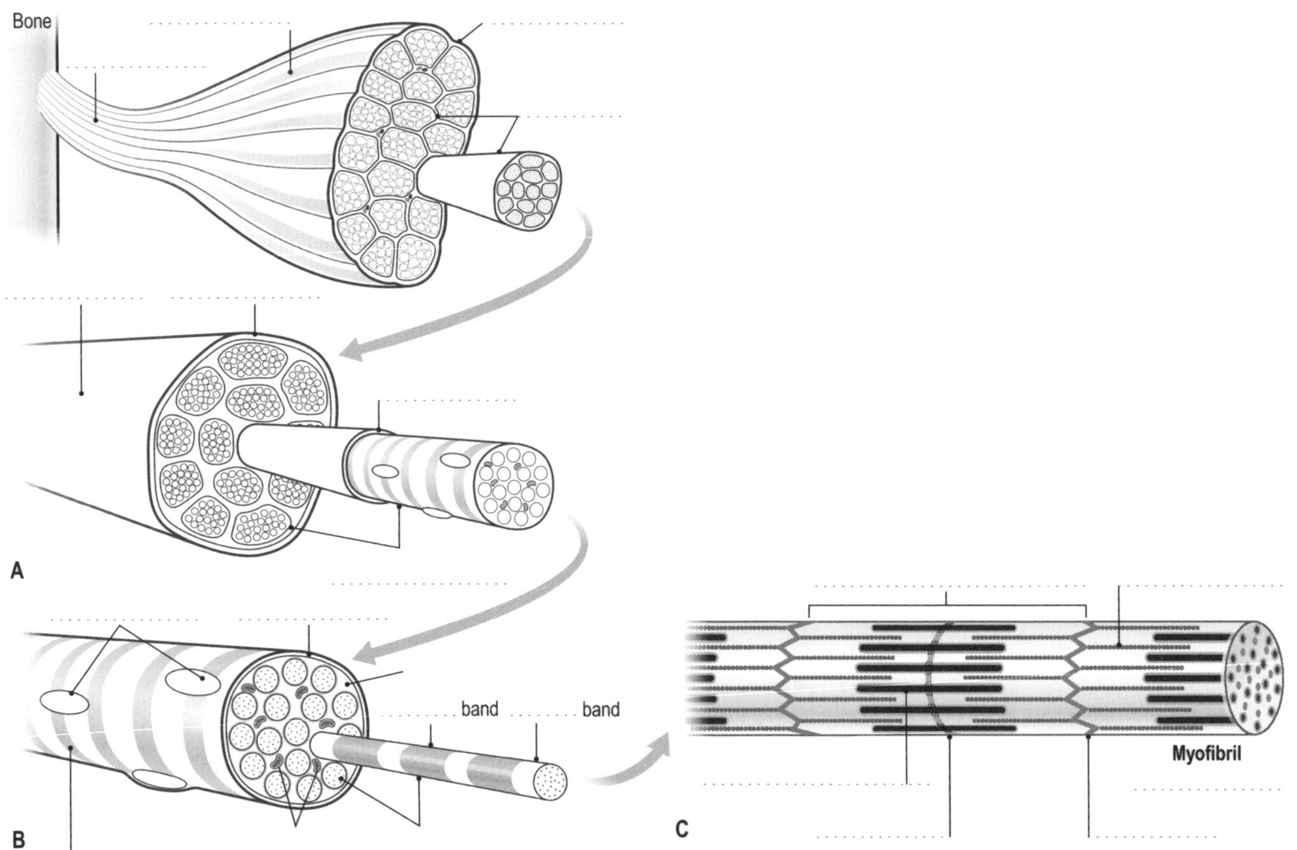

Figure 16.13 Levels of organisation within a skeletal muscle. (A) A skeletal muscle and its connective tissue. (B) A muscle fibre (cell). (C) A myofibril.

56. Colour and label the muscles of the back shown on Figure 16.14.

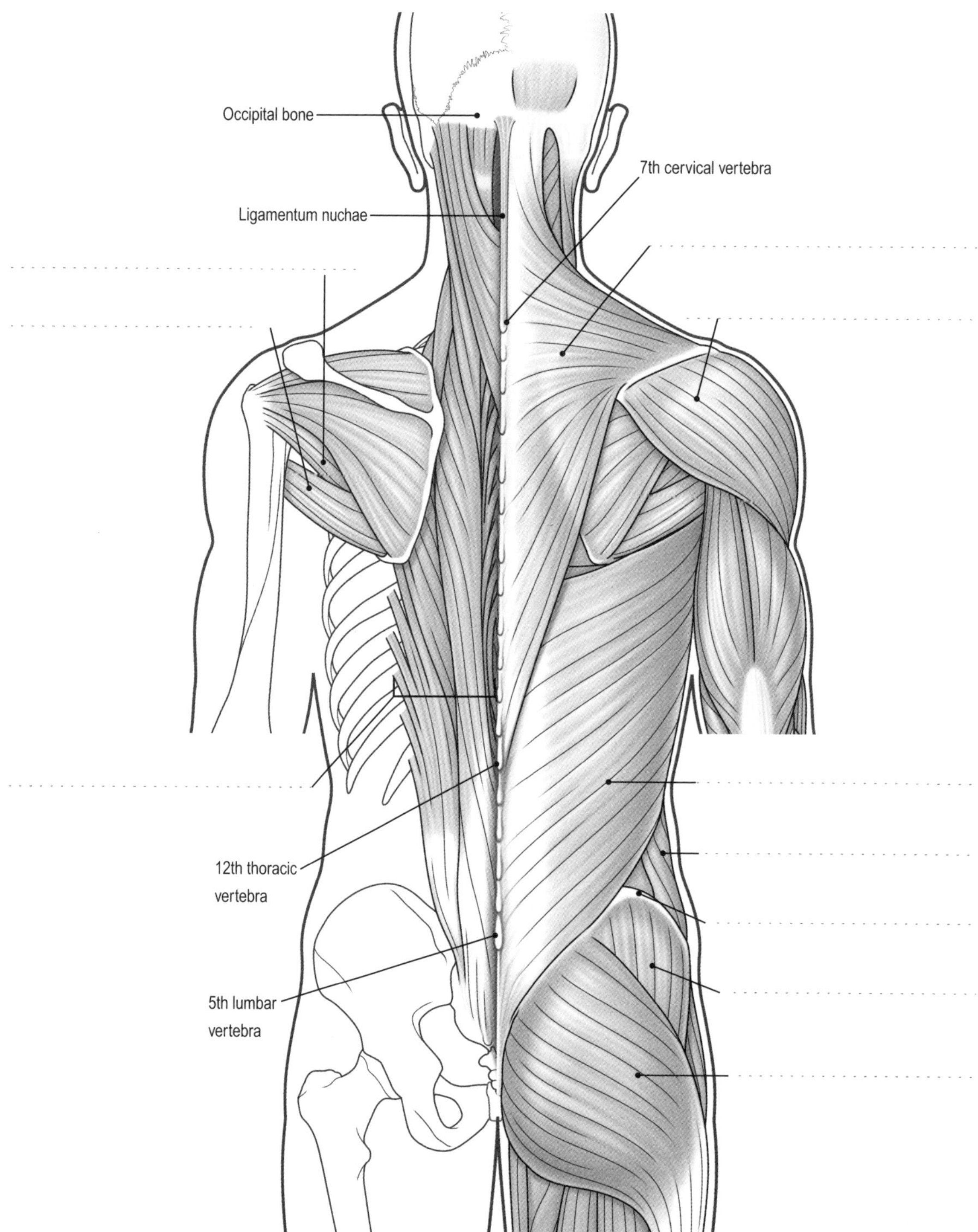

Figure 16.14 The main muscles of the back, posterior view

57. Colour and label the muscles of the shoulder and upper limb shown on Figure 16.15.

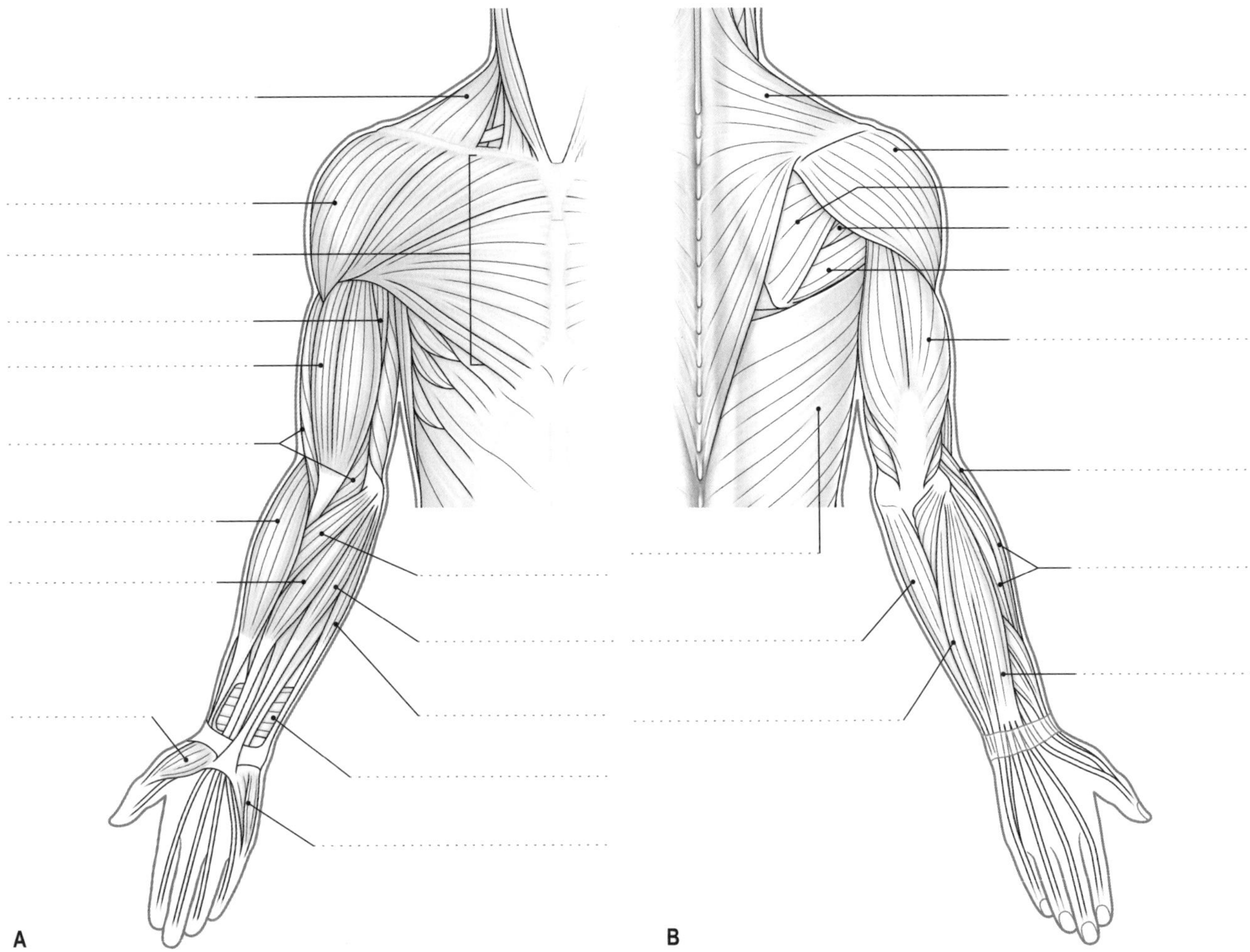

Figure 16.15 The main muscles of the right shoulder and upper limb. (A) Anterior view. (B) Posterior view

58. Colour and label the muscles of the lower limb shown on Figure 16.16.

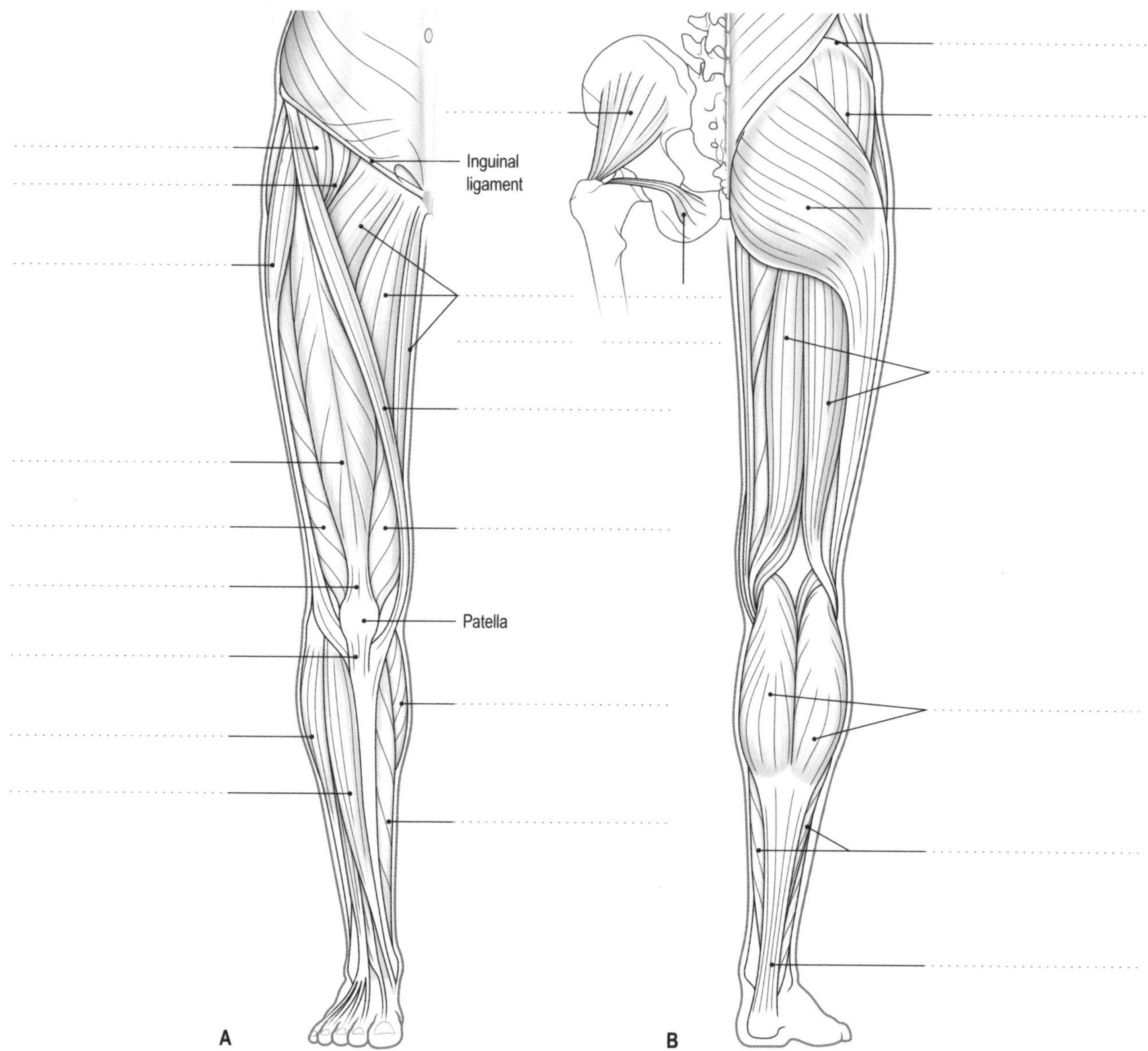

Figure 16.16 The main muscles of the right lower limb. (A) Anterior view. (B) Posterior view

59. Colour and label the muscles of the female pelvic floor shown on Figure 16.17.

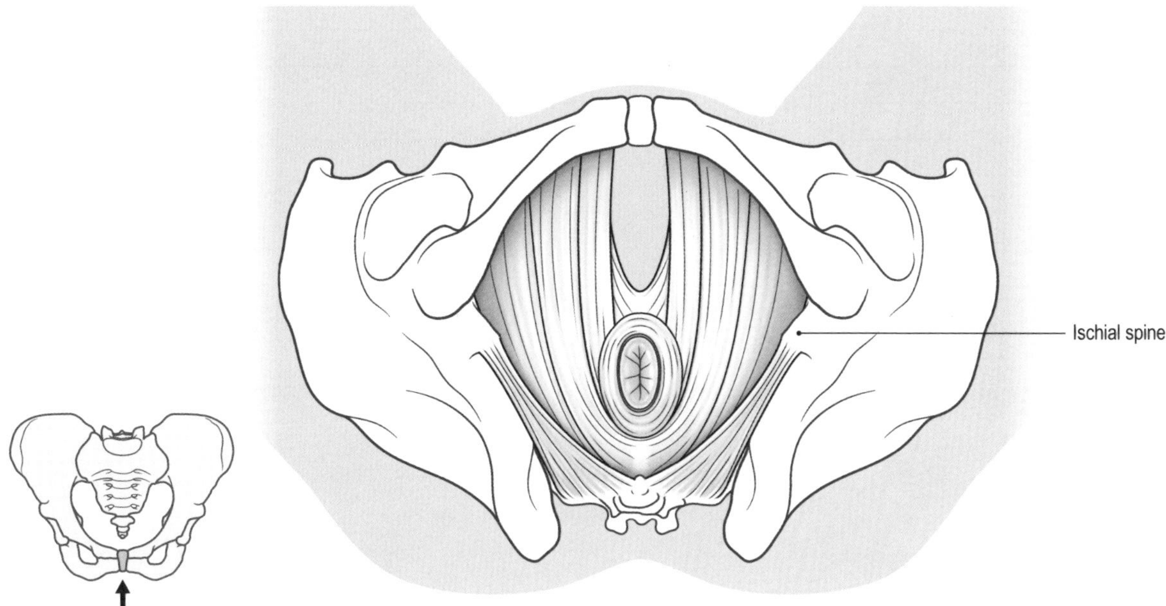

Figure 16.17 The muscles of the female pelvic floor

COMPLETION

60. The following paragraph describes the sliding filament theory. Complete it by filling in the blanks.

The functional unit of a skeletal muscle cell is the __________. At each end of this unit are lines called ___-lines. Within the unit are two types of filament, thick filaments (made of ________), and thin ones, made of ________. When the muscle cell is relaxed, these two filaments are not connected to each other. Contraction is initiated when an electrical impulse, called an ____ ______________________________, passes along the cell membrane (also called the ______________________________ ______) of the muscle cell and penetrates deep into the sarcoplasm via the network of ______________________________ that run through the cell. This electrical stimulation causes ____________________ ions to be released from the ______ ______________________________________ within the cell; these ions cause links, called ____________________ ____________, to form between the thick and thin filaments. The filaments pull on each other, which causes the functional unit to __________________ in length, pulling the ___________ at either end towards one another. If enough units are stimulated to contract at the same time, the entire _____________ will also ______________________________.

Table 16.4 Functions of muscles of the face and neck

Muscle	Paired/unpaired	Function
Occipitofrontalis		
Levator palpebrae superioris		
Orbicularis oculi		
Buccinator		
Orbicularis oris		
Masseter		
Temporalis		
Pterygoid		
Sternocleidomastoid		Contraction of one side:
		Contraction of both sides:
Trapezius		

61. Complete Table 16.4 to outline the functions of the muscles of the face and neck.

DEFINITIONS

Define the following terms, which all relate to muscle physiology:

62. Isotonic contraction ____________________

63. Isometric contraction ____________________

64. The origin of a muscle ____________________

65. Antagonistic pair ____________________

MCQs

66. Which of the following muscles flexes the knee (choose all that apply)? ______
    a. Quadriceps femoris
    b. Sartorius
    c. Gastrocnemius
    d. Hamstrings

67. When the rectus abdominis contracts, which movement occurs? ______
    a. The trunk twists to the side
    b. The shoulders move towards the knees
    c. The back flexes
    d. The scapulae are pulled backwards

68. The triceps has three heads (origins). Which of the following is true? ______
    a. All three heads originate on the scapula.
    b. Two heads originate on the humerus and one on the clavicle.
    c. One head originates on the humerus, one on the clavicle and one on the scapula.
    d. Two heads originate on the humerus and one originates on the scapula.

69. Which of the following is NOT a muscle of the pelvic floor? ______
    a. External anal sphincter
    b. Levator ani
    c. Psoas
    d. Coccygeus

70. Which muscle contributes to shoulder rotation, flexion, extension, abduction and adduction? ______
    a. Deltoid
    b. Trapezius
    c. Latissimus dorsi
    d. Pectoralis major

71. The calcaneal tendon attaches which muscle to which bone? ______
    a. Soleus to tibia
    b. Hamstrings to tibia
    c. Rectus femoris to hip
    d. Gastrocnemius to heel bone

72. The flexor retinaculum: ______
    a. Is also known as the 'funny bone' of the elbow
    b. Is one of the longitudinal bands of connective tissue stabilising the vertebral column
    c. Encloses a number of tendons and their sheaths in the wrist
    d. Is one of the cruciate ligaments stabilising the knee joint

17 Introduction to genetics

Genetics is the study of genes, which direct the function of body cells, and transmit hereditary information from one generation to the next (heredity).

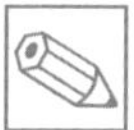

COMPLETION

1. The paragraph below describes the structure and function of DNA. Complete the paragraph by filling in the blanks.

The nucleus contains the body's ________________ material, in the form of DNA, which is built from nucleotides, each made up of three components: a _________ group, the sugar _____________ and one of four _____________. DNA is a double strand of nucleotides that resembles a ________________, or twisted ladder. DNA and associated proteins called ________________ are coiled together, forming a substance called__________________. In preparation for cell division, the DNA becomes very tightly coiled and can be seen as ________________ under the microscope. There are _____ pairs of them in most human cells. Each consists of many functional subunits called ________________. Any given type of cell uses only part of the whole genetic code, also called the _____________, to carry out its specific activities. Each ____________ contains the genetic code, or instructions, for the synthesis of one __________________, that could, for example, be an ____________ needed to catalyse a particular chemical _______________, a hormone, or it may form part of the structure of a cell. The coded instructions have to be transferred to the ___________ of the cell, because that is where the organelles that make protein, the _____________________, are found. DNA itself does not transfer, but a copy of the genetic code is made in the form of _______________, which leaves the ____________. When its instructions have been read and the new protein synthesised, the copy is destroyed.

2. The following paragraph relates to autosomal inheritance. Complete it by crossing out the incorrect options in bold.

All nucleated body cells, with the exception of spermatozoa and ova, contain **23/46/92** chromosomes, arranged in pairs. One chromosome of each pair is inherited from the mother and one from the father, so there are **two/four** copies of each gene in the cell. Two chromosomes of the same pair are called **homologues/homozygotes/autosomes**, and the genes are present in paired sites called **chromatids/traits/alleles**.

When the paired genes are identical, they are called **homozygous/heterozygous**, but if they are different forms they are called **homozygous/heterozygous**. Dominant genes are always **present on the maternal chromosome/expressed over recessive genes/found in pairs**. Individuals homozygous for a dominant gene **can/cannot** pass the recessive form on to their children, and individuals heterozygous for a gene **can/cannot** pass on either form of the gene to theirs.

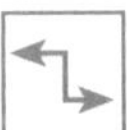 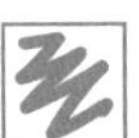 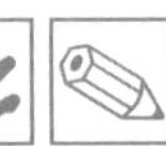

MATCHING, COLOURING AND COMPLETION

3. Figure 17.1 shows a section of DNA. Using the key, colour and match the sugar and phosphate constituents of the back bone.
4. Complete the base sequence on strand 1 in Figure 17.1 by drawing in and colouring the bases to complement strand 2.
5. Using the base sequence for the DNA in Strand 1 in Table 17.1, work out the corresponding sequence:
   a. in strand 2 of the DNA molecule, and
   b. of a piece of mRNA made from this DNA

Use this information to complete Table 17.1.

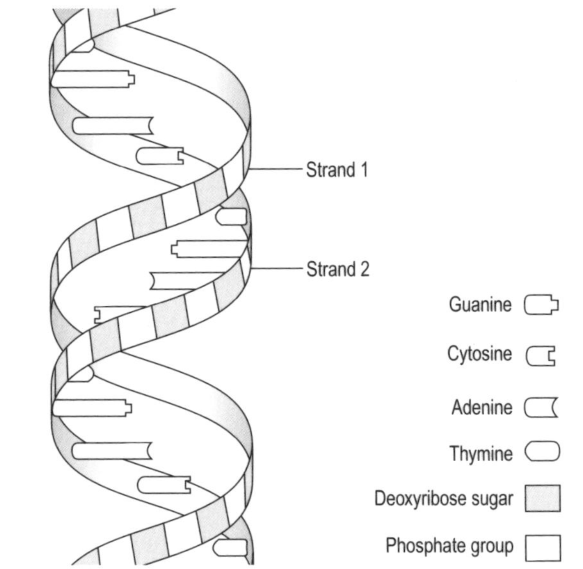

Figure 17.1 Deoxyribonucleic acid (DNA)

Table 17.1 The DNA code

DNA Strand 1	C	C	G	T	A	A	C	T	C	A	A	T	G	T
DNA Strand 2														
mRNA														

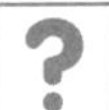

POT LUCK

6. Of the following eight statements, only four are correct. Identify the incorrect statements and write the corrected version in the spaces provided.
   a. Translation takes place in the nucleus.
   b. The base code in DNA is read in triplets.
   c. A codon is a piece of DNA carrying information.
   d. Stop and start codons initiate and terminate protein synthesis.
   e. All new proteins made by a cell must be used within that cell.
   f. All body cells contain an identical copy of the genome.
   g. In each cell, genes whose function is not required are kept switched off.
   h. Proteins are built on ribosomes in the cytoplasm.

- ______________________________
- ______________________________
- ______________________________
- ______________________________

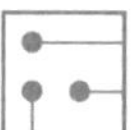

LABELLING

7. Figure 17.2 shows the mechanism of protein synthesis from reading the DNA code to assembly of the new protein. Label the structures indicated.

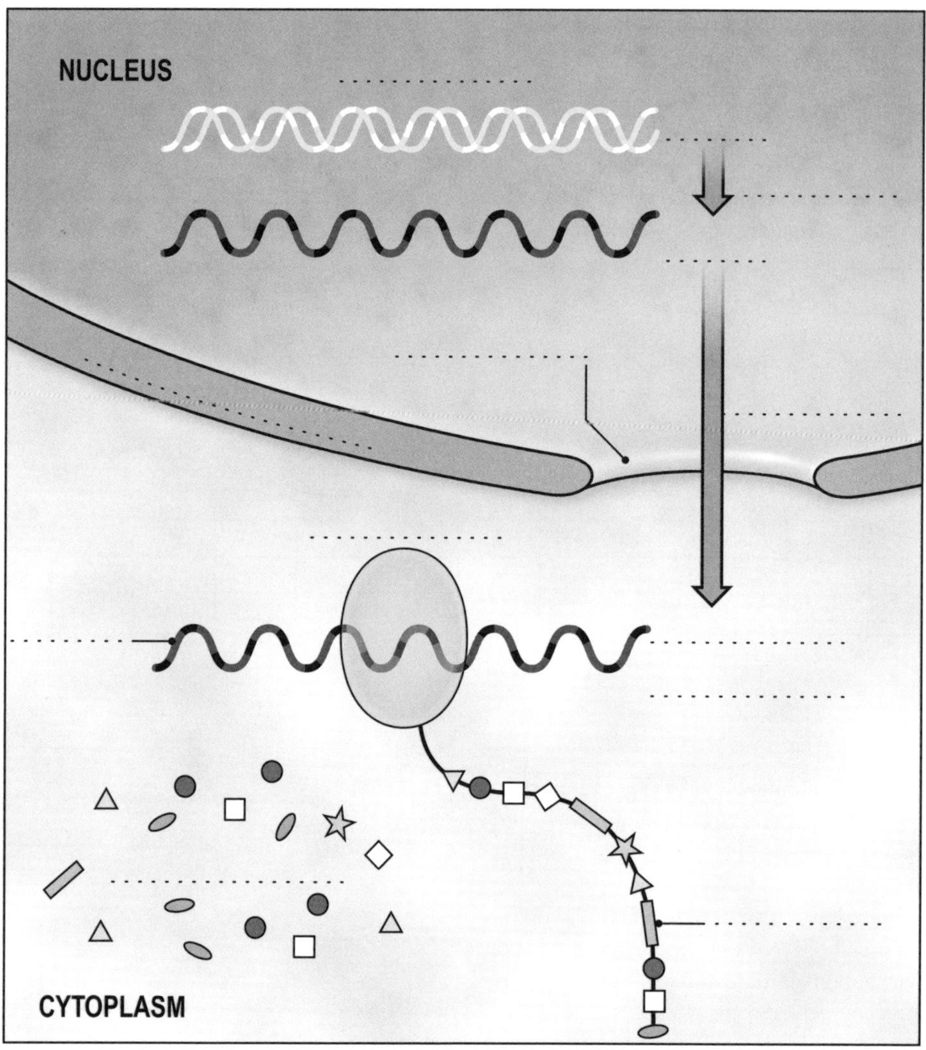

Figure 17.2 The relationship between DNA, RNA and protein synthesis

Box 17.1 Punnett square showing all possible genetic combinations in children of parents both heterozygous for the ability to roll their tongue. *T*, dominant gene;*t*, recessive gene.

	Father's genes	
Mother's genes		

Box 17.2 Punnett square showing all possible genetic combinations in children of a mother homozygous blue-eyed mother and heterozygous brown-eyed father. *B*, brown eyes;*b*, blue eyes.

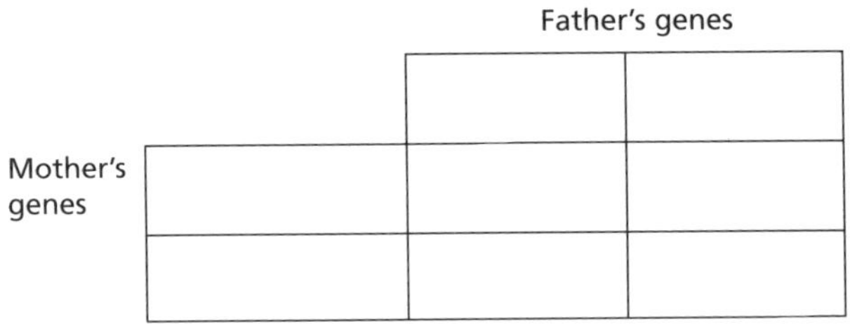

Box 17.3 Punnett square showing all possible genetic combinations in children of a colour-blind mother and a normally sighted father. *B*, normal gene;*b*, colour-blind gene.

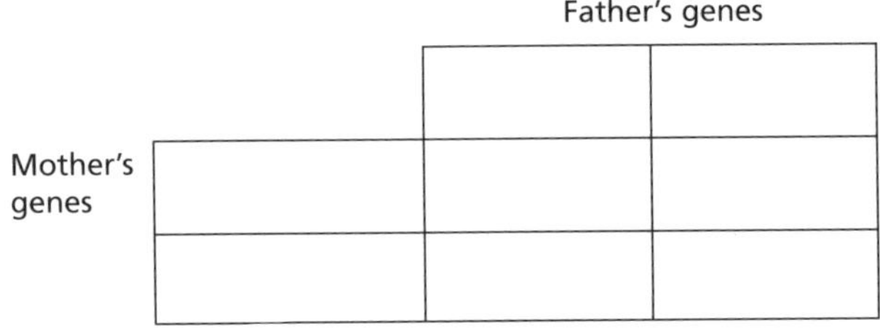

COMPLETION

8. Punnett squares are used to work out the possible combinations of a particular gene in the children of parents whose genetic makeup is known. Complete the Punnett square (Box 17.1) to illustrate the possible combinations of the gene that controls tongue rolling in the children of parents both heterozygous for the ability to roll their tongue. Use T = dominant gene, which codes for the ability to tongue roll and t = recessive gene, which codes for an inability to roll the tongue.

9. Which of the genotypes above will give a tongue-rolling child? ______________________

____

10. Which of the genotypes in Box 17.1 are homozygous?

____

11. Complete the Punnett square (Box 17.2) to illustrate the possible combinations of genes in the children of a mother homozygous for the recessive gene for blue eyes and a father homozygous for the dominant gene for brown eyes. Use B = brown eyes and b = blue eyes.

12. If the parents have four children, one each of the genotypes above, how many blue-eyed children will they have? ______________________

____

____

13. Red–green colour blindness is inherited on the X chromosome (sex linkage). Complete the Punnett square (Box 17.3), to show the possible combinations of genes in the children of a colour-blind mother and a normally sighted father. Don't forget to include the sex chromosomes (XX and XY); use B = normal gene and b = colour-blind gene as superscripts, such as X^B.

14. What is the male-to-female ratio in the children above?

____

15. What percentage of the sons will be colour blind?

____

16. What term is used to describe the genetic condition of the daughters? ______________________

MCQS

17. A diploid cell has: _______
    a. 23 chromosomes
    b. No nucleus
    c. 22 pairs of autosomes
    d. Two X chromosomes

18. Which of the following describes the structural hierarchy of the genetic material of the cell, starting with the largest? _______
    a. DNA, gene, nucleotide, chromosome
    b. Gene, chromosome, DNA, nucleotide
    c. Chromosome, gene, DNA, nucleotide
    d. Nucleotide, DNA, chromosome, gene

19. Of the X and Y chromosomes, which of the following statements is not true? _______
    a. These are the sex chromosomes
    b. In the cell karyotype, they are pair number 23
    c. Gametes carry one or the other
    d. They carry no genes of significance.

20. Genes: _______
    a. Normally exist in pairs, called alleles
    b. Are not found in red blood cells or skeletal muscle cells
    c. Carry information that codes for carbohydrate production
    d. Always exist in the same form at each locus

21. A telomere is: _______
    a. A collection of genes coding for related traits
    b. DNA at each end of the chromosome, 'sealing' it
    c. The region of the chromosome where chromatids are joined
    d. The name given to the sugar, base and nucleotide units from which DNA is built

22. Which of the following is true regarding genetic mutations? _______
    a. Mutations are common
    b. Most mutations are lethal to the cell
    c. Mutations are always permanent
    d. Mutations are commonly caused by bacterial infections

23. Other than the nucleus, DNA is found in the: _______
    a. Ribosomes, which produce the proteins coded by DNA
    b. Cytosol, which condenses into chromosomes for cell replication
    c. Endoplasmic reticulum, which produces enzymes for protein packaging
    d. Mitochondria, which is inherited from the mother

24. Lack of telomerase in older adults leads to: _______
    a. Uncontrolled cell multiplication
    b. Shorter and more fragile chromosomes
    c. An inability to express individual genes correctly
    d. Reduced capacity to repair DNA

25. In meiosis, which of the following is false? _______
    a. Two divisions occur
    b. Four daughter cells are produced
    c. Crossing over produces new combinations of genes
    d. The daughter cells are identical to one another

18 The reproductive systems

The male and female reproductive systems produce sex cells (spermatozoa and ova) which transmit the parent's genetic material to the next generation. At fertilisation, a spermatozoan and an ovum combine to form a zygote, which can then develop within the female reproductive tract into a new human being. This chapter will test your understanding of reproductive anatomy and physiology.

FEMALE REPRODUCTIVE ANATOMY AND PHYSIOLOGY

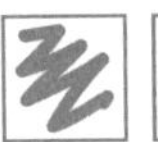 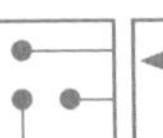 

COLOURING, LABELLING AND MATCHING

1. Figure 18.1 shows the female reproductive organs and some associated structures in the pelvis. Label the structures indicated and colour and match the following:

- ○ Bladder
- ○ Peritoneum
- ○ Pubic symphysis
- ○ Sigmoid colon
- ○ Rectum
- ○ Vertebrae

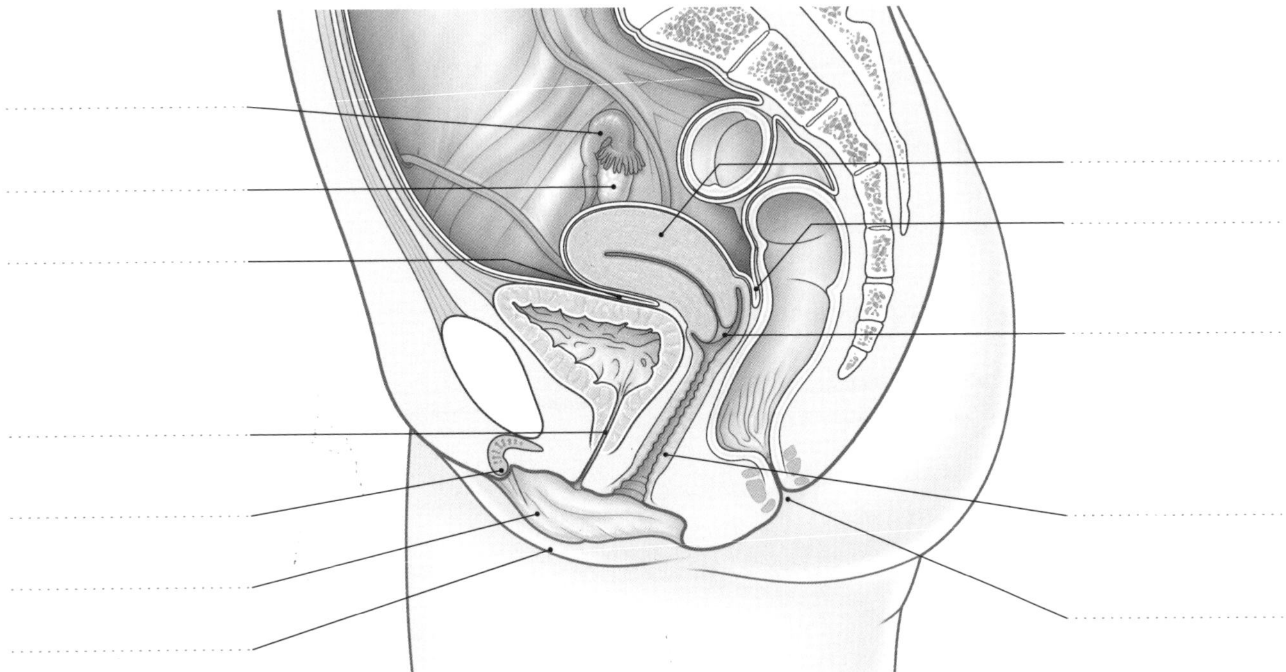

Figure 18.1 Lateral view of the female reproductive organs and associated structures

2. Figure 18.2 shows the internal female reproductive organs. Label the structures indicated and colour and match the following:

- ○ Ovary
- ○ Round ligament
- ○ Broad ligament
- ○ Ovarian ligament
- ○ Suspensory ligament of ovary
- ○ Uterosacral ligament

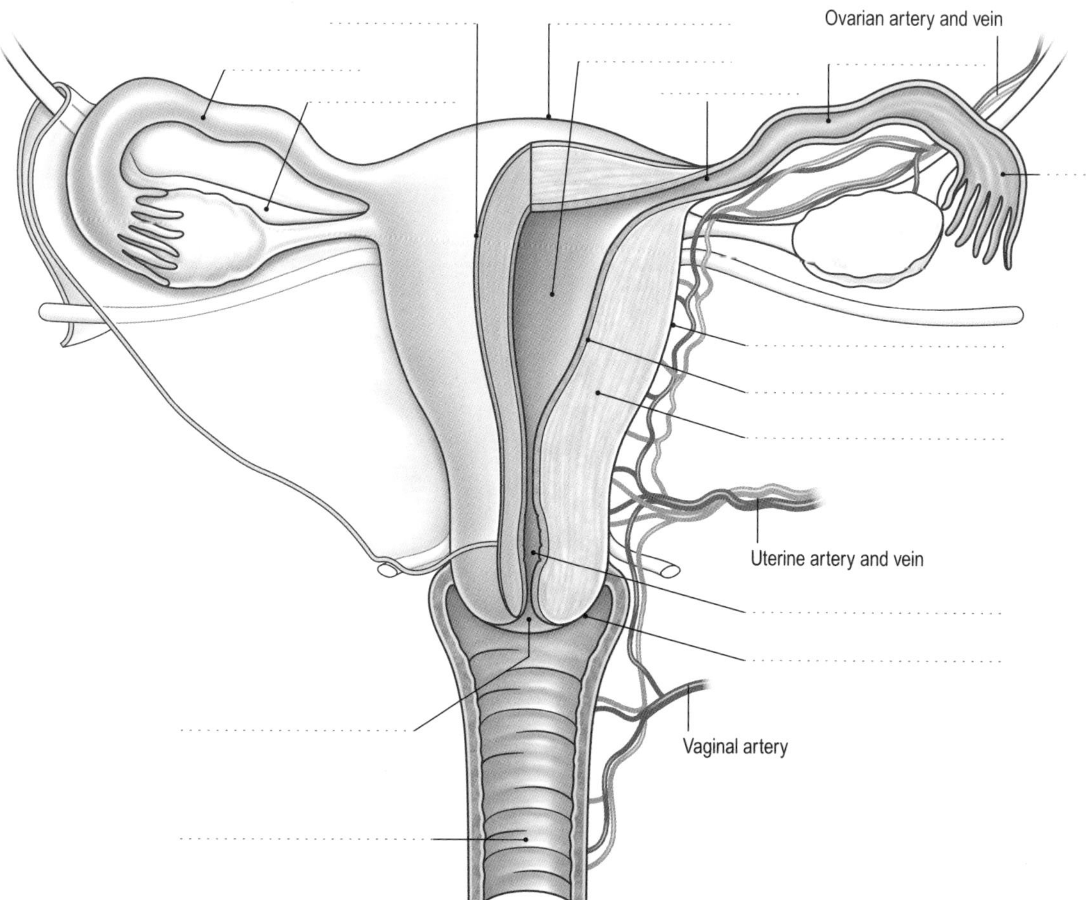

Figure 18.2 Frontal view of the female reproductive organs

3. Figure 18.3 shows the main stages of development of a single ovarian follicle. Colour, match and label the structures listed below at each stage of the process:

- ○ Primordial follicles
- ○ Developing follicles
- ○ Mature ovarian (Graafian) follicle
- ○ Developing ovum within a follicle
- ○ Developing corpus luteum
- ○ Fully formed corpus luteum
- ○ Fibrous corpus albicans

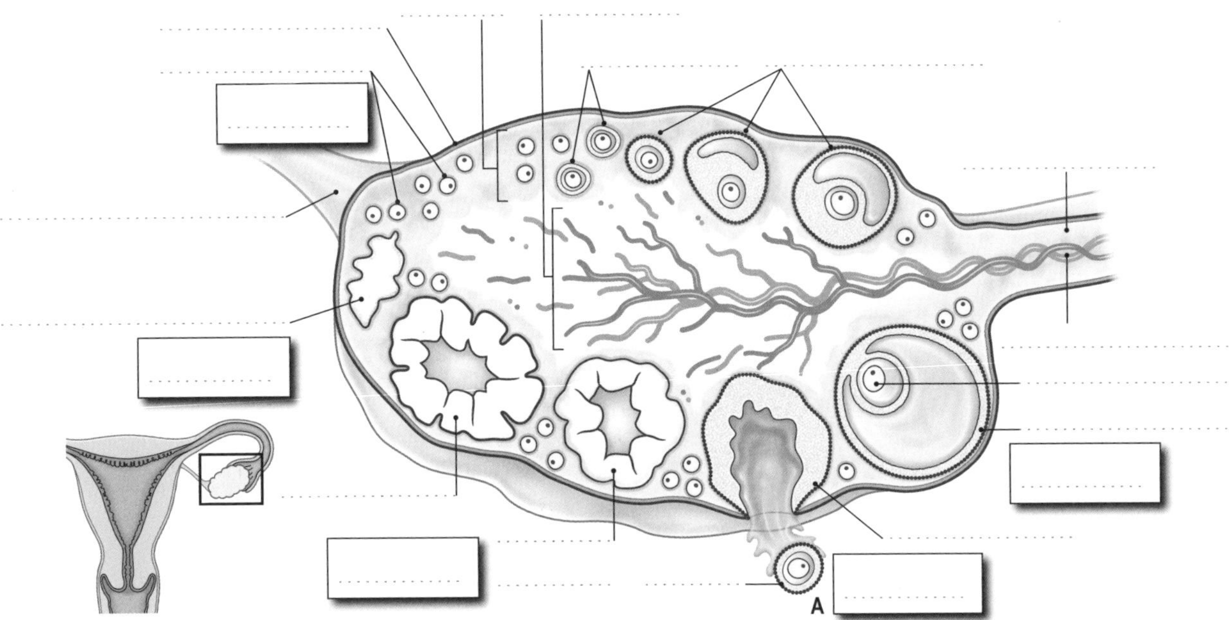

Figure 18.3 Stages of follicular development in the ovary

4. On Figure 18.3, indicate the times during an average ovarian cycle that each of these stages would be reached by completing the time scale in the open boxes around the ovary.

5. Name the process taking place at A.

____

6. A surge of which hormone triggers event A?

____

7. Complete Figure 18.3 by labelling the remaining structures indicated.

POT LUCK

8. List the main changes that take place in the female body during puberty:

- ____
- ____
- ____
- ____
- ____
- ____

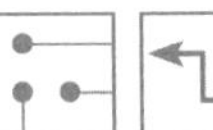

LABELLING AND MATCHING

Figure 18.4 represents various body changes during one menstrual cycle. Each part of the figure summarises a subcycle involving different tissues and organs. Complete the figure as instructed below.

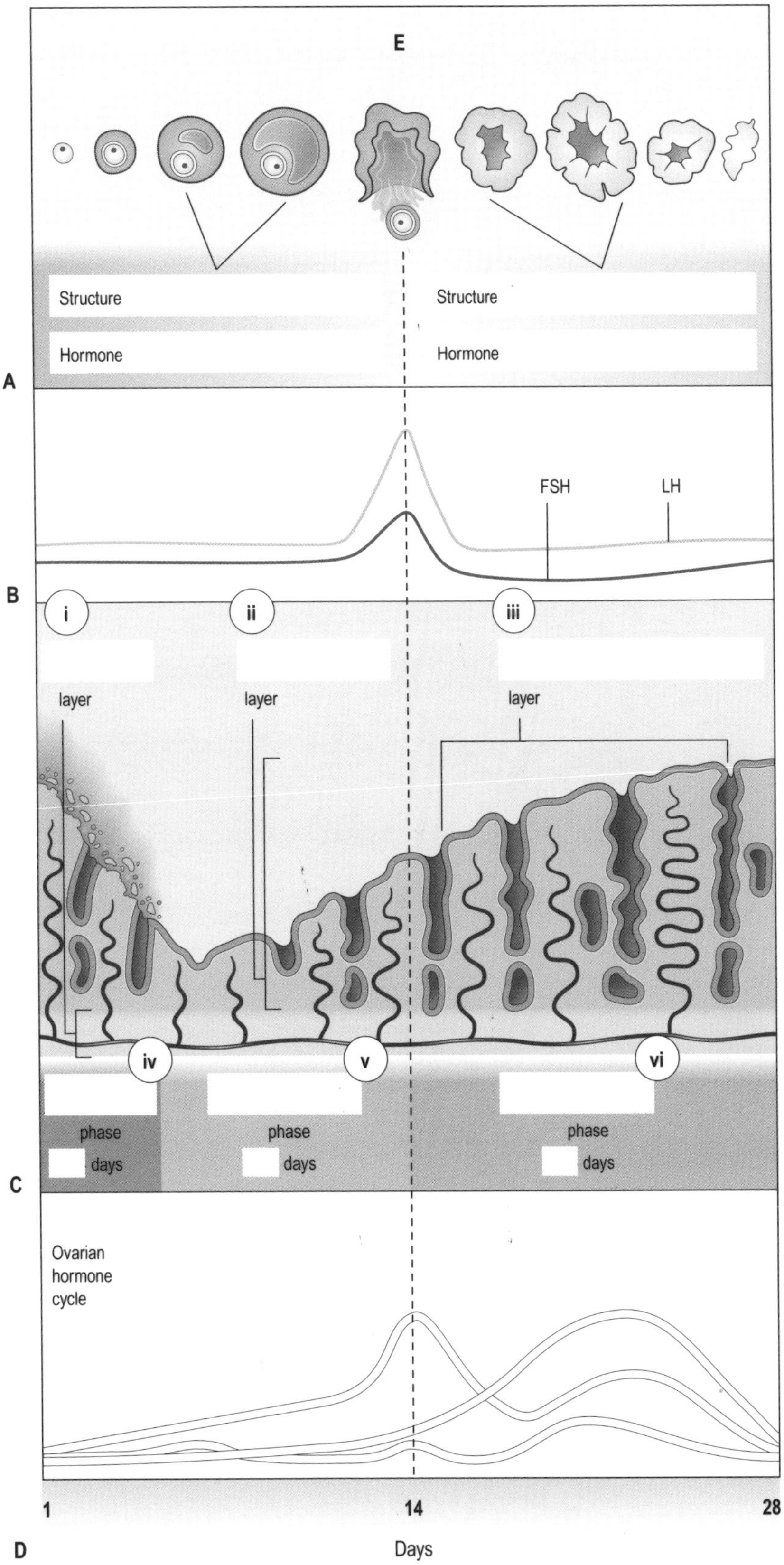

Figure 18.4 Summary of one female menstrual cycle

9. Figure 18.4A summarises the ovarian cycle. Identify event E.

____

10. Identify the two main hormones and the structures in the ovary that synthesise them before and after event E by labelling the boxes in Figure 18.4A.

11. Fig. 18.4B shows the release of follicle-stimulating hormone (FSH) and luteinising hormone (LH). Which endocrine gland secretes them?

____

12. Which of these two hormones is responsible for event E?

____

13. Fig. 18.4C shows the uterine cycle. Label the diagram to show the layers of the endometrium (i, ii and iii), the phases of the uterine cycle and the length of time spent in each phase (iv, v and vi).

14. Fig. 18.4D shows the ovarian hormone cycle. Identify the three hormones that are represented by the curves in the diagram by colouring and matching each line using the key below:

○ ____

○ ____

○ ____

15. What is the function of the hormone shown in D whose levels remain significantly lower than the other two?

____

____

16. This menstrual cycle has not resulted in pregnancy. Why do the levels of the two most abundant hormones fall in the second half of the cycle?

____

____

17. Explain why, should pregnancy occur, the levels of these two hormones would not fall but would continue to rise, and remain high during pregnancy.

____

____

____

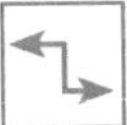

MATCHING

18. Match the key choices below, all related to the developmental stages of pregnancy, to the appropriate items in list A. (Take care – you will not need all the key choices.)

List A

Blastocyst ____________	Gestation ____________
Embryo ____________	Fetus ____________
Trophoblast ____________	Zygote ____________

Key choices:

a. The period between ovulation and birth
b. The developing baby between fertilisation and 8 weeks
c. Contributes significantly to placental development
d. The cell formed at fertilisation
e. The cell formed at ovulation
f. A hollow ball of cells
g. The developing baby between 8 weeks postfertilisation and birth
h. Usually formed in the uterine tube
i. Implants in the endometrium
j. The term describing the baby at term
k. Nourished by the placenta
l. Pregnancy
m. Contains between 70 and 100 cells
n. The term applied to a baby at its fourth week of development

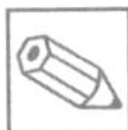

COMPLETION

19. The breast is a hormonally responsive organ and its reproductive function is controlled by a number of important hormones. Complete Table 18.1 to identify these hormones.

Table 18.1 The effect of hormones on the breast

Statement	Hormone(s)
Stimulates body growth and development in puberty	
Initiates release of milk	
Stimulates production of milk	
Stimulates growth and development in pregnancy	

MCQs

20. With regard to the female external genitalia, what is the vestibule? _______
    a. The distal third of the vagina and the vaginal opening
    b. The triangle of skin between the base of the labia minora to the anal opening
    c. The external structures enclosed by the labia majora
    d. The structures lying between the thighs, including the labia and the base of the mons pubis but excluding the anal opening

21. Which of the following is true concerning the uterine tubes? (Choose all that apply) _______
    a. They are covered by the round ligament
    b. They make direct contact with the ovaries at their lateral ends
    c. They are supplied with blood by the uterine arteries
    d. Fertilisation normally takes place here

22. Montgomery's tubercles are: ______
    a. Sebaceous glands
    b. Lactiferous ducts
    c. Glandular tissue
    d. Ligamentous bands

23. How many lobes are found, on average, in the breast? ______
    a. 2
    b. 10
    c. 20
    d. 25

24. Between menarche and menopause, the healthy female: _______
    a. Continues to produce new ova
    b. Is better protected than the male against cardiovascular disease by high levels of progesterone
    c. Is protected against osteopenia by high levels of oestrogen
    d. Is likely to be fertile approximately twice a month

25. Which of the following is associated with the female menopause? _______
    a. The ovary stops producing new ova
    b. High circulating levels of FSH and LH
    c. Inhibin levels steadily rise
    d. Enlargement of the breasts as milk ducts are replaced with fibrous tissue

26. At what stage of intrauterine life is a beating heart seen in the developing baby? _______
    a. 24 hours
    b. 1 week
    c. 2 weeks
    d. 4 weeks

27. Which of the following is true with regard to reproductive function in older women? _______
    a. The female menopause begins later than in the male.
    b. Vaginal secretions tend to increase, which in turn increases the risk of infection.
    c. Oestrogen levels in the post-menopausal female rise in an attempt to stimulate the failing ovaries.
    d. Blood cholesterol levels in the female tend to rise after menopause.

MALE REPRODUCTIVE ANATOMY AND PHYSIOLOGY

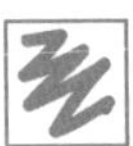 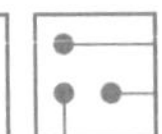

COLOURING, LABELLING AND MATCHING

28. Figure 18.5 shows the male reproductive organs and some associated tissues. Label the structures indicated and colour, match and label the following using the key below:

- ○ Peritoneum
- ○ Urinary bladder
- ○ Sigmoid colon
- ○ Rectum
- ○ Vertebrae

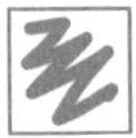 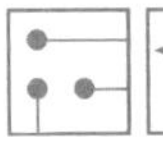

COLOURING, LABELLING AND MATCHING

29. Figure 18.6 is a section through the testis, showing its internal structure. Colour and match the different layers around the testis and the sections of tubule within using the key below, and label the remaining structures indicated.

- ○ Skin
- ○ Cremaster muscle
- ○ Tunica vaginalis
- ○ Tunica albuginea
- ○ Septum formed by connective tissue
- ○ Convoluted seminiferous tubules
- ○ Straight seminiferous tubules
- ○ Efferent ductules

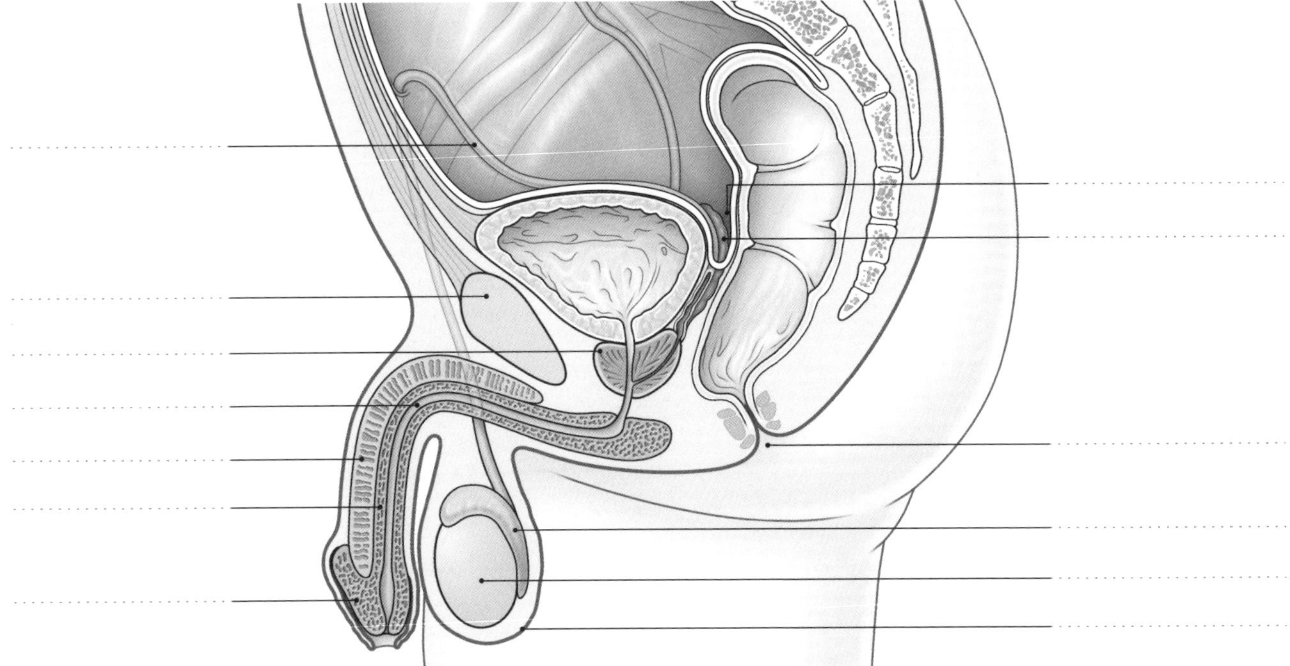

Figure 18.5 Lateral view of the male reproductive organs and associated structures

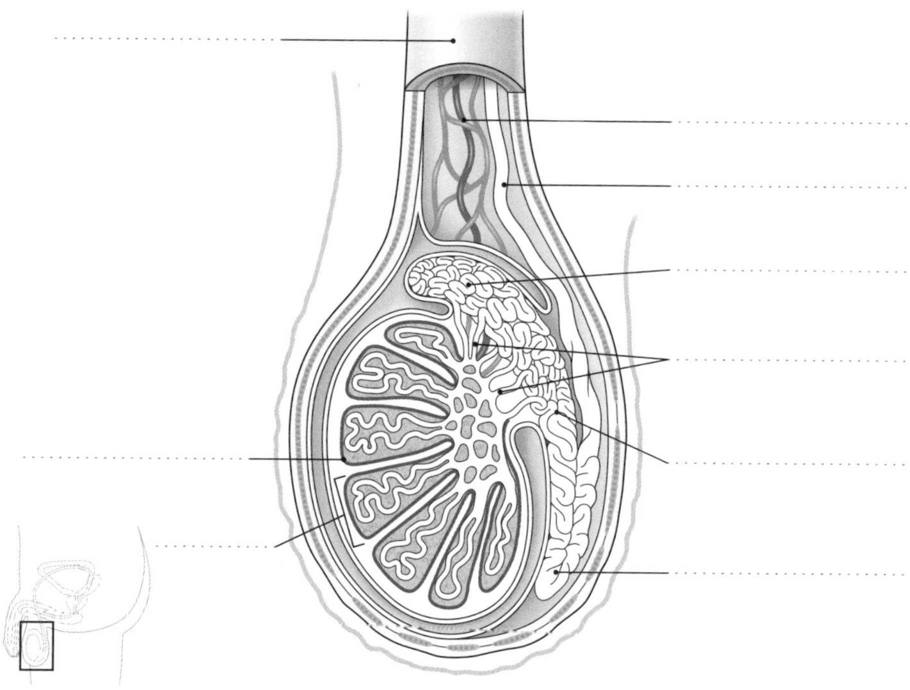

Figure 18.6 A section through the testis, showing its coverings and the origin of the deferent duct through the prostate gland and associated structures

MCQs

30. Which part of the spermatozoan contains its DNA? ___________
    a. Nucleus
    b. Head
    c. Body
    d. Tail

31. What is the normal composition of semen? ___________
    a. 30% sperm, 50% prostatic fluid, 20% seminal fluid
    b. 5% sperm, 80% prostatic fluid, 15% seminal fluid
    c. 50% sperm, 10% prostatic fluid, 40% seminal fluid
    d. 10% sperm, 30% prostatic fluid, 60% seminal fluid

32. What is the function of the epididymis? ___________
    a. Secretion of testosterone
    b. Spermatozoa production
    c. Maturation of spermatozoa
    d. Propulsion of semen through the reproductive tract

33. Which of the following is true of the prostate gland? ___________
    a. It secretes a clotting enzyme to thicken the semen in the vagina
    b. It generally reduces in size with age, contributing to reduced male fertility in older age
    c. It encloses the vas deferens, and can obstruct urine flow in older men
    d. It secretes fructose as an energy source for the spermatozoa

1 Anatomy and organisation of the body

Answers

1. See Figure 1.1

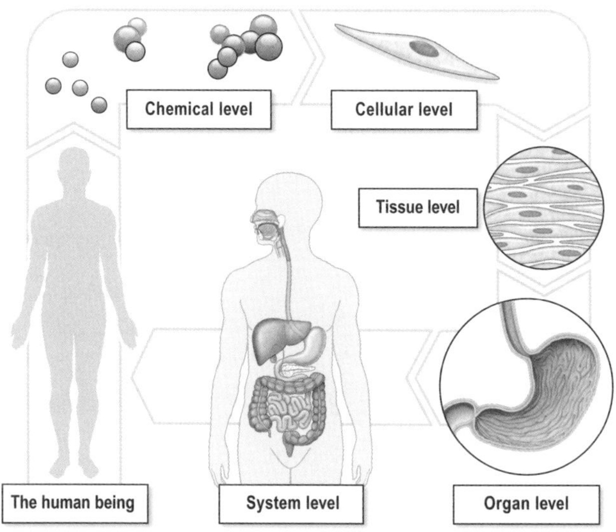

Figure 1.1

2.

Table 1.1 Levels of structural complexity and their characteristics

Level of structural complexity	Characteristics
The human being	Comprises many systems that work interdependently to maintain health
Organ level	Carries out a specific function and is composed of different types of tissue
Cellular level	Smallest independent units of living matter
System level	Consists of one or more organs and contributes to one or more survival needs of the body
Chemical level	Atoms and molecules that form the building blocks of larger substances
Tissue level	Group of cells with similar structures and functions

3. and 4. See Figure 1.2

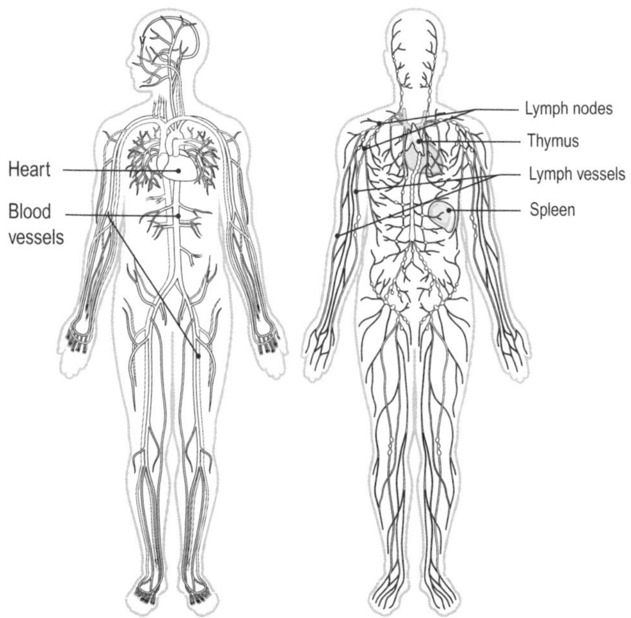

Figure 1.2

5. and 6. See Figure 1.3

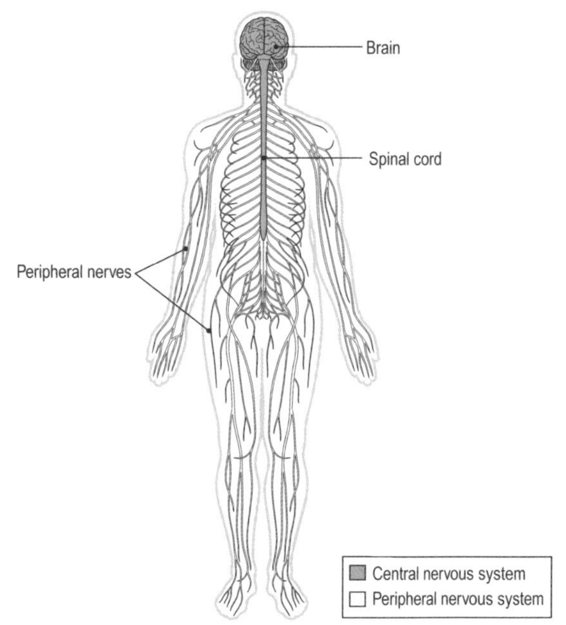

Figure 1.3

7. Reflex action.
8. See Figure 1.4

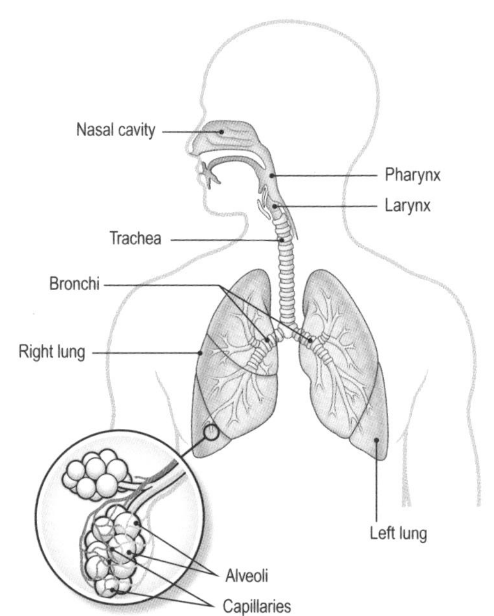

Figure 1.4

9. Oxygen and carbon dioxide.
10. and 11. See Figure 1.5.

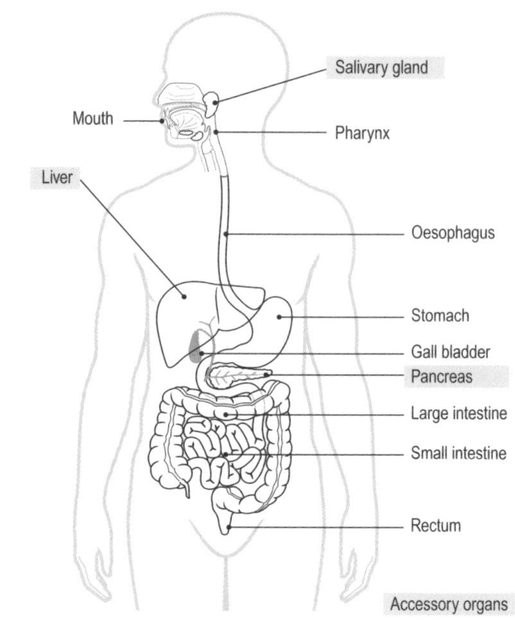

Figure 1.5

12. See Figure 1.6.

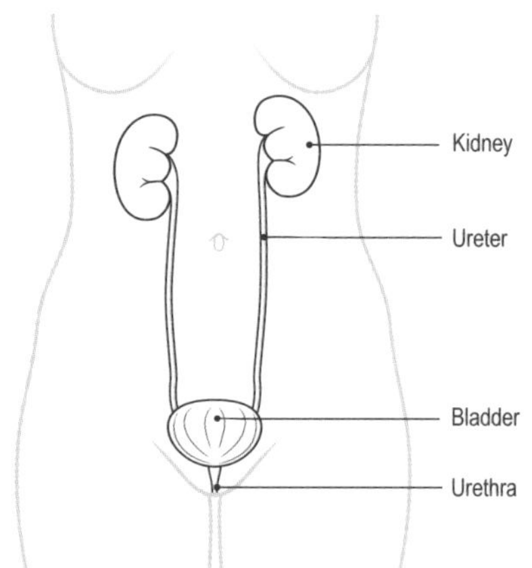

Figure 1.6

13. and 14. See Figure 1.7.

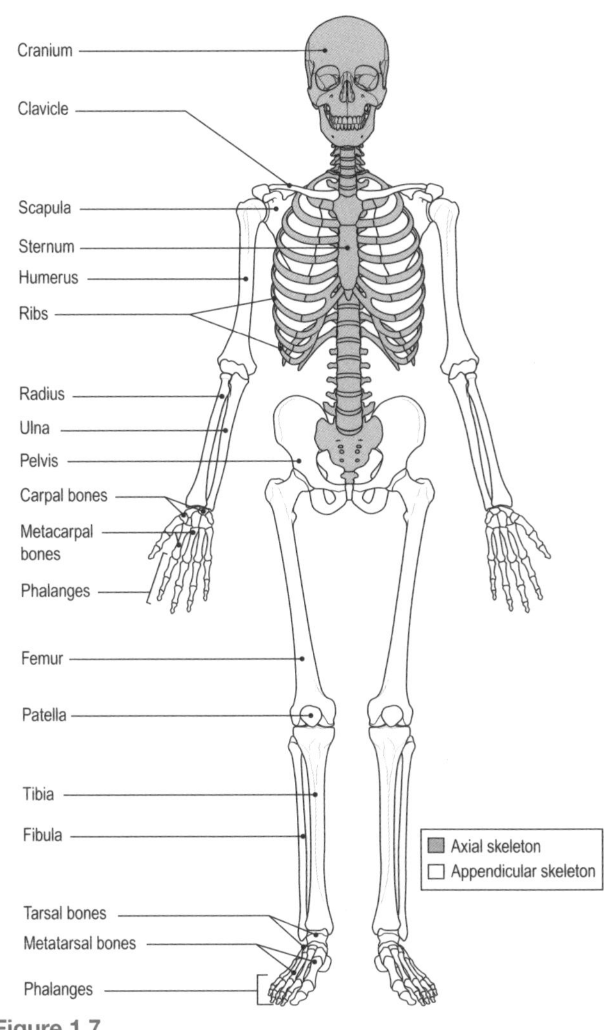

Figure 1.7

15. See Figure 1.8.

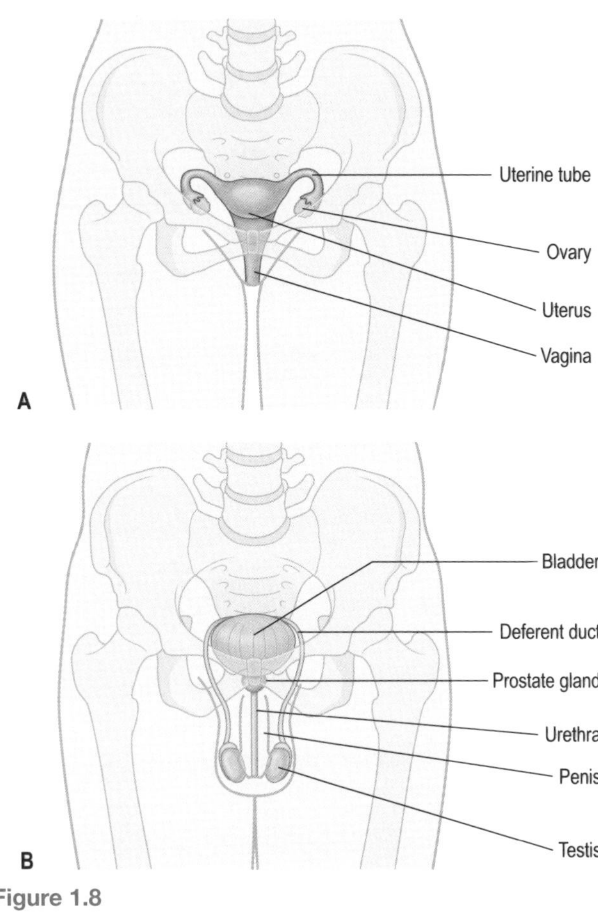

Figure 1.8

16. The childbearing years begin at **puberty** and end at the **menopause.** During this time, an **ovum** matures in the ovary about every **28** days. If **fertilisation** takes place, the zygote embeds itself in the **uterus** and grows to maturity during pregnancy or **gestation,** in about **40** weeks. If fertilisation does not occur, it is expelled from the body along with the **uterine lining,** accompanied by bleeding, called **menstruation.**

17. The endocrine system consists of a number of **glands** in various parts of the body. The glands synthesise and secrete chemical messengers called **hormones** into the **bloodstream.** These chemicals stimulate **target organs/ tissues.** Changes in hormone levels are usually controlled by **negative feedback** mechanisms. The endocrine system, in conjunction with part of the **nervous** system, controls **involuntary** body function. Changes involving the latter system are usually **fast,** whereas those of the endocrine system tend to be **slow** and precise.

18.

Table 1.2 The common and special senses

Common senses	Special senses
Pain	Sight
Touch	Hearing
Heat	Balance
Cold	Smell
	Taste

19. and 20. See Figure 1.9.

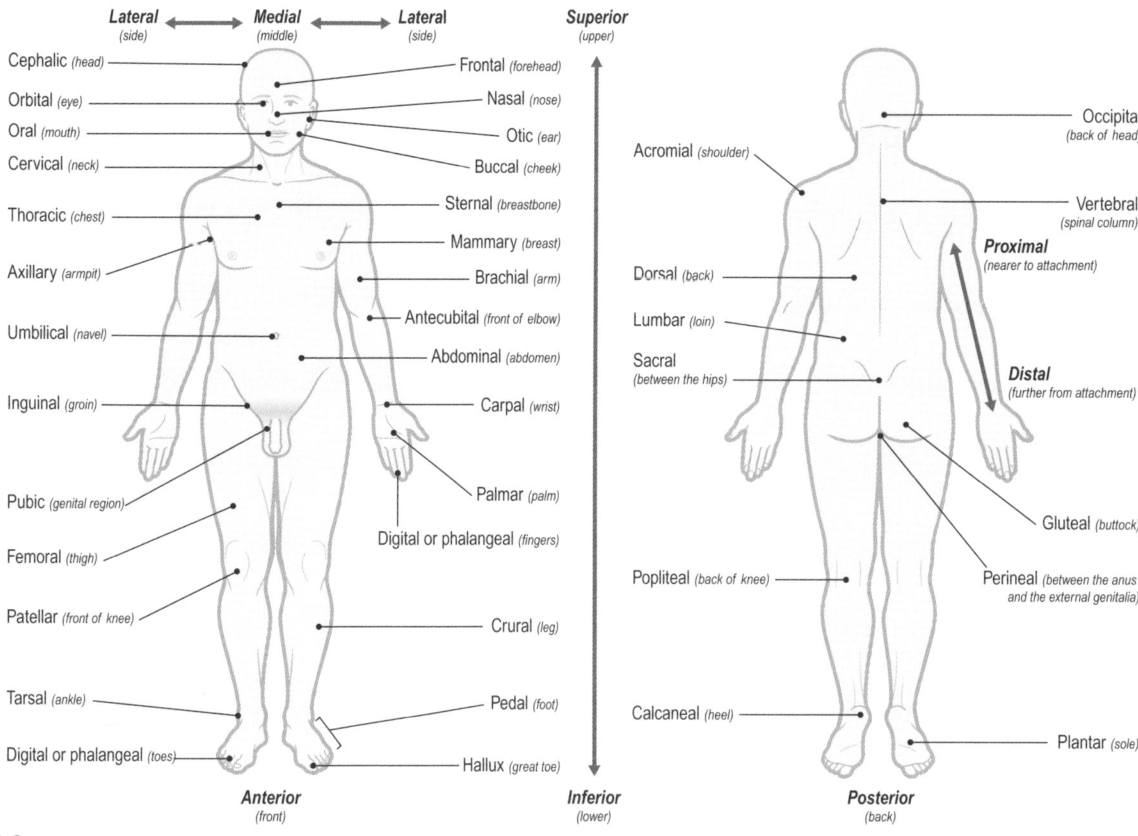

Figure 1.9

21. A. Median plane. B. Frontal (coronal) plane.
C. Transverse plane.

22. See Figure 1.11.

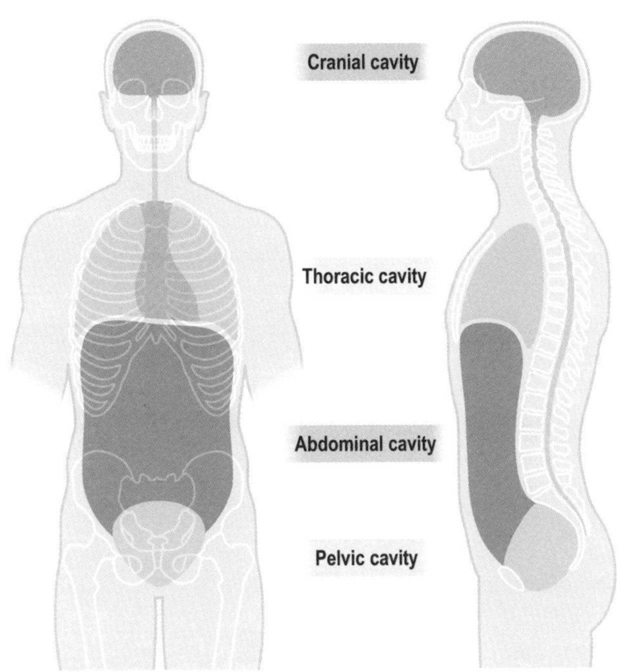

Figure 1.11

23.

Table 1.3 Contents of the body cavities

Cranial cavity	Thoracic cavity
Brain	Alveoli Bronchi Heart Oesophagus Lungs
Abdominal cavity	**Pelvic cavity**
Appendix Adrenal glands Duodenum Gall bladder Kidneys Liver Pancreas Small intestine Spleen Stomach Transverse colon	Ovaries Seminal vesicles Sigmoid colon Uterus Urinary bladder

24. Plasma.
25. Arteries.
26. 65–75.
27. Cranium and face.
28. Clavicle and scapula
29. Femur, tibia, fibula, patella, 7 tarsal bones, 5 metatarsal bones and 14 phalanges.
30. Filtering of microorganisms and other material from lymph.
31. Nonspecific defence mechanisms, such as the skin, mucus from mucous membranes and gastric juices, provide protection against a wide range of invaders, whereas specific defence mechanisms afford protection against one particular invader (an antigen), and the response is through the immune system.
32. **a.** The humerus is **lateral** to the heart. **b.** The vertebrae are **posterior** to the kidneys. **c.** The phalanges are **distal** to the ulna. **d.** The skull is **superior** to the vertebral column. **e.** The greater omentum is **anterior** to the small intestine. **f.** The appendix is **inferior** to the stomach. **g.** The patella is **proximal** to the tarsal bones. **h.** The scapulae are **lateral** to the sternum.
33. **a.** Building up or synthesis of large and complex chemical substances. **b.** Breaking down of large chemical substances into smaller ones.
34. c.
35. d.
36. a.
37. a. and d.
38. b.
39. c.

2 Physiological chemistry and processes

Answers

1–3.

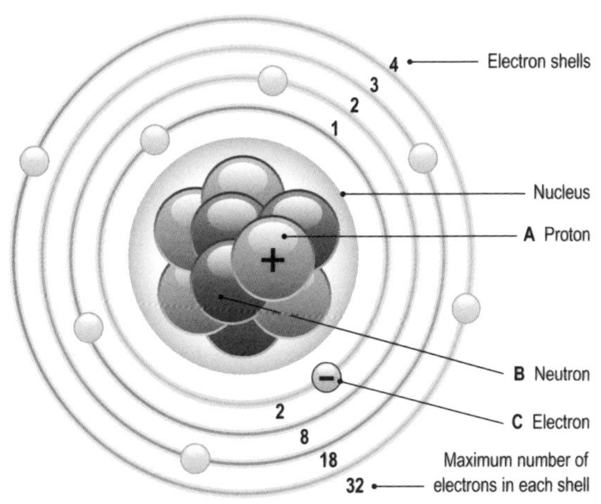

4.

Table 2.1 Characteristics of subatomic particles

Particle	Mass	Electric charge	Location in atom
Proton	1 unit	1 positive	Within the nucleus
Neutron	1 unit	Neutral	Within the nucleus
Electron	Negligible	1 negative	Orbits the nucleus

5.

Table 2.2 Chemical bonds

Characteristic	Ionic bonds	Covalent bonds
Gives rise to charged particles (ions)	✓	
Most common bond		✓
Atoms transfer their electrons.	✓	
Links sodium and chloride in a molecule of sodium chloride	✓	
Stable bond		✓
Atoms share their electrons.		✓
There is no change in the number of protons or neutrons.	✓	✓
The weaker of the two bonds	✓	
Links hydrogen and oxygen in a water molecule		✓

6.

Table 2.3 Characteristics of some important biological molecules

Characteristic	Carbohy-drates	Pro-teins	Nucleo-tides	Lipids
Building blocks are amino acids		✓		
Contain carbon	✓	✓	✓	✓
Molecules joined with glycosidic linkages	✓			
Used to build genetic material	✓		✓	
Building blocks are monosaccharides.	✓			
Contain glycerol				✓
Contain hydrogen	✓	✓	✓	✓
Molecules joined together with pep-tide bonds		✓		
Strongly hydro-phobic				✓
Built from sugar unit, phosphate group and base			✓	
Enzymes are made from these.		✓		
Contain oxygen	✓	✓	✓	✓

7. Carbohydrates are mainly used to provide **energy** for body cells. The carbohydrate used by cells for this purpose is the monosaccharide **glucose,** which is carried to all body cells in the **bloodstream.** An excess of this monosaccharide can be stored as **glycogen**, mainly in the liver. It can also be converted to **fat** and stored in adipose tissue. The carbohydrates **deoxyribose** and **ribose** are integral components of DNA and RNA, respectively. Some carbohydrates are exposed on cell membranes as recognition and binding molecules called **receptors**, which allow the cell to interact with other cells and extracellular molecules.

8. The lipids are a varied group of substances and include certain **hormones,** such as steroids. Chemically, they are all **hydrophobic**, meaning water repelling. In the form of **phospholipids**, they are the main component of the cell membrane, making a **double** layer separating the cell contents from the extracellular environment. The steroid derivative **cholesterol** stabilises cell membranes. Vitamins **A**, **D**, **E**, and **K** are lipids.

   Fats are a form of lipid and store energy in **adipose** tissue. The alternative name for fats is **triglycerides.** Compared to energy release from a molecule of glucose, breaking down fat produces **more** energy. Subcutaneous fat **insulates** the body, and internal fat **protects** internal organs. Fats from animal sources are classified as **saturated** and are usually **solid** at room temperature.

9. **a.** 7.0; **b.** 1.5; **c.** 8.3; **d.** 13; **e.** 3.5; **f.** 7.4; **g.** 6.0; **h.** 3.0.

10. c; 11. d; 12. b; 13. c; 14. b; 15. c; 16. b; 17. d; 18. d

19. Lungs and kidneys

20. An excess of hydrogen ions or an excessive decrease in the pH of a body fluid or tissues.

21. CO_2 (carbon dioxide) + H_2O (water) $\rightleftharpoons$ H_2CO_3 (carbonic acid) $\rightleftharpoons$ H^+ (hydrogen ion) + HCO_3^- (bicarbonate ion).

22. Insulin; haemoglobin; antibodies; enzymes; collagen.

23. Enzymes are **proteins** that are used in the body to **increase** the reactivity of active chemicals on which the body's metabolism depends. They are not themselves normally used up in the reactions in which they participate and are usually fairly **specific** in the reactions they control. They can either cause two or more molecules to bind together (**a synthetic reaction**) or cause the breaking up of a molecule into smaller groups (**a catabolic or breakdown reaction**). The molecule(s) entering the reaction are called **reactants** and they bind to a reactive site on the enzyme molecule called the **active site.** Some reactions require the presence of a **cofactor**, which promotes binding of the enzyme to the other participating molecules. They are bound for only a fraction of a second but, when they are released, the reaction has occurred, and the new forms of the reactants are now called **products.**

24. The **external** environment surrounds the body and provides the oxygen and nutrients its cells require. The **internal** environment is the medium in which the body cells exist. Cells are bathed in **interstitial** fluid, also known as **tissue** fluid. The cell **membrane** provides a potential barrier to substances entering or leaving the cell. This property is known as **selective permeability.**

25. The composition of the internal environment is maintained within narrow limits, and this fairly constant state is called **homeostasis.** In systems controlled by negative feedback mechanisms, the effector response **reverses** the effect of the original stimulus. When body temperature falls below the preset level, specialised temperature-sensitive nerve endings act as **detectors** and relay this information to cells in the hypothalamus of the brain that form the **control centre.** This results in the activation of **effector** responses, which raise body temperature. When body temperature returns to the **normal** range again, the temperature-sensitive nerve endings no longer stimulate the cells in the hypothalamus, and the heat-conserving mechanisms are switched off.

26. Shivering; narrowing of the blood vessels supplying the skin (vasoconstriction).

27. Water and electrolyte concentrations, pH of body fluids, blood glucose levels, blood pressure, blood and tissue oxygen and carbon dioxide levels.

28. It is an amplifier or cascade system in which the stimulus progressively increases the response until stimulation ceases.

29. 60%

30. Cytoplasm, potassium, ATP.

31. Figure 2.2 demonstrates osmosis, which refers specifically to the movement of **water** molecules down their **concentration** gradient. The force driving this is called osmotic **pressure.** In A, the red blood cell has not changed in size. This tells you that the solution is **isotonic** – that is, the concentration of water in the suspending solution is **the same as** the cell, and **there is no net water movement.** In B, the red blood cell has swollen. This tells you that the solution is **hypotonic** – that is, the concentration of water in the suspending solution is **higher than** the cell and **more water is moving into the cell than out of it.** In C, the red cell has shrunk. This tells you that the solution is **hypertonic** – that is, the concentration of water in the suspending solution is **less than** the cell, and **more water is moving out of the cell than into it.**

   The movement of water in A, B and C will proceed until **equilibrium** is reached, and water concentrations on either side of the red blood cell membrane are **equal/stable.**

32. a 33. c 34. a 35. d 36. b

37. and 38.

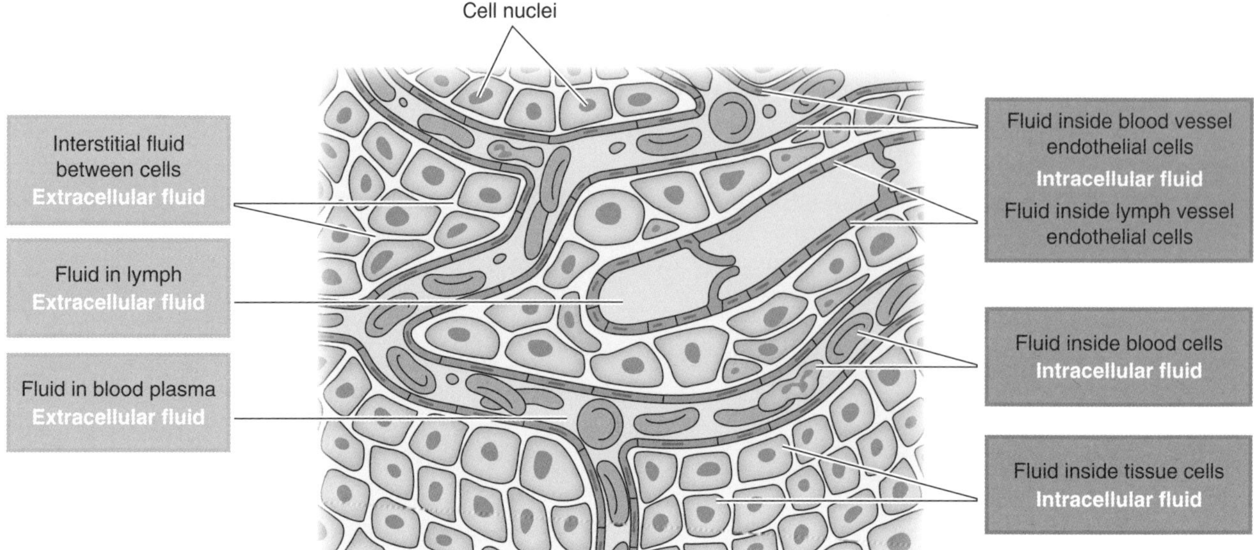

3 Cells and tissues
Answers

1. and 2.

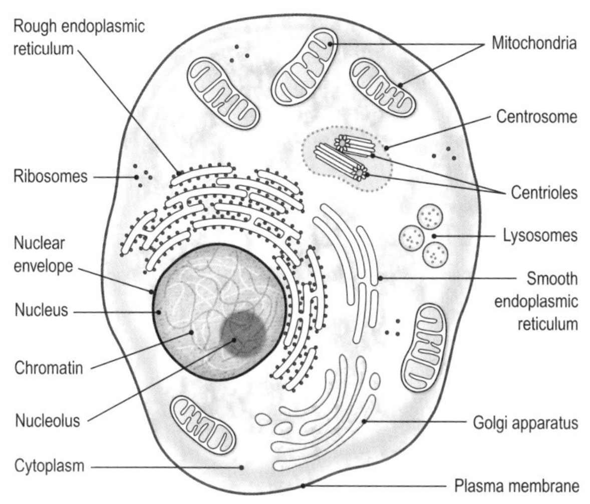

Figure 3.1

3. and 4. See Fig. 3.2. All cells are lightly shaded, and the nuclei are darkly shaded.

5. Urinary bladder.

6. **a.** Lines tissues, providing a thin and smooth membrane. **b.** Absorption and secretion, may be ciliated, such as in the upper respiratory tract. **c.** Allows stretching – for example, as the bladder fills with urine.

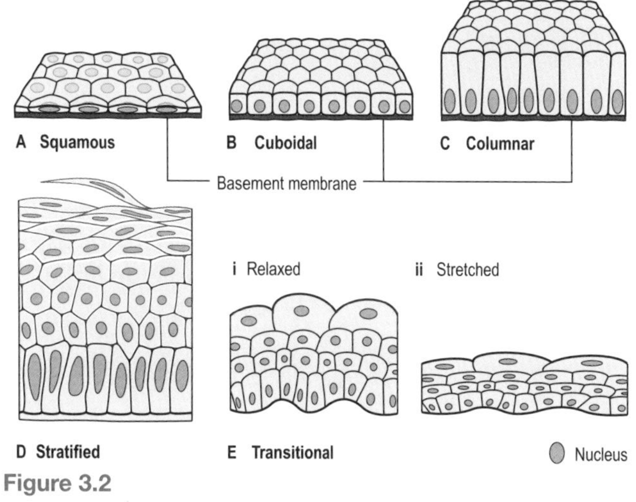

Figure 3.2

7. and 8. See Fig. 3.3.

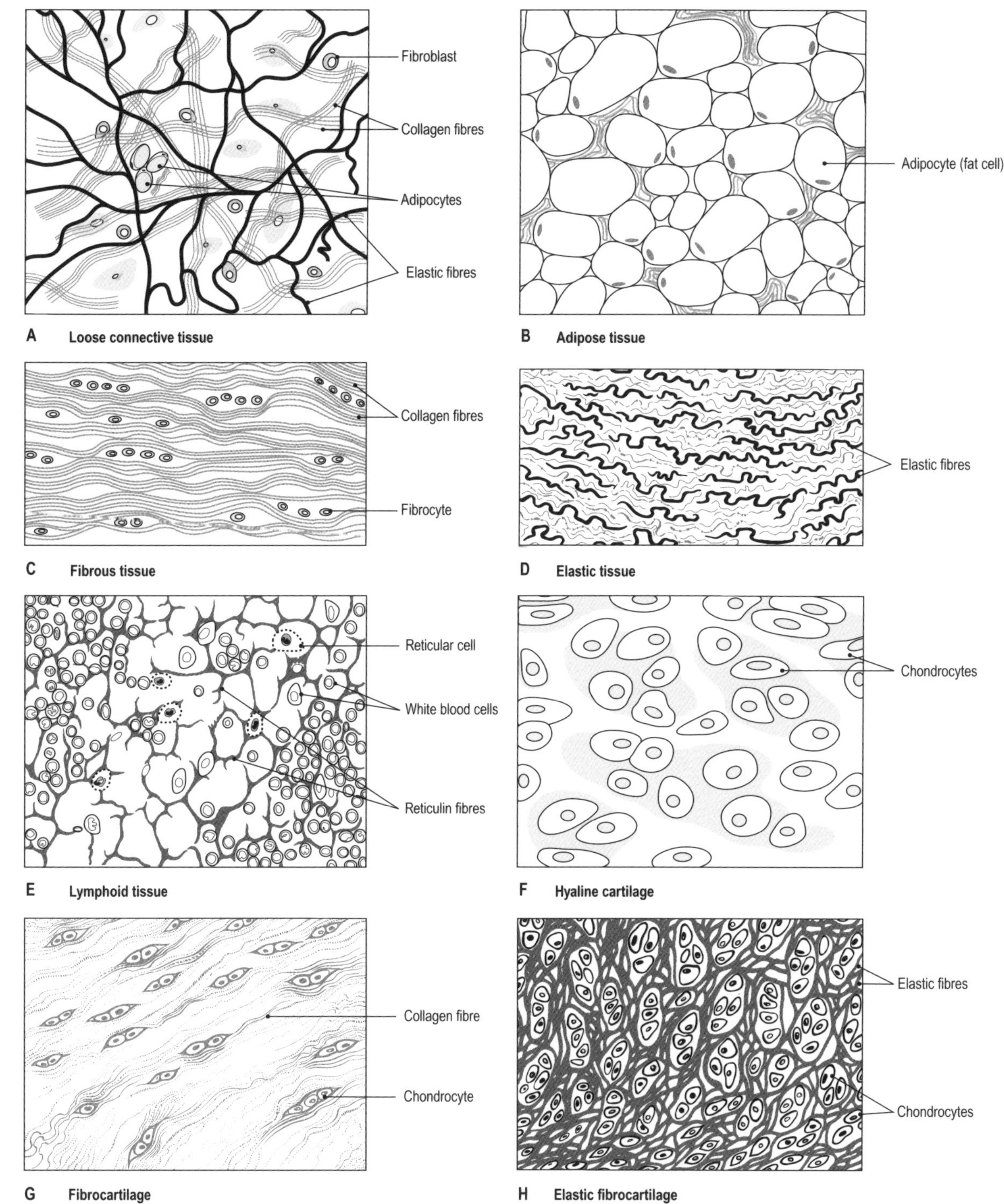
Fibroblast
Collagen fibres
Adipocytes
Elastic fibres
A Loose connective tissue
Adipocyte (fat cell)
B Adipose tissue
Collagen fibres
Fibrocyte
C Fibrous tissue
Elastic fibres
D Elastic tissue
Reticular cell
White blood cells
Reticulin fibres
E Lymphoid tissue
Chondrocytes
F Hyaline cartilage
Collagen fibre
Chondrocyte
G Fibrocartilage
Elastic fibres
Chondrocytes
H Elastic fibrocartilage

Figure 3.3

9. and 10. See Fig. 3.4.

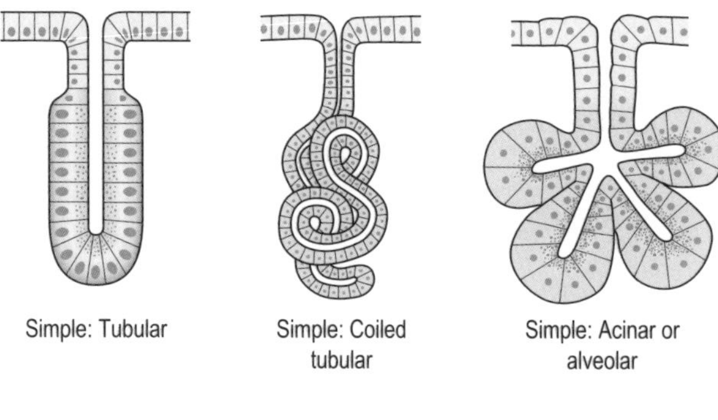

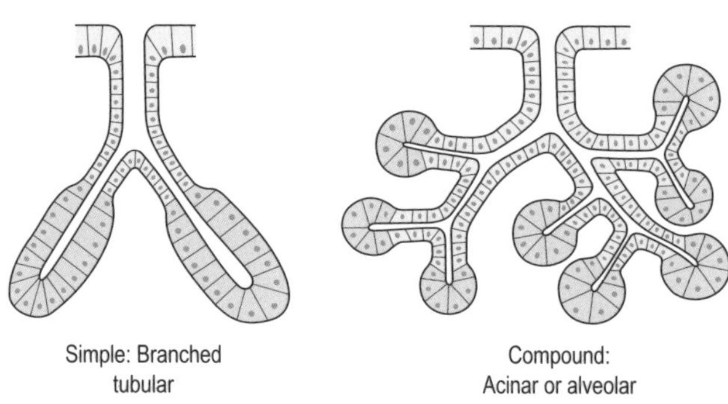

Figure 3.4

11.

Table 3.1 Intracellular organelles and their functions

Organelle	Function
Nucleus	The largest organelle; directs the activities of the cell
Mitochondria	Sites of aerobic respiration, often described as the powerhouse of the cell
Ribosomes	Tiny granules consisting of RNA and protein, which synthesise proteins for use within cells
Rough endoplasmic reticulum	Manufactures proteins exported from cells
Smooth endoplasmic reticulum	Synthesises lipids and steroid hormones
Golgi apparatus	Flattened membranous sacs that form membrane-bound vesicles
Lysosomes	Vesicles that contain enzymes for the breakdown of substances, such as fragments of old organelles
Microfilaments	Tiny strands of protein that provide the structural support and shape of a cell
Microtubules	Contractile proteins involved in the movement of cells and of organelles within cells

12. Transfer of large particles across the plasma membrane into the cell occurs by **phagocytosis**, and smaller particles enter by **pinocytosis.** The particles are engulfed by extensions of the **plasma membrane** that enclose them, forming a membrane-bound **vacuole.** Then **lysosomes** adhere to the cell membrane, releasing **enzymes** that **digest** the contents. Extrusion of waste materials by the reverse process is called **exocytosis.**

13. Most body cells have **46** chromosomes and divide by **mitosis.** The daughter cells of mitosis are genetically **identical.** The formation of gametes takes place by **meiosis** and the daughter cells are genetically **different.** The period between two cell divisions is known as the **cell** cycle, which has two stages, the M phase and the interphase. The **interphase** is the longer stage. The interphase has **three** separate stages. Most cell growth takes place during the **first** gap phase; the chromosomes replicate during the **S phase.**

14. Muscle cells are also called **fibres.** Muscle tissue has the property of **contractility**, which brings about movement, both within the body and of the body itself. This requires a blood supply to provide **oxygen**, **calcium** and **nutrients** and to remove **wastes.** The chemical energy needed is derived from **adenosine triphosphate (ATP).**

    Skeletal muscle is also known as **voluntary** muscle because **contraction** is under conscious control. When examined under the microscope, the cells are roughly **cylindrical** in shape and may be as long as **35** cm. The cells show a pattern of clearly visible stripes, also known as **striations.** Skeletal muscle is stimulated by **motor** nerve impulses that originate in the brain or spinal cord and end at the **neuromuscular junction.**

    Smooth muscle has the intrinsic ability to **contract** and **relax**, a property known as automaticity (e.g. **peristalsis**), but it can also be stimulated by **autonomic** nerve impulses, some **hormones** and **local metabolites.**

    Cardiac muscle is found only in the wall of the **heart**, which has its own **pacemaker** system, meaning that this tissue contracts in a coordinated manner, without external stimulation. **Autonomic** nerve impulses and some **hormones** influence the activity of this type of muscle.

15. Mucous membrane is sometimes referred to as the **mucosa.** It forms the moist lining of body tracts, such as the **alimentary**, **respiratory** and **genitourinary** tracts. The membrane consists of **epithelial** cells, some of which produce a secretion called **mucus.** This sticky substance is present in the alimentary tract, where it **lubricates** the contents, and in the respiratory system, where it traps **inhaled particles.**

16. The plasma membrane consists of two layers of phospholipids, with some **protein** molecules embedded in them. The **lipid** cholesterol is also present. Membrane

proteins are involved in the transport of substances across the plasma membrane. The phospholipid molecules have a head that is electrically charged and hydrophilic (meaning water **loving**) and a tail that has no charge and is hydrophobic. The phospholipid bilayer is arranged like a sandwich, with the hydrophilic heads on the **outside** and the hydrophobic tails on the **inside.** These differences also influence the passage of substances across the cell membrane.

17. **a.** Increase in the size of cells. **b.** This occurs when cells divide more quickly than previously, increasing cell numbers (and which may lead to the development of tumours). **c.** Decrease in cell size or the number of cells.
18. Apoptosis is normal genetically programmed cell death, during which an ageing cell at the end of its life cycle shrinks, and its remaining fragments are phagocytosed, without any inflammatory reaction. Necrosis is cell death resulting from a lack of oxygen (ischaemia), injury or pathological process; the plasma membrane ruptures, releasing the intracellular contents and triggering the inflammatory response.
19. a, d.
20. b.
21. c.
22. a.
23. a, c, d.
24. b.
25. b.
26. c.
27. d.
28. a.
29. b.
30. c.

4 The blood

Answers

1. A: plasma. B: cellular fraction.
2. A: serum. B: blood clot.
3. Clotting proteins
4. and 5.

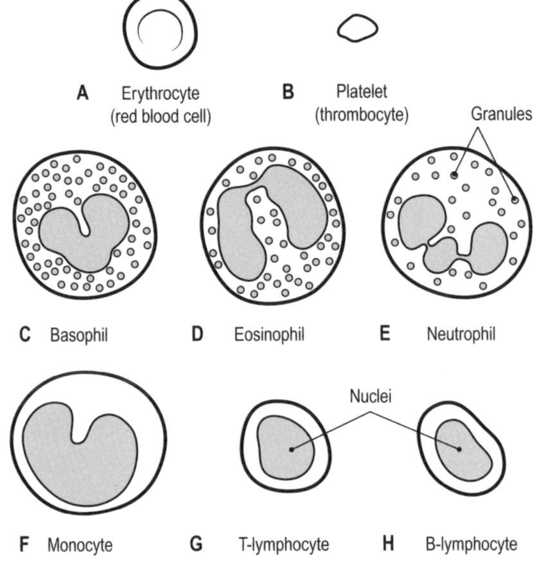

6. Without a nucleus, erythrocytes cannot divide: this allows their numbers to be controlled by the rates of production and destruction.

7. a. 11, 12, 13, 17, 18, 19, 20
   b. 3, 8, 12, 17, 18
   c. 1, 4, 17, 18
   d. 4, 7, 14, 17, 18
   e. 4, 6, 17, 18
   f. 5, 9, 16, 17, 18
   g. 5, 9, 10, 15, 17, 18
   h. 2, 5, 9, 10, 15, 17, 18.

8.

Table 4.1 Components of plasma

Descriptive phrase	Component
These chemicals travel from the gland of origin to distant tissues.	Hormones
These provide the building blocks for new tissue proteins.	Amino acids
These molecules are also called immunoglobulins.	Antibodies
90%–92% of plasma is this.	Water
This substance is needed for haemoglobin synthesis.	Iron
An important non-nitrogenous waste is carried as this.	Bicarbonate ion
A general term for ions, such as phosphate in body fluids.	Electrolyte
This is needed for healthy bones and teeth.	Calcium
This is the principal fuel source for body cells.	Glucose
This is mainly responsible for blood viscosity.	Albumin

9. A. Kidneys secrete erythropoietin into the blood. B. Bone marrow increases erythropoiesis. C. Red blood cell numbers rise. D. Increased blood oxygen-carrying capacity reverses tissue hypoxia.

10.

Table 4.2 The ABO system of blood grouping

Blood group	Type of antigen present on red cell surface	Type of antibody present in plasma	Can safely donate to:	Can safely receive from:
A	A	Anti-B	A, AB	A, O
B	B	Anti-A	B, AB	B, O
AB	A, B	Neither	AB	AB, A, B, O
O	Neither	Anti-A, Anti-B	O, A, B, AB	O

11. a. Ayesha
b. Both A and B antigens: he is blood group AB
c. All three could theoretically donate, because Harold's AB blood doesn't have anti-A or anti-B antibodies to react with their red cells
d. No. Ayesha (group A) has A antigens on her red cells. Hassan (group O) makes both anti-A and anti-B antibodies, and so would react to Ayesha's cells.
e. B
f. Hassan, in theory, could donate to all the others because he has neither A nor B antigens on his red blood cells to stimulate a reaction from their antibodies.

12. Oxygen (O_2) + haemoglobin (Hb) $\leftrightarrow$ oxyhaemoglobin (HbO_2)

13. The life span of red blood cells is usually about **120** days. Their breakdown, also called **haemolysis**, is carried out by phagocytic **reticuloendothelial** cells found mainly in the **liver**, **spleen** and **bone marrow.** Their breakdown releases the mineral **iron**, which is kept by the body and stored in the **liver.** It is used to form new **haemoglobin.** The protein released is converted to the intermediate **biliverdin**, and then to the yellow pigment **bilirubin**, before being bound to plasma protein and transported to the **liver**, where it is excreted in the **bile.**

14. b; 15. d; 16. a; 17. c; 18. d; 19. b; 20. d; 21. d; 22. a; 23. c; 24. a; 25. a

5 The cardiovascular system

Answers

1. and 2.

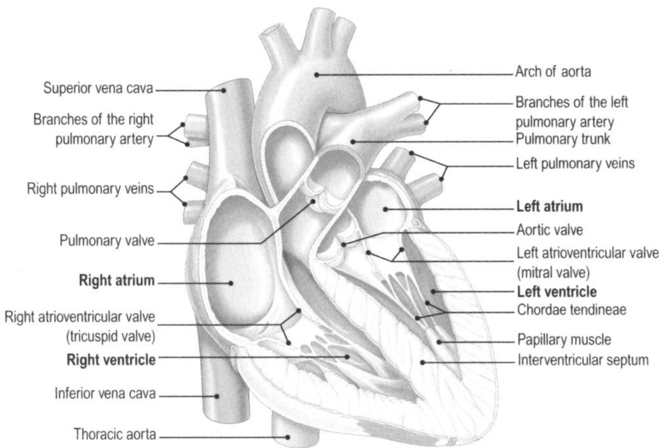

Figure 5.1 Interior of the heart – answer version

3.

4. Left ventricle; it has the highest workload of all the heart chambers because it pumps blood into the systemic circulation

5. a. myocardium; b. serous pericardium; c. fibrous pericardium; d. endocardium; e. serous pericardium; f. fibrous pericardium; g. endocardium; h. myocardium; i. serous pericardium; j. myocardium; k. endocardium; l. endocardium.

6. Lungs, which are covered with the pleural membrane, and the peritoneal cavity, lined with the peritoneum.

7.

8. b; 9. c; 10. b; 11. c; 12. d; 13. d; 14. c

15. The heart pumps blood into two separate circulatory systems, the **pulmonary** circulation and the **systemic** circulation. The **right** side of the heart pumps blood to the lungs, whereas the **left** side of the heart supplies the rest of the body. The **capillaries** are the sites of exchange of nutrients, gases and wastes. Tissue wastes, including

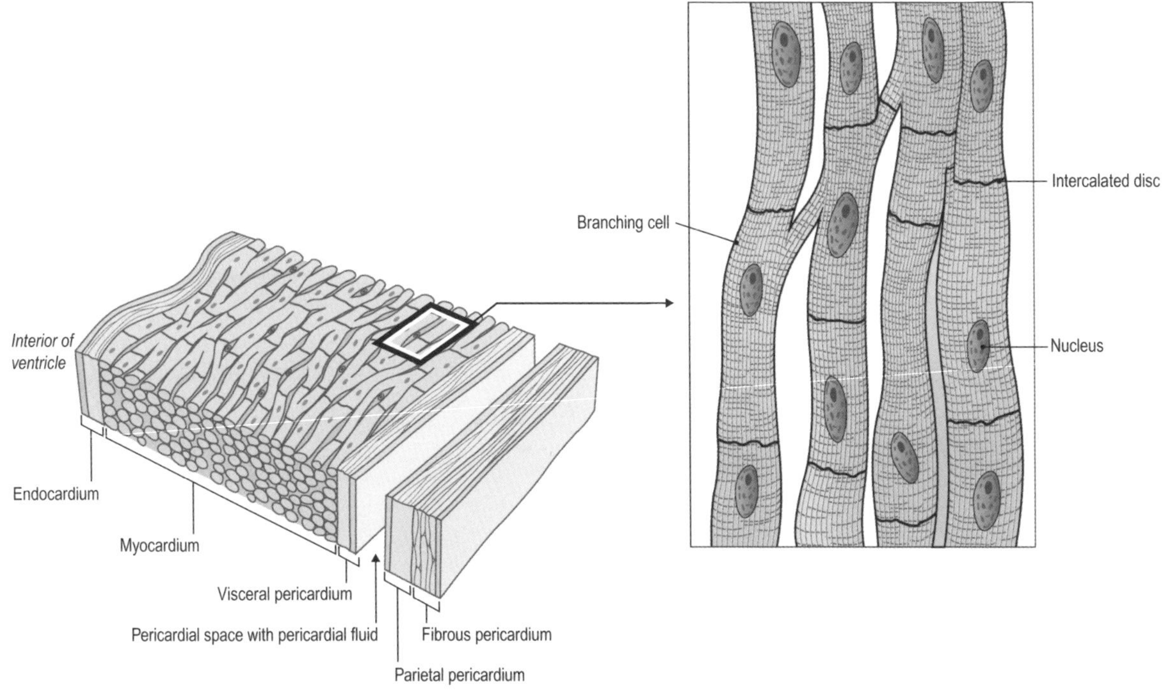

Figure 5.2 Layers of the heart wall – answer version

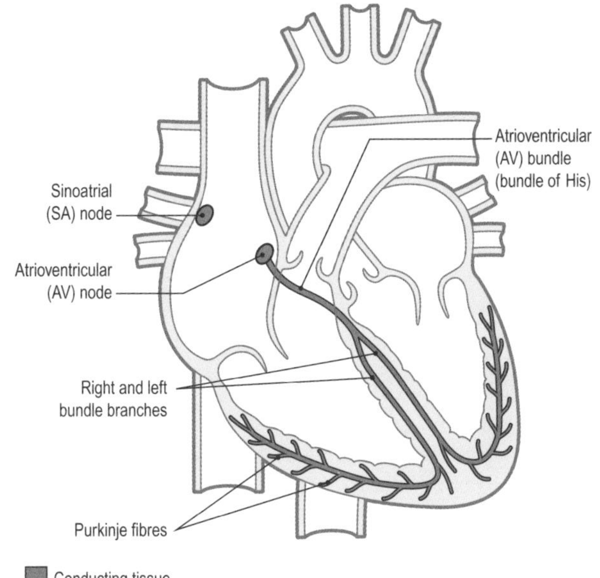

Figure 5.3 Conduction system of the heart – answer version

carbon dioxide, pass into the **bloodstream** and the tissues are supplied with **oxygen** and **nutrients.** By definition, a blood vessel returning blood to the heart is called a **vein** and a blood vessel carrying blood from the heart is an **artery.**

16. Blood leaving the right ventricle first enters the **pulmonary trunk**, which passes upwards close to the aorta and divides into the right **pulmonary artery** and the left **pulmonary artery** at the level of the fifth thoracic vertebra. Each of these branches goes to the corresponding **lung** and enters these organs in the area called the **hilum/root.** Within the tissues, the vessels divide and subdivide, giving a network of many millions of tiny **capillaries**, across the walls of which gases exchange. Blood draining these structures then passes through veins of increasing diameter, which finally unite in the **pulmonary vein**, which carries the blood back to the **left atrium** of the heart.
17. A: vessel lumen; B: tunica externa; C: tunica intima; D: tunica media
18. B (tunica externa): v, vi; C (tunica intima): i, iv; D (tunica media): ii, iii

19. and 20.

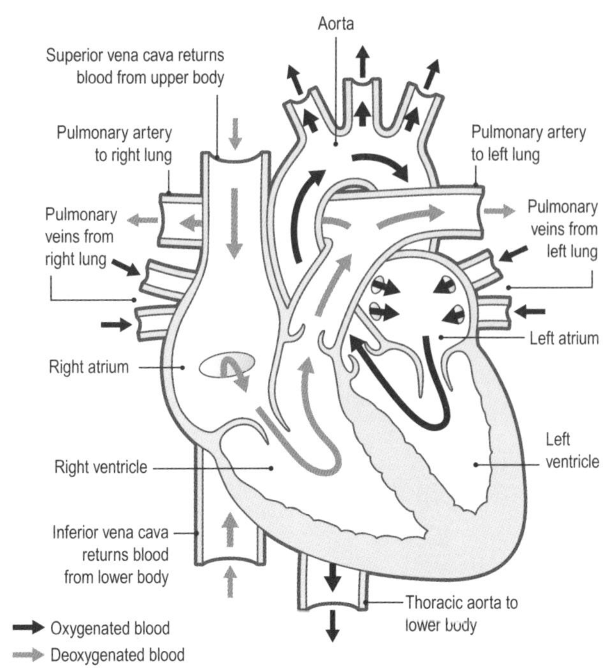

Figure 5.5 Direction of blood flow through the heart – answer version

21.

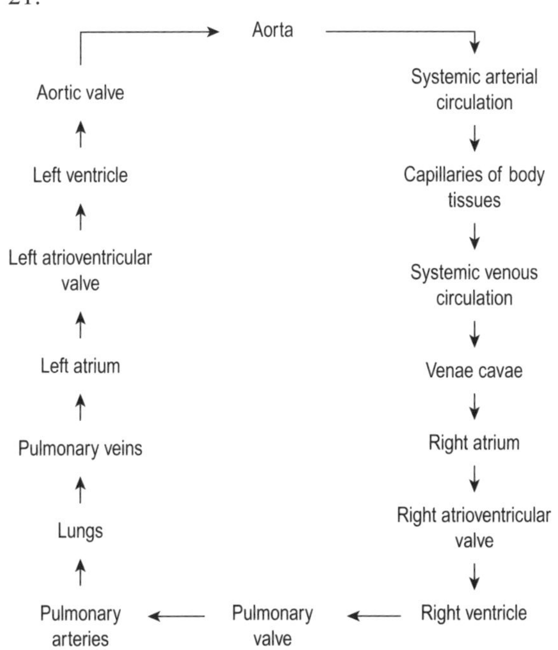

22.

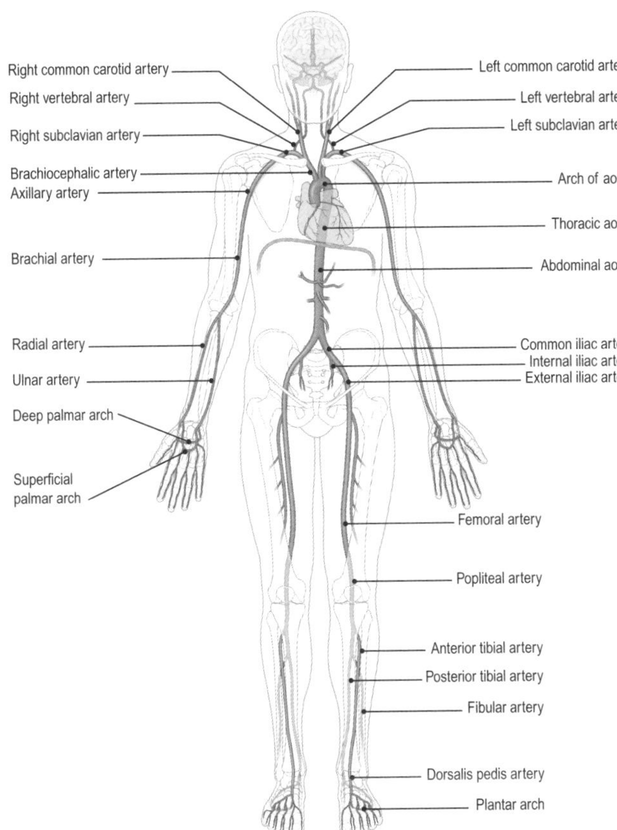

Figure 5.6 Aorta and main arteries – answer version

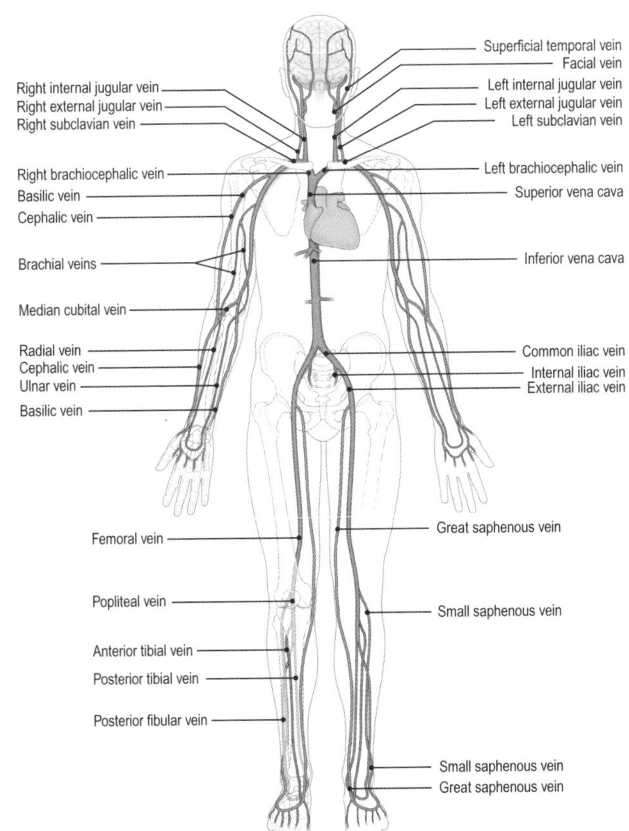

Figure 5.7 The venae cavae and main veins – answer version

23. and 24.

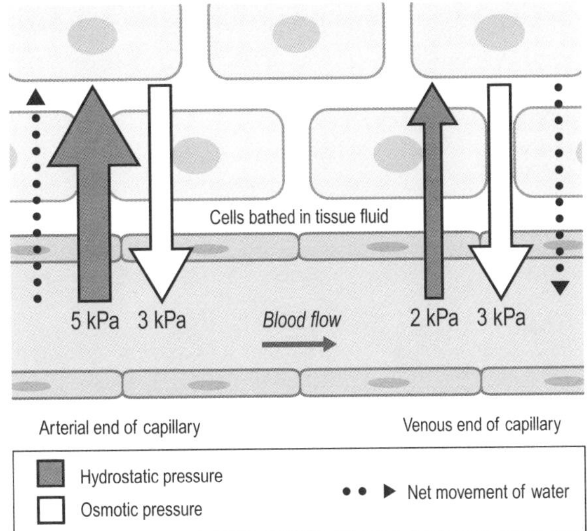

Figure 5.8 Effect of capillary pressures on water movement across capillary walls – answer version

25. and 26.

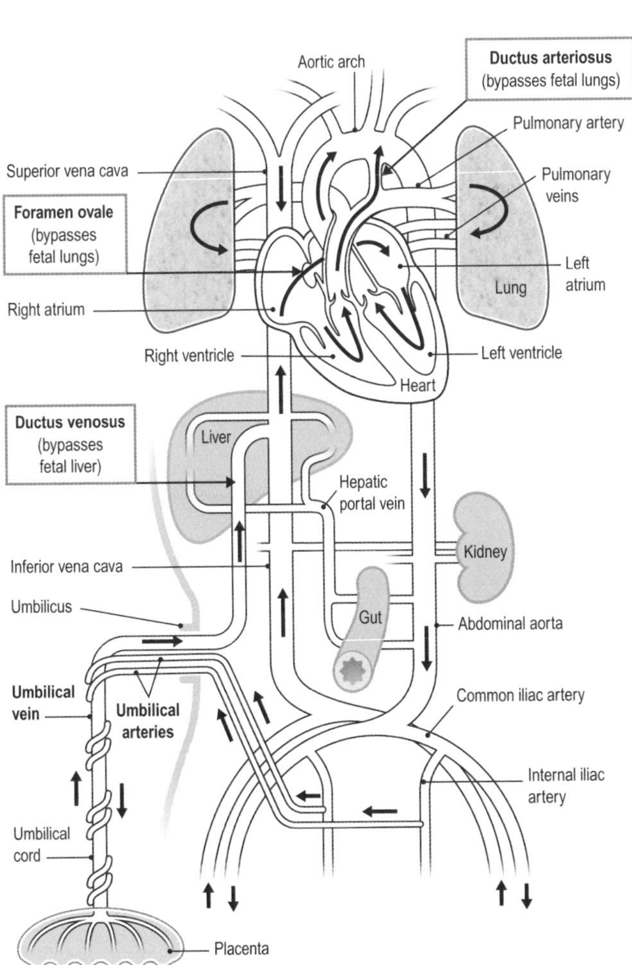

Figure 5.9 The fetal circulation – answer version

27. Descending aorta, common iliac artery, external iliac artery, femoral artery, popliteal artery, anterior tibial artery, dorsalis pedis artery, digital arteries, digital veins, dorsal venous arch, anterior tibial vein, popliteal vein, femoral vein, external iliac vein, common iliac vein, inferior vena cava.

28.

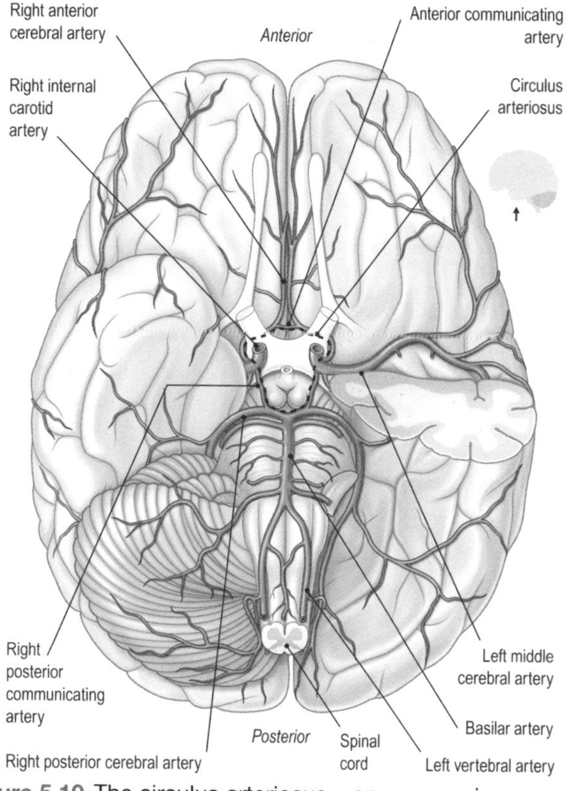

Figure 5.10 The circulus arteriosus – answer version

29. b; 30. a; 31. a; 32. c, d; 33. c; 34. b;
35. b; 36. b, d; 37. a; 38. b

39. 40. and 41. See Fig. 5.11: answer version.

42. and 43. See Fig. 5.12: answer version.

44. b, d and e are true.
a. The QRS complex is bigger than the P wave because there is more muscle in the **ventricles** than in the **atria.**
c. The T wave represents **ventricular** relaxation.
f. The waves on the ECG are generated by the **electrical activity of the myocardium.**
g. The P wave shows atrial **depolarisation.**
h. The delay between the P and QRS components represents the time taken for the impulse to spread from the **atria to the ventricles.**

45. a, b, g.

46. c, d, f, g, h.

47. Vasodilation: a, b, d, f, g, i, m; vasoconstriction: c, e, h, j, k, l, n.

48. Autoregulation means **local** control of blood flow. For example, **increased** metabolic activity increases blood flow to a tissue. Cooler tissues receive **less** blood than warmer ones and blood vessels in warmer tissues **dilate** to **increase** blood supply. Oxygen and carbon dioxide levels are important in autoregulation; hypoxia **increases** blood flow to a capillary bed. The changes in blood vessel diameter controlling blood flow are mediated by the release of chemicals such as histamine, which is **vasodilating** in action, and nitric oxide, a potent and **short**-lived mediator that **increases** blood flow to organs. On the other hand, adrenaline, also called **epinephrine**, from the adrenal **medulla** and angiotensin II are powerful **vasoconstrictors.**

49. The baroreceptor reflex is important in the **moment to moment** control of blood pressure. It is controlled by the cardiovascular centre found in the **medulla oblongata**, which receives and integrates information from baroreceptors, chemoreceptors and higher centres in the brain. Baroreceptors are receptors sensitive to blood pressure and are found in the **carotid arteries/aorta.** A **rise** in blood pressure activates these receptors, which respond by increasing the activity of **parasympathetic** nerve fibres supplying the heart; this **slows the heart down** and returns the system towards normal. In addition to this, **sympathetic** nerve fibres supplying the blood vessels are **inhibited**, which leads to **vasodilation**, again returning the system towards normal (note that most blood vessels have little or no **parasympathetic** innervation).

On the other hand, if the blood pressure **falls**, baroreceptor activity is decreased, and this also triggers compensatory mechanisms. This time, **sympathetic** activity is increased, which leads to an **increase** in heart rate; in addition, cardiac contractile force is **increased.** The blood vessels respond with **vasoconstriction**; this is mainly due to **increased** activity in **sympathetic** fibres. These measures lead to a restoration of blood pressure towards normal.

In addition to the activity of the baroreceptors described above, chemoreceptors in the **carotid bodies/aorta** measure the pH of the blood. An increase in **carbon dioxide** content of the blood decreases pH and **stimulates** these receptors, leading to an **increase** in stroke volume and heart rate and a general **vasoconstriction**; this **increases** blood pressure. Other control mechanisms include the renin–angiotensin system, which is involved in **long-term** regulation; activation **increases** blood volume, thereby **increasing** blood pressure.

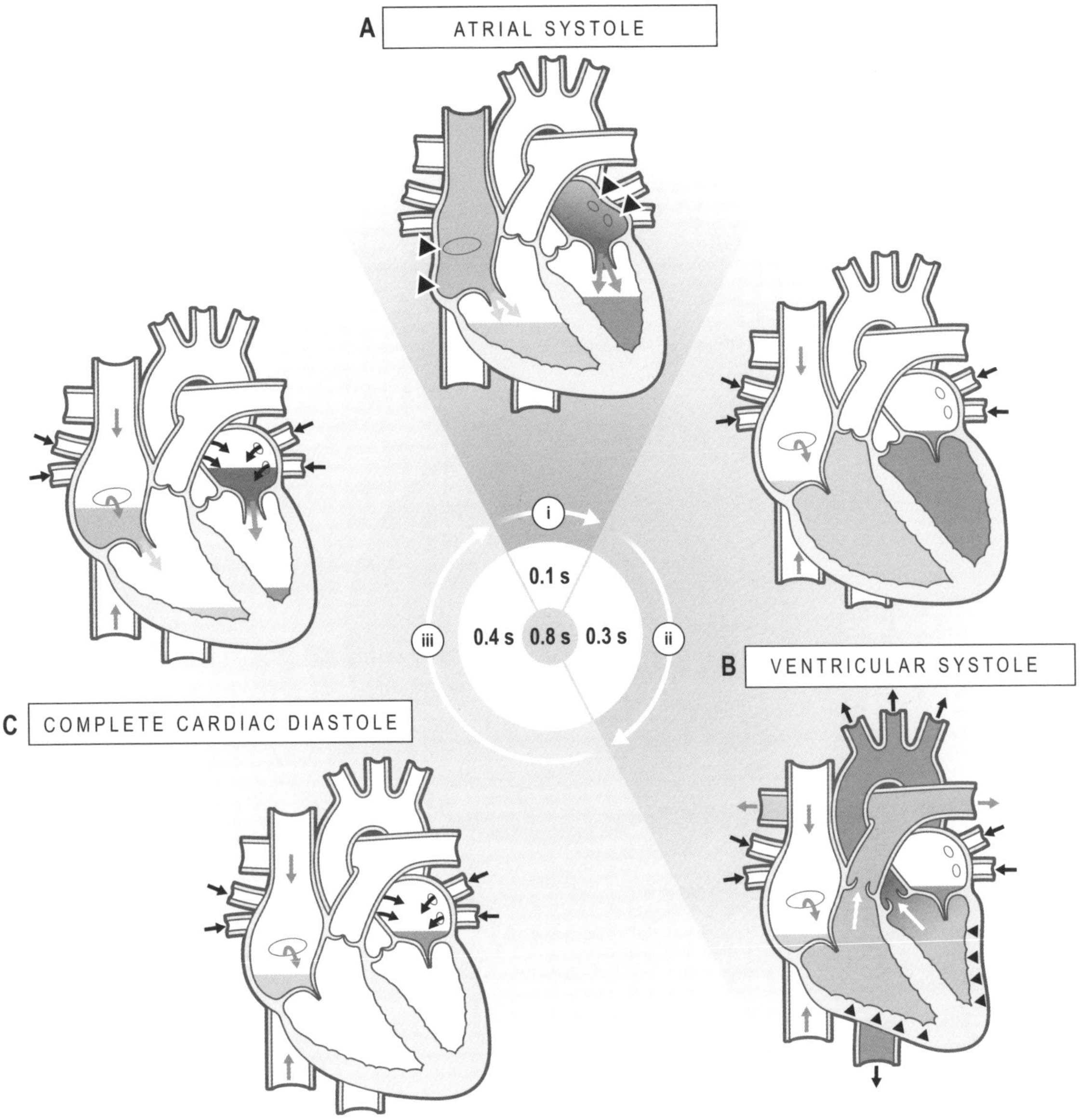

A ATRIAL SYSTOLE

B VENTRICULAR SYSTOLE

C COMPLETE CARDIAC DIASTOLE

i 0.1 s

ii 0.3 s

iii 0.4 s

0.8 s

A Atria contract Aortic/pulmonary valves closed Atrioventricular valves open Ventricles relaxed	**B** Atria relaxed Aortic/pulmonary valves open Atrioventricular valves closed Ventricles contract	**C** Atria and ventricles relaxed Aortic/pulmonary valves closed Atrioventricular valves open

Figure 5.11 One complete cardiac cycle – answer version

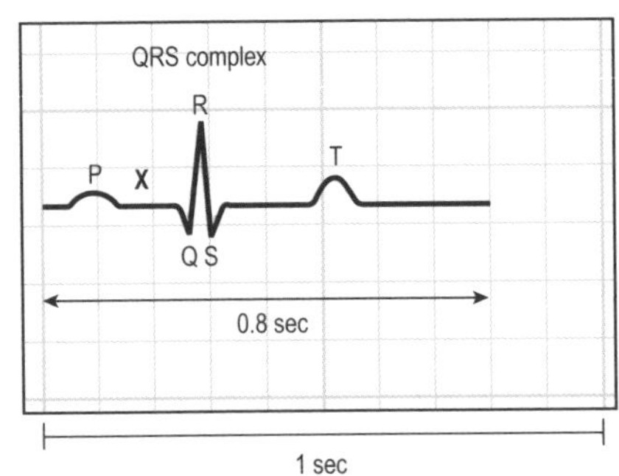

Figure 5.12 The electrocardiogram – answer version

50. 5.625 litres.

51. 83.3 mL.

52. 100 beats per minute.

53. d; 54. b; 55. c; 56. b; 57. a; 58. c; 59. c; 60. a; 61. d; 62. c; 63. a; 64. b; 65. c; 66. a, d; 67. b, c

6 The lymphatic system

Answers

1. and 2.

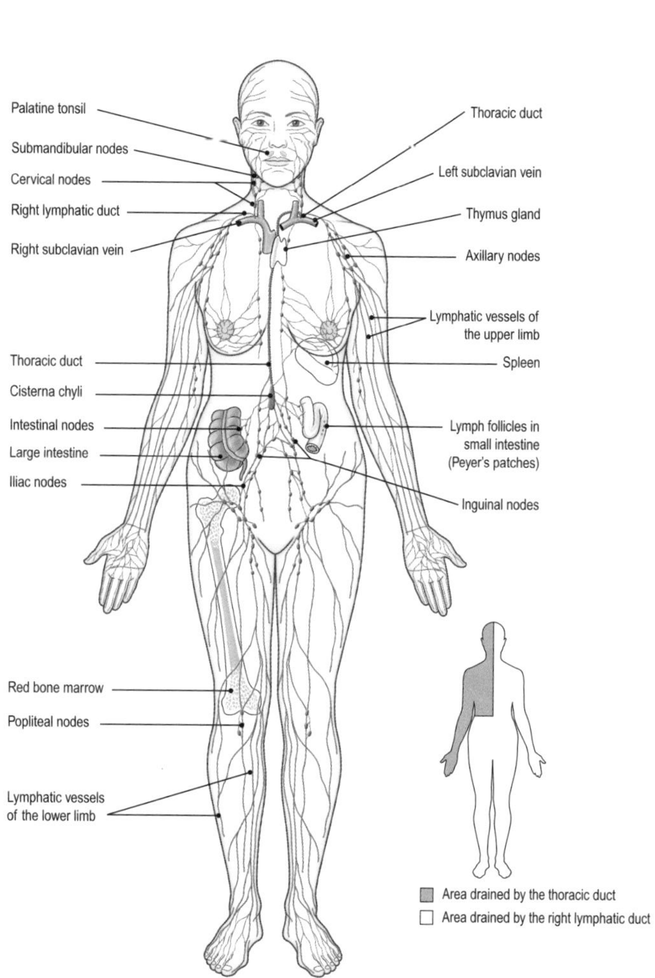

Figure 6.1 The lymphatic system – answer version

3. and 4.

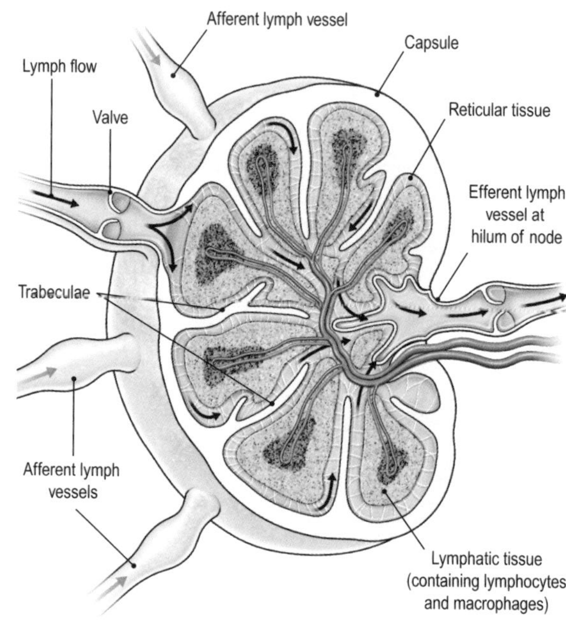

Figure 6.2 Section of a lymph node – answer version

5. 8–10 litres

6.

Table 6.1 Characteristics of lymph nodes, spleen and thymus

Spleen	Thymus	Lymph node
Largest lymphatic organ	Maximum weight usually 30–40 g	Size from pinhead to almond-sized
Lies immediately below the diaphragm	Lies immediately behind the sternum	Distributed throughout lymphatic system
Stores blood	Secretes the hormone thymosin	Phagocytoses cellular debris
Oval in shape	Made up of two narrow lobes	Bean-shaped
Synthesises red blood cells in the fetus	Where T-lymphocytes mature	Site of multiplication of activated lymphocytes
Red blood cells destroyed here	At its maximum size at puberty	Filters lymph

7. The smallest lymphatic vessels are called **capillaries.** One significant difference between them and the smallest blood vessels is that they **originate in the tissues**; their function is to drain the lymph, containing **white blood cells**, away from the interstitial spaces. Most tissues have a network of these tiny vessels, but one notable exception is **bone tissue.** The individual tiny vessels join up to form larger ones, which now contain **three** layers of tissue in their walls, similar to veins in the cardiovascular system. The inner lining, the **endothelial** layer, covers the valves, which **regulate flow of lymph.** As vessels progressively unite and become wider and wider, eventually they empty into the biggest lymph vessels of all, the **thoracic duct and the right lymphatic duct.** The first one of these drains the **right side of the body above the diaphragm.** The second drains the **lower part of the body and the upper left side above the diaphragm.**

8. b; 9. c; 10. d; 11. c; 12. b; 13. a; 14. c; 15. a; 16. d; 17. B; 18. c; 19. a; 20. c; 21. b

7 The nervous system
Answers

1.

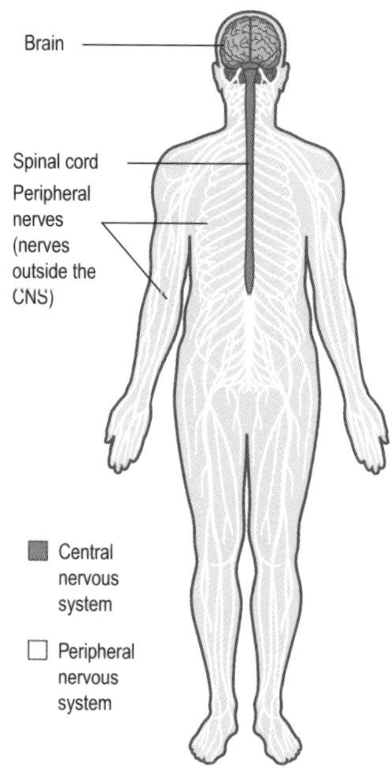

Figure 7.1

2. Brain, spinal cord.
3. The peripheral nervous system has two functionally distinct divisions. One relays information along **afferent** nerves towards the central nervous system; this is the **sensory** division. The **motor** division transmits impulses from the brain and spinal cord to effector organs along **efferent** nerves. Some of these nerves transmit impulses to **skeletal** or voluntary muscles enabling control of **movement** and maintenance of **balance.**

   Smooth and cardiac muscle as well as **glands** are **effector** organs of the **autonomic** nervous system, which has two complementary divisions. The **sympathetic** division prepares the body for 'fight or flight' while the **parasympathetic** division enables the body to 'rest and repair'.

4., 5. and 6. See Figure 7.2. Arrow shows the direction of impulse transmission.

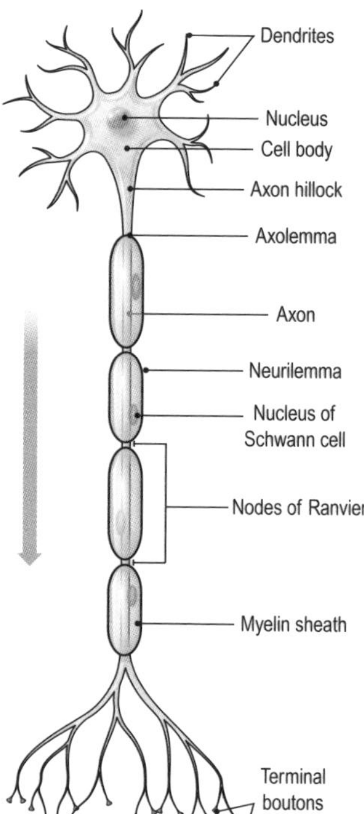

Figure 7.2

7., 8. and 9. See Figure 7.3. Arrows show the direction of impulse transmission.

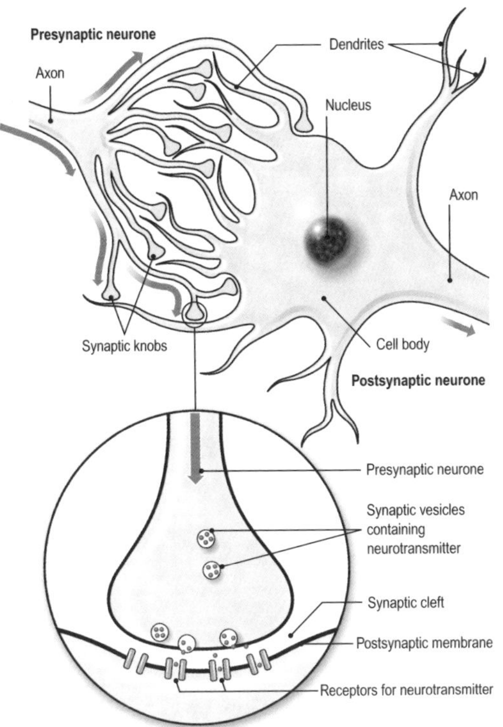

Figure 7.3

10. Transmission of the **action potential**, or impulse, is due to movement of **ions** across the nerve cell membrane. In the resting state, the nerve cell membrane is **polarised** due to differences in the concentrations of ions across the plasma membrane. This means that there is a different electrical charge on each side of the membrane, which is called the resting **membrane potential.** At rest, the charge outside the cell is **positive** and inside it is **negative.** The principal ions involved are **sodium** and **potassium.** In the resting state, there is a continual tendency for these ions to diffuse down their **concentration gradients.** During the action potential, sodium ions flood **into** the neurone, causing **depolarisation.** This is followed by **repolarisation**, when potassium ions move **out of** the neurone. In myelinated neurones, the insulating properties of the **myelin sheath** prevent the movement of ions across the membrane when this is present. In these neurones, impulses pass from one **node of Ranvier** to the next and transmission is called **saltatory conduction.** In unmyelinated fibres, impulses are conducted by the process called **simple propagation (or continuous conduction).** Impulse conduction is faster when the mechanism of transmission is **saltatory conduction** than when it is **simple propagation.** The diameter of the neurone also affects the rate of impulse conduction – the **larger** the diameter, the faster the conduction.

11. d.

12. c.

13. b.

14. c.

15. c.

16. a. Astrocytes; b. microglia; c. oligodendrocytes; d. astrocytes; e. ependymal cells; f. oligodendrocytes; g. astrocytes.

17. Protects the brain from potentially toxic substances and chemical variations in the blood.

18. Supports the brain in the cranial cavity; maintains uniform pressure around the brain and spinal cord; protects the brain and spinal cord by acting as a shock absorber between the brain and cranial bones; keeps the brain and spinal cord moist and may allow exchange of substances between CSF and nerve cells.

19. and 20.

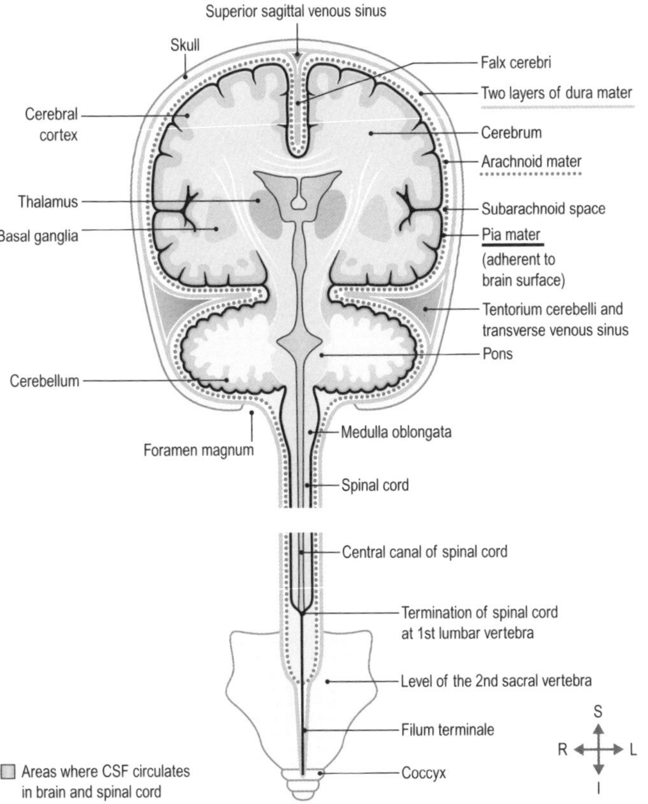

Figure 7.4

21. and 22.

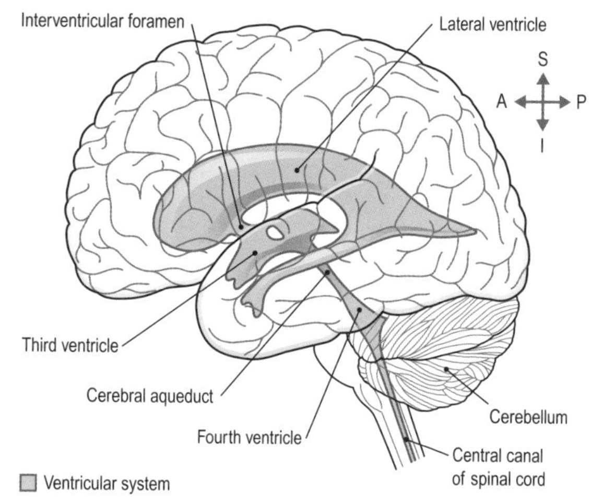

Figure 7.5

23. and 24.

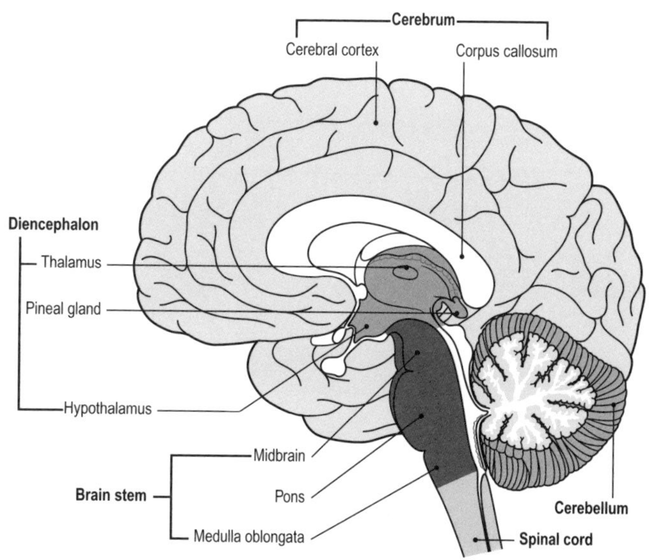

Figure 7.6

25. and 26.

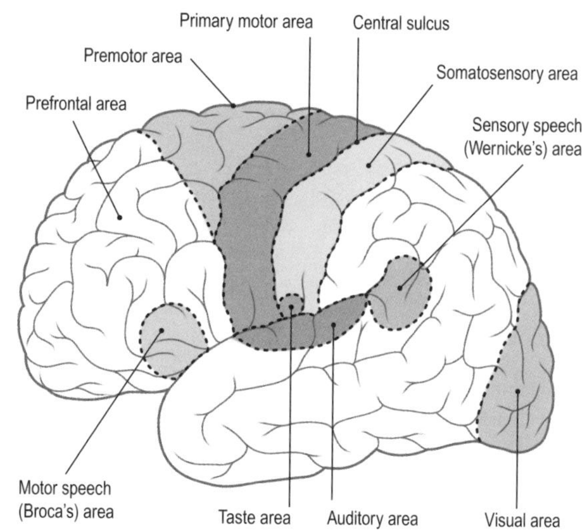

Figure 7.7

27.

Table 7.1 Characteristics of the meninges

Characteristic	Dura mater	Arachnoid mater	Pia mater
Consists of two layers of fibrous tissue	✓		
Consists of fine connective tissue			✓
A delicate serous membrane		✓	
The subdural space lies between these two layers	✓	✓	
Surrounds the venous sinuses	✓		
The subarachnoid space separates these two layers		✓	✓
Forms the filum terminale			✓
CSF is found in the space between these two layers		✓	✓
Equivalent to the periosteum of other bones	✓		

28. This is the largest part of the brain and is divided into left and right cerebral **hemispheres.** Deep inside, the two parts are connected by the **corpus callosum**, which consists of **white** matter. The superficial layer of the cerebrum is known as the **cerebral cortex** and consists of **nerve cell bodies** or **grey** matter. The deeper layer consists of **axons** and is **white** in colour. The cerebral cortex has many furrows and folds that vary in depth. The exposed areas are the convolutions or **gyri** and they are separated by **sulci**, also known as fissures, which increase the surface area of the cerebrum.

29. The primary motor area lies in the **frontal** lobe immediately anterior to the **central** sulcus. The cell bodies are **pyramid-shaped** and stimulation leads to contraction of **skeletal** muscle. Their nerve fibres pass downwards through the **internal capsule** to the **medulla,** where they cross to the opposite side and then descend in the spinal cord. These neurones are the upper motor neurones. They synapse with the lower motor neurones in the **spinal cord,** and lower motor neurones terminate at a **neuromuscular junction.** This means that the motor area of the right hemisphere controls skeletal muscle movement on the **left** side of the body.

    In the motor area of the cerebrum, body areas are represented **upside down,** and the proportion of the cerebral cortex that represents a particular part of the body reflects its **complexity of movement.**

    The motor speech (Broca's) area lies in the **frontal** lobe and controls the movements needed for speech. The right hemisphere is dominant in **left-handed** people.

30. a. Selective awareness, which blocks or transmits sensory information to the cerebral cortex, such as a crying child; b. coordination of voluntary movement, posture and balance; c. relays and distributes information from most parts of the brain to the cerebral cortex; simple recognition (not perceptions) of some senses and thought to be involved in processing of some emotions.

31. b, c, d.

32. a, b, d.

33. d.

34. d.

35. b

36. c.

37. a, b, d.

38. a, c.

39. d.

40. c.

41., 42. and 43. See Fig. 7.8.

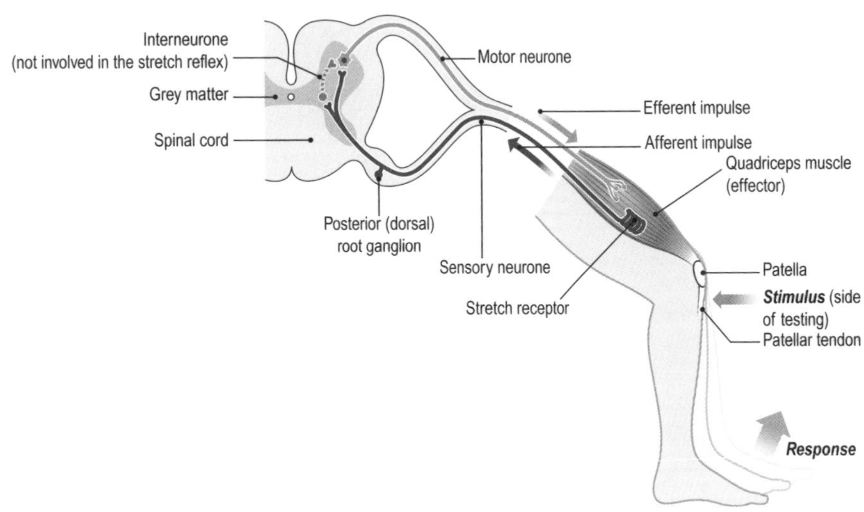

Figure 7.8

44. Within the peripheral nervous system, there are **31** pairs of spinal nerves and **12** pairs of cranial nerves. These nerves are composed of either **sensory** nerve fibres conveying afferent impulses to the **brain** from **sensory** organs or **motor** nerve fibres that transmit efferent impulses from the **brain** to **effector** organs. Some nerves, known as **mixed** nerves, contain both types of fibres.

45. It is a site where spinal nerves are regrouped before going on to their destination, meaning that damage to one spinal nerve does not cause loss of function of an area.

46. a. Intercostal; b. Phrenic; c. Sciatic; d. Pudendal; e. Pudendal.

47. Sciatic nerve.

48., 49. and 50. See Fig. 7.9.

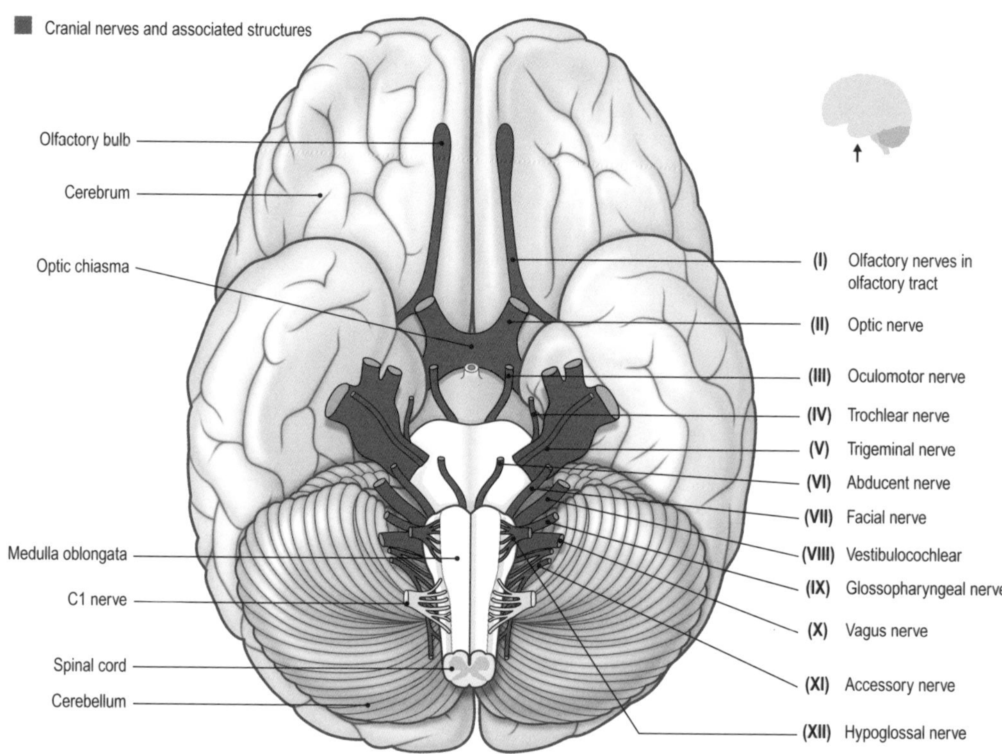

Figure 7.9

51., 52., 53. and 54. See Fig. 7.10

55. Increased heart rate and cardiac contractility, dilation of the coronary arteries, bronchodilation and increased metabolic rate.

56. Noradrenaline released at the synapses by stimulation of the sympathetic nervous system is quickly inactivated. Adrenaline and noradrenaline are released from the adrenal medulla into the bloodstream and travel around the body to target tissues and organs, prolonging and sustaining the effects of sympathetic stimulation.

57. The parasympathetic nervous system **decreases** the heart rate and **decreases** the force of cardiac contraction. In the lungs its effects include mild **bronchoconstriction** that **decreases** airflow to the alveoli. It **stimulates** secretion of saliva and gastric juice. Peristalsis in the digestive tract is **increased.** This action on the gastrointestinal **smooth** muscle **increases** the rate at which gastrointestinal contents pass along and is facilitated by **relaxation** of its sphincters. In the liver, storage of glucose is promoted by **increasing** its conversion to **glycogen.**

58. b, c, d.

59. c.

60. b.

61. a.

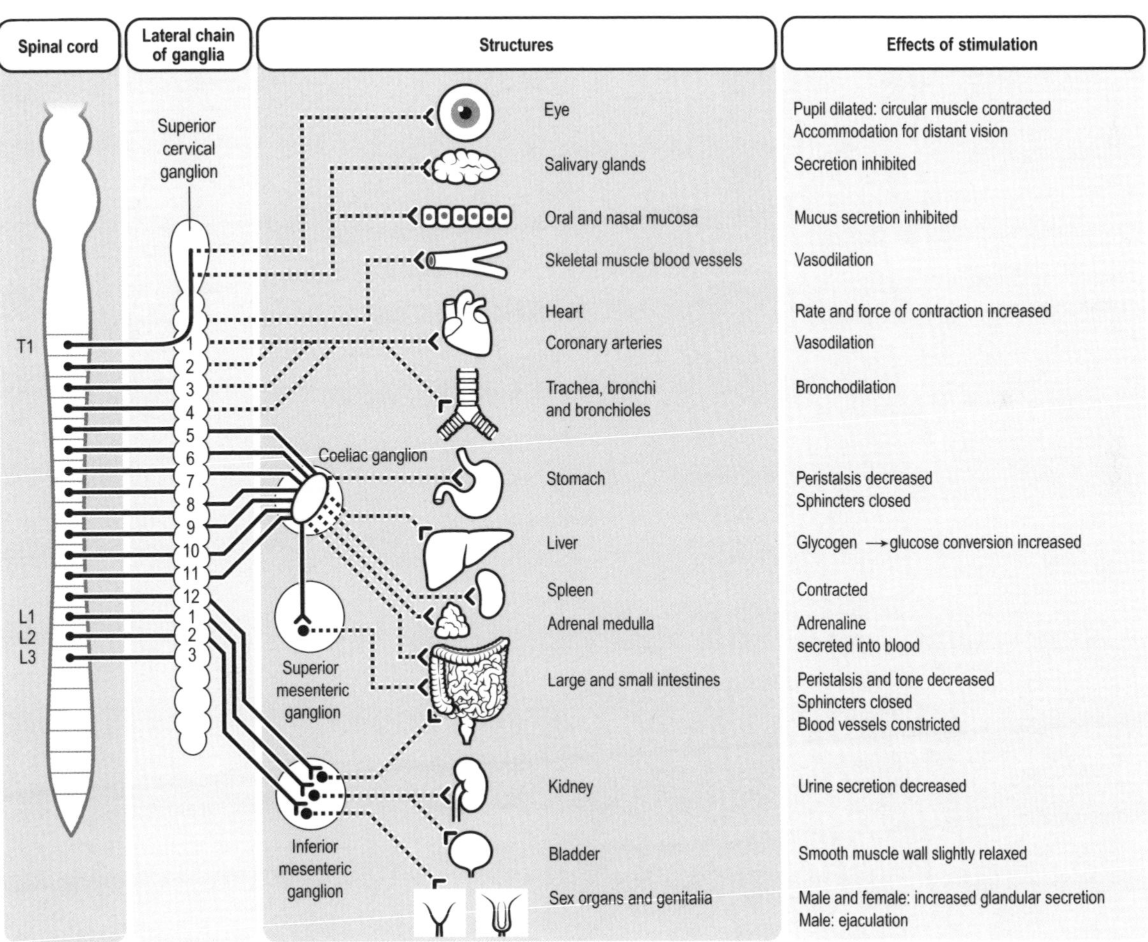

Figure 7.10

8 The special senses

Answers

1. and 2.

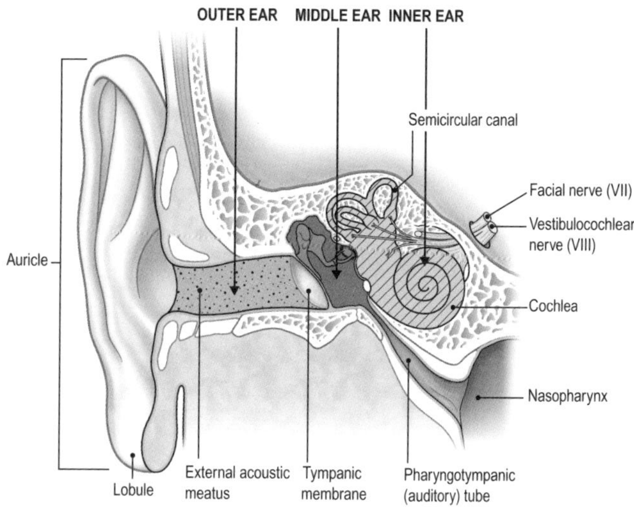

Figure 8.1

3. Cerumen (ear wax).

4.

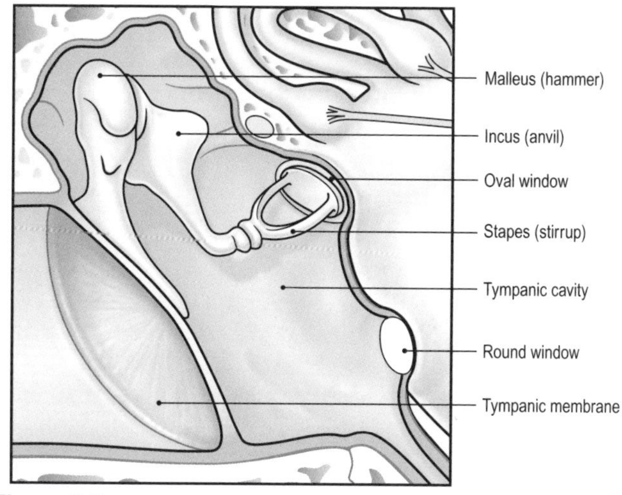

Figure 8.2

5. and 6. See Fig. 8.3

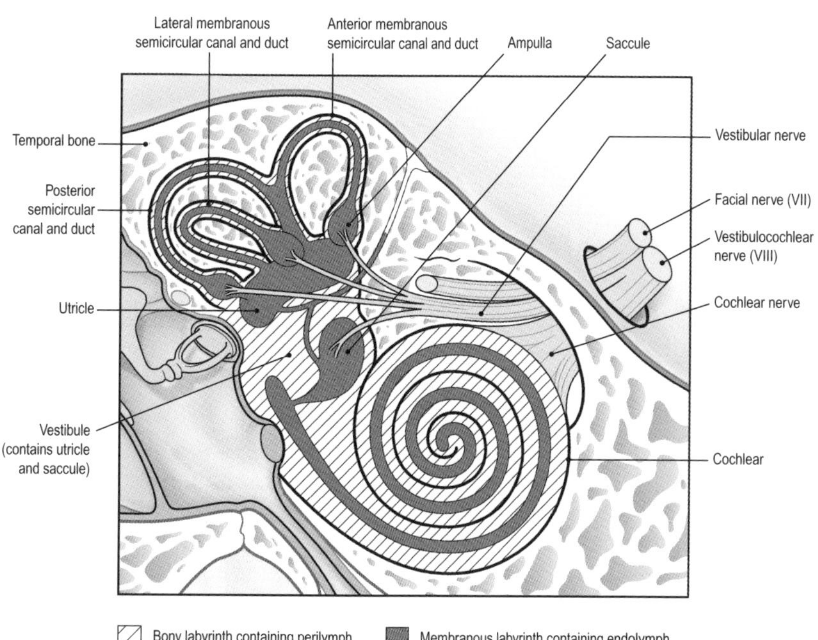

Figure 8.3

7. Vestibule.
8. A sound produces **waves/vibrations** in the air. The auricle **collects** and **directs** them along the **auditory canal** to the **tympanic membrane (eardrum).** The vibrations are **transmitted** and **amplified** through the middle ear by movement of the **(auditory) ossicles.** At its medial end, movement of the **stapes** in the **oval** window sets up fluid waves in the **perilymph** of the scala vestibuli. Most of this pressure is transmitted into the **cochlear duct**, resulting in a corresponding fluid wave in the **endolymph.** This stimulates the auditory receptors in the **hair** cells in the organ of hearing, the **spiral organ (of Corti).** Stimulation of the auditory receptors results in the generation of **nerve impulses** that travel to the brain along the **cochlear/auditory** part of the **vestibulocochlear** nerve. The fluid wave is extinguished by vibration of the membrane of the **round** window.
9. The organs involved with balance are found in the **inner** ear. They are the three **semicircular** canals, one in each plane of space, and the vestibule, which comprises two parts, the **saccule** and the utricle. The canals, like the cochlea, are composed of an outer bony wall and inner membranous ducts. The membranous ducts contain **endolymph** and are separated from the bony wall by **perilymph.** They have dilated portions near the vestibule called ampullae containing hair cells with sensory nerve endings between them. Any change in the position of the head causes movement in the endolymph and perilymph. This stimulates the hair cells and nerve impulses are generated. These travel in the vestibular part of the vestibulocochlear nerve to the **cerebellum** via the **vestibular** nucleus. Perception of body position occurs because the cerebrum coordinates impulses from the eyes and proprioceptors in addition to those from the cerebellum.

10. and 11. See Fig. 8.4.

12. Adipose (fat) tissue.
13. See Fig. 8.5.

14., 15. and 16. See Fig. 8.6.

17. About 6 metres.
18. See Fig. 8.7.
19. The visual cortex that lies in the occipital lobe of the cerebrum.
20. Internally, the eye is divided into **three** compartments by the iris and the lens: the **vitreous, anterior** and **posterior** chambers. The largest is the **vitreous** chamber, which lies behind the lens and fills the **eyeball.** It contains **vitreous humour**, a soft, colourless, transparent substance with a **jelly-like** consistency.

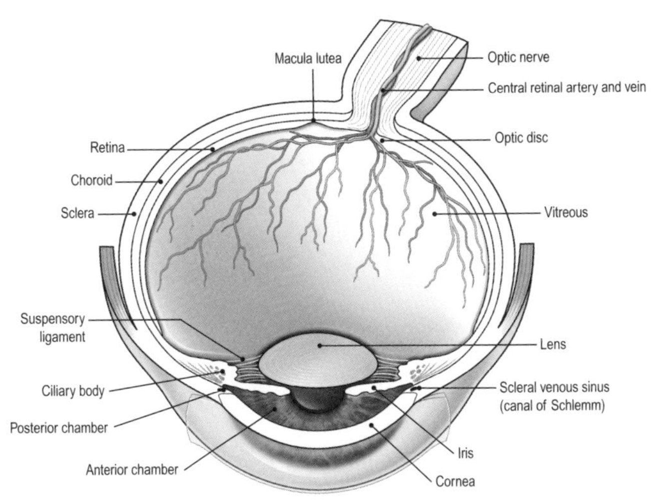

Figure 8.4

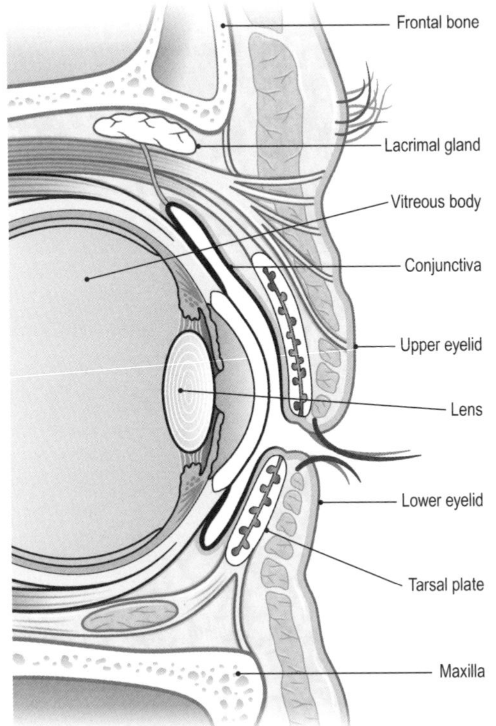

Figure 8.5

The **posterior** chamber lies between the lens and the iris, and the **anterior** chamber between the iris and the cornea. These two chambers are filled with another clear substance called **aqueous humour/fluid**, whose consistency is **watery/liquid.** This substance is secreted into the **posterior** chamber by the **ciliary glands** and drains back into the circulation via the **scleral venous sinus** (canal of **Schlemm**). Because there is continuous production and drainage, the intraocular pressure remains fairly constant. The structures in the front of the eye,

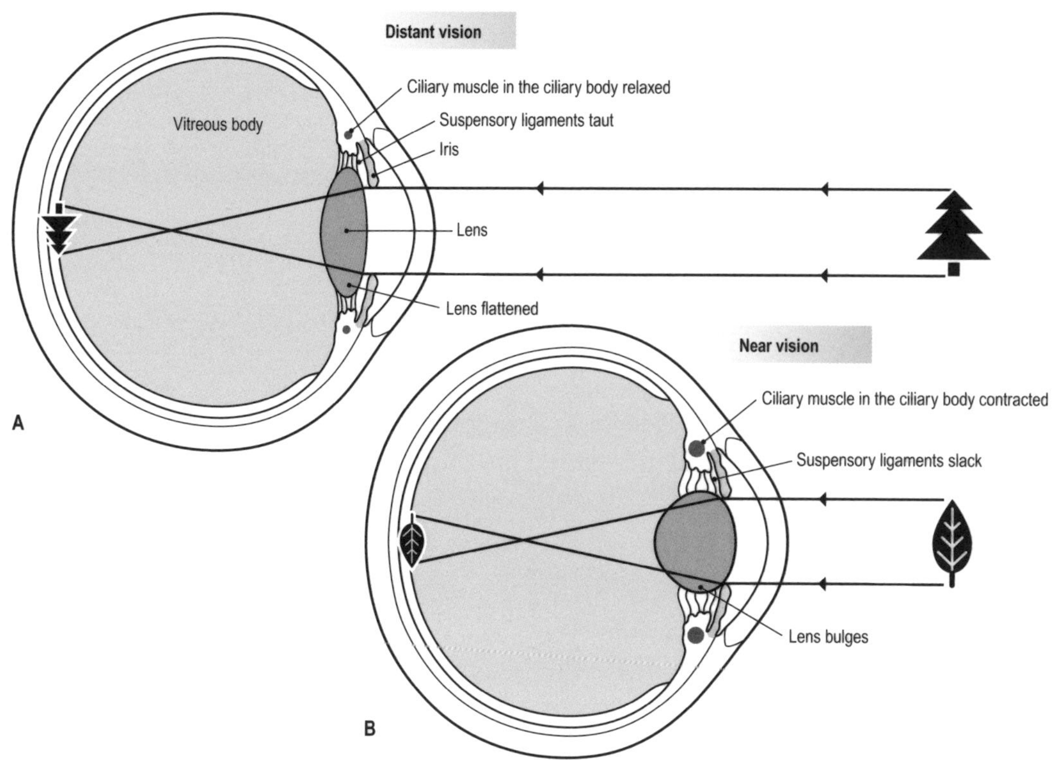

Figure 8.6

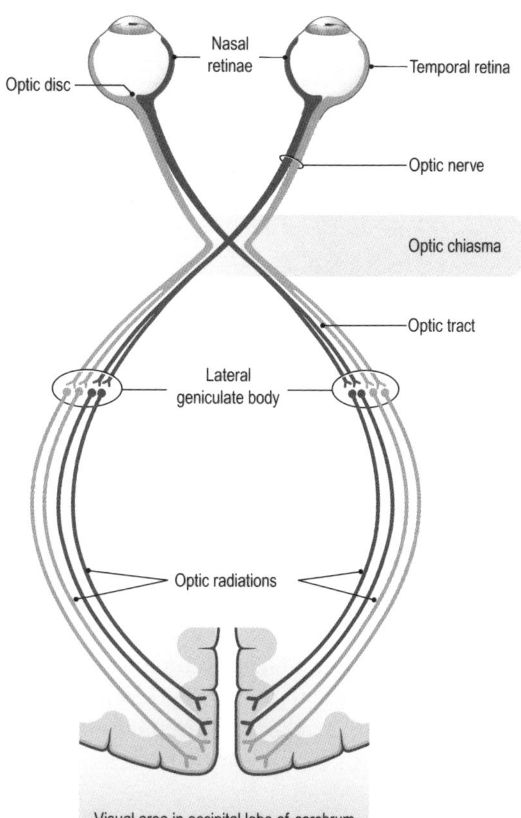

Figure 8.7

including the cornea and the lens, are supplied with nutrients by the **aqueous humour/fluid.**

21. The retina lines the **eyeball.** Near the centre of the posterior part is the **macula lutea**, or yellow spot. In the centre of the yellow spot is the **fovea centralis**, which has only one type of light-sensitive receptor, the **cone.** The area where the optic nerve leaves the retina is the **optic disc**, also known as the **blind spot.**
22. The amount of light entering the eye is controlled by the **size** of the pupils. In a bright light they are **constricted** and in darkness they are **dilated.** The iris consists of two layers of smooth muscle – contraction of the circular fibres causes **constriction** of the pupil, whereas contraction of the radiating fibres causes **dilation.** The autonomic nervous system controls the size of the pupil – sympathetic stimulation causes **dilation**, whereas parasympathetic stimulation causes **constriction** of the pupil.
23. Lacrimal glands.
24. Water, mineral salts, antibodies, lysozyme.
25. Washing away irritants; the bactericidal enzyme lysozyme prevents infection; the oily secretion from the tarsal glands delays evaporation and prevents drying of the conjunctiva; nourishment of the cornea.

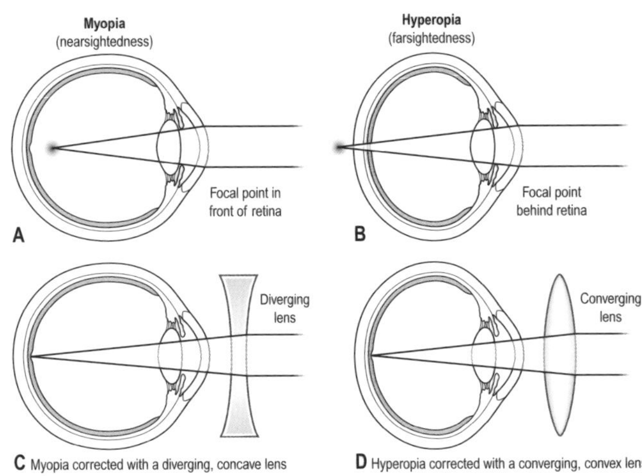

Figure 8.8

26. All odorous materials give off **volatile** molecules that are carried into the nose in the inhaled air and stimulate the olfactory **chemoreceptors.** When currents of air are carried to the **roof of the nasal cavity**, the smell receptors are stimulated, setting up impulses in the olfactory nerve endings. These pass through the cribriform plate of the **ethmoid bone** to the olfactory bulb. Nerve fibres that leave the olfactory bulb form the olfactory tract. This passes posteriorly to the olfactory lobe of the **cerebrum or cerebral cortex**, where the impulses are interpreted and odour is perceived.
27. c.
28. c.
29. c.
30. c.
31. c.
32. b.
33. a, c.
34. d.
35. a.
36. Nearsightedness – the eyeball is too long, resulting in focusing of distant images in front of the retina; close objects are focused normally.
37. Farsightedness – the eyeball is too short, causing a near image to be focused behind the retina; distant objects are focused normally.

38. and 39. See Fig. 8.8.

9 The endocrine system

Answers

1.and 2.

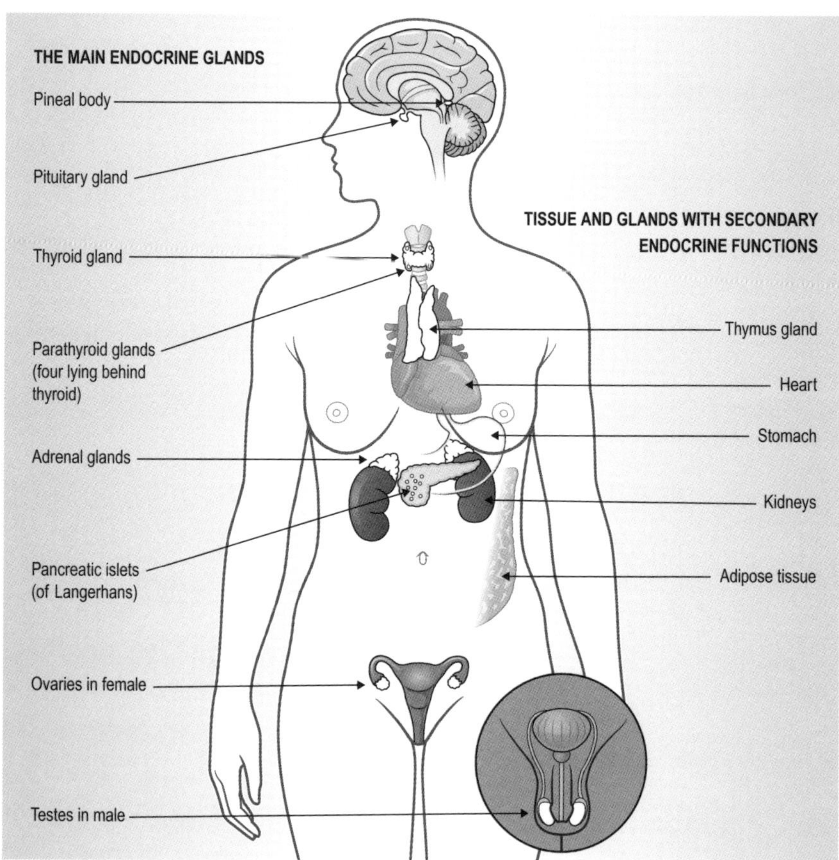

Figure 9.1

3. Hormones are formed by glands or tissues that **secrete** them into the **bloodstream** and are transported to their **target organ/tissue.** When a hormone arrives at its site of action, it binds to specific molecular groups on the cell membrane called **receptors.** Homeostasis of the **internal** environment is maintained partly by the nervous system and partly by the endocrine system. The former is concerned with **fast** changes, whereas those that involve the endocrine system are **slow** and more precise. Chemically, hormones fall into two groups – protein-based and **lipid**-based. Hormones in the first group are **water**-soluble and include **insulin**, **glucagon** and **adrenaline.** The latter group includes **steroids** and **thyroid hormones.**

4.

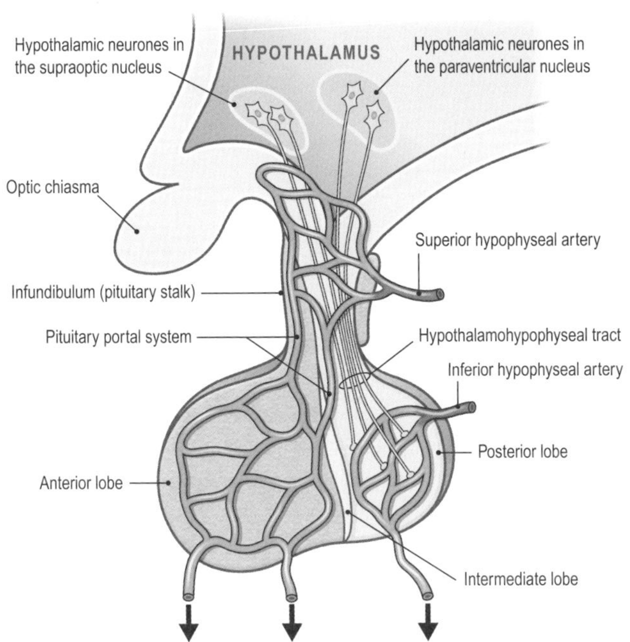

Figure 9.2

5. Oxytocin and antidiuretic hormone (ADH).

6. Oxytocin.

7.

Table 9.1 Summary of the hormones secreted by the anterior pituitary gland

Hormone	Abbreviation	Function
Growth hormone	GH	Regulates metabolism, promotes tissue growth – especially bone
Thyroid-stimulating hormone	TSH	Stimulates growth and activity of the thyroid gland
Adrenocorticotropic hormone	ACTH	Stimulates the adrenal glands to secrete glucocorticoids
Prolactin	PRL	Stimulates milk production in the mammary glands
Follicle-stimulating hormone	FSH	Males: Stimulates production of sperm in the testes Females: Stimulates secretion of oestrogen in the ovaries, maturation of ovarian follicles, ovulation
Luteinising hormone	LH	Males: Stimulates secretion of testosterone in the testes Females: Stimulates secretion of progesterone by the corpus luteum

8. Negative feedback means that any movement of such a control system away from its normal set point is negated (reversed). If a variable rises, negative feedback brings it down again and if it falls, negative feedback brings it back up to its normal level. The response to a stimulus therefore reverses the effect of that stimulus, keeping the system in a steady state and maintaining homeostasis.

9. A. Anterior lobe of pituitary gland. B. Target gland

10. i. Releasing hormones. ii. Trophic hormones. iii. Raised. iv. Lowered.

11. An increase in the rate of urine production is called **diuresis.** ADH is secreted by the **posterior** pituitary gland; its main effect is to **decrease** urine output. It does this by **increasing** the permeability of the **distal** convoluted tubules and **collecting** ducts in the nephrons to **water**, thereby increasing its reabsorption from the filtrate. ADH secretion is stimulated by increased **osmotic pressure** of the blood, which is detected by **osmo**receptors in the hypothalamus – for example, during **dehydration** and **haemorrhage (shock).** In more serious situations, ADH also causes **contraction** of smooth muscle, causing **vasoconstriction** in small arteries. This has a pressor effect – that is, it increases **blood pressure** – reflecting the alternative name of this hormone, **vasopressin.**

12.

Table 9.2 Effects of abnormal secretion of thyroid hormones

Body function affected	Hypersecretion of T_3 and T_4	Hyposecretion of T_3 and T_4
Metabolic rate	Increased	Decreased
Weight	Loss	Gain
Appetite	Good	Poor, anorexia
Mental state	Anxious, excitable, restless	Depressed, lethargic, mentally slow
Scalp	Hair loss	Brittle hair
Heart	Tachycardia, palpitations, atrial fibrillation	Bradycardia
Skin	Warm and sweaty	Dry and cold
Faeces	Loose – diarrhoea	Dry – constipation
Eyes	Exophthalmos	None

13. and 14. See Fig. 9.3.

15. The adrenal glands are situated on the **upper** pole of each kidney. The outer part of the gland is the **cortex** and **is** essential for life. The adrenal **cortex** secretes steroid hormones which are formed from **cholesterol.** There are **three** groups of steroid hormones. The main group is

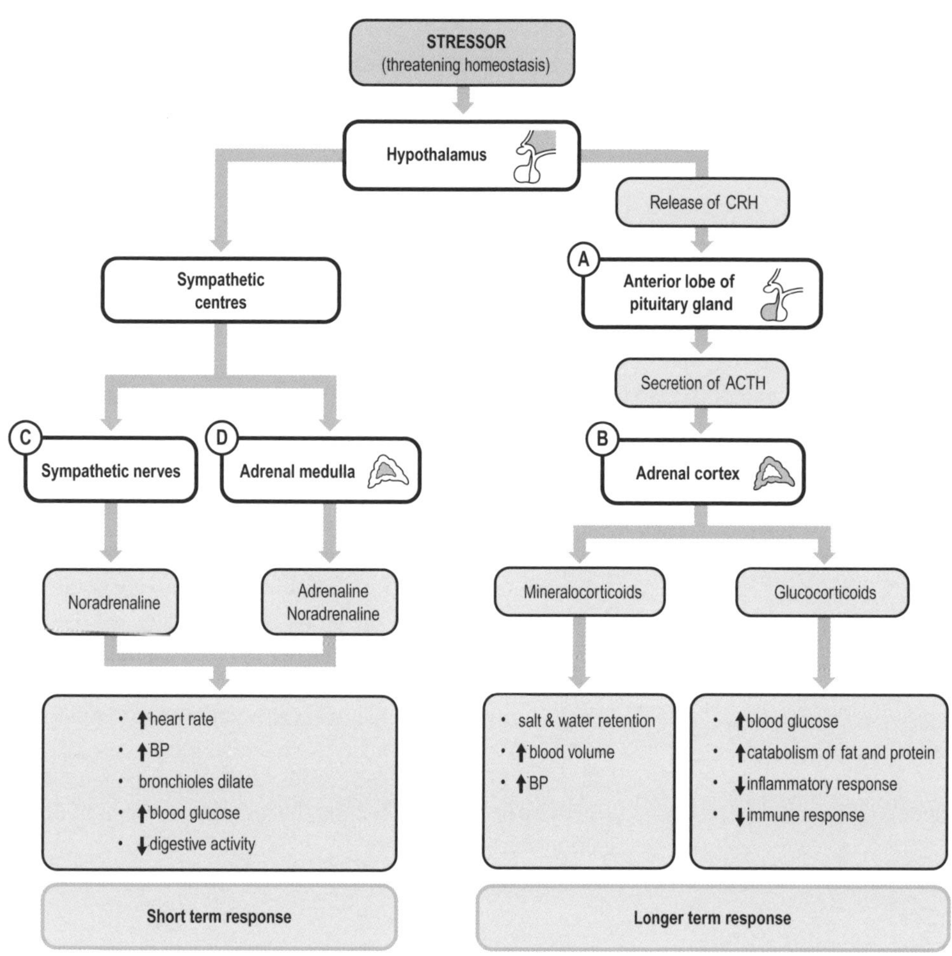

Figure 9.3

the **glucocorticoids.** The adrenal **medulla** secretes the hormones adrenaline and noradrenaline, which occurs in response to stimulation of the **sympathetic** nervous system.

16. a. T; b. F; c. T; d. F; e. T.

17. There are **four** parathyroid glands located on **the posterior lobes** of the thyroid gland. They secrete parathyroid hormone; blood calcium levels regulate its secretion. When they **fall**, secretion of PTH is increased and vice versa. The main function of PTH is to **increase** the blood calcium level. This is achieved by **increasing** the amount of calcium absorbed from the small intestine and reabsorbed from the renal tubules. If these sources do not provide adequate calcium levels, the PTH stimulates **osteoclasts** (bone destroying cells) and calcium is released into the blood from **bones.** Normal blood calcium levels are needed for muscle **contraction**, blood clotting and nerve impulse transmission.

18. a. beta (β); alpha (α); delta (δ).

19. a. T; b. F; c. T; d. F; e. F; f. T; g. F; h. T.

20. a, b, c.

21. a.

22. a.

23. c, d.

24. c.

25. b

26. c, d.

27. a, b, c.

28. c.

29. a, b, c.

10 The respiratory system

Answers

1. and 2.

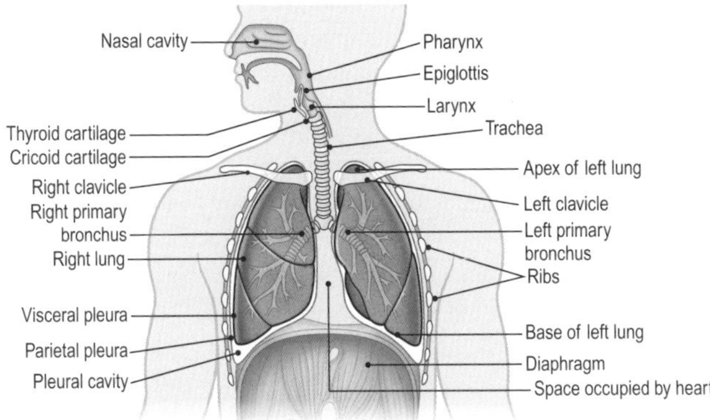

Figure 10.1

3. and 4.

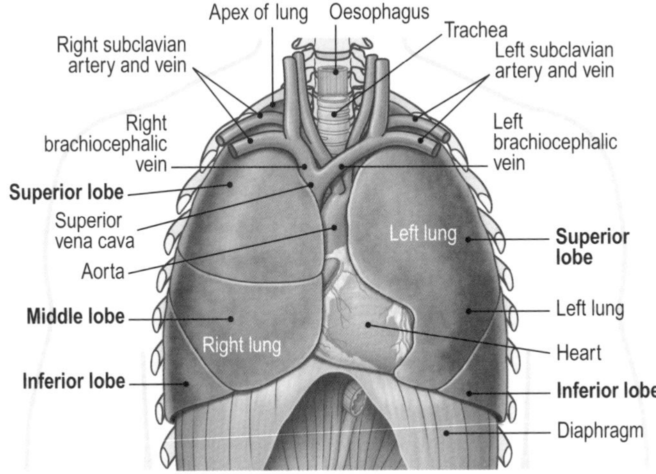

Figure 10.2

5.

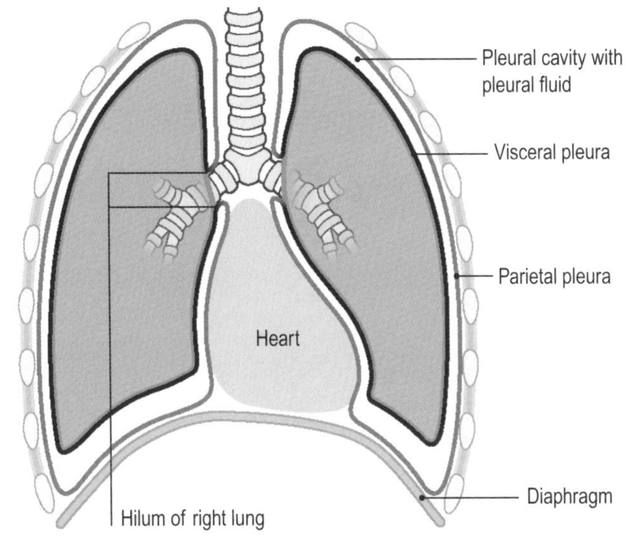

Figure 10.3

6. Pleural fluid, a phospholipid fluid that allows the pleura to slide over one another and permit comfortable expansion and recoil of the lungs during breathing
7. Pulmonary arteries and veins; lymphatic vessels; nerves

8. and 9.

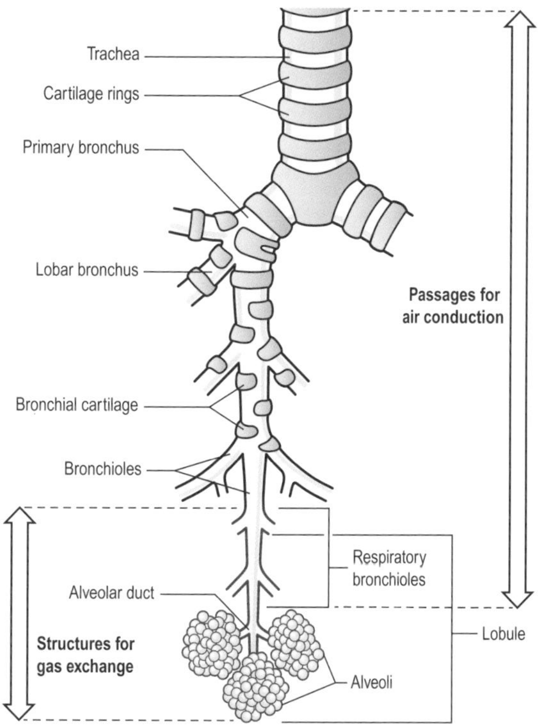

Figure 10.4

9. Arrow X: structures involved in gas exchange; arrow Y: passageways for conduction of air but not gas exchange

10.

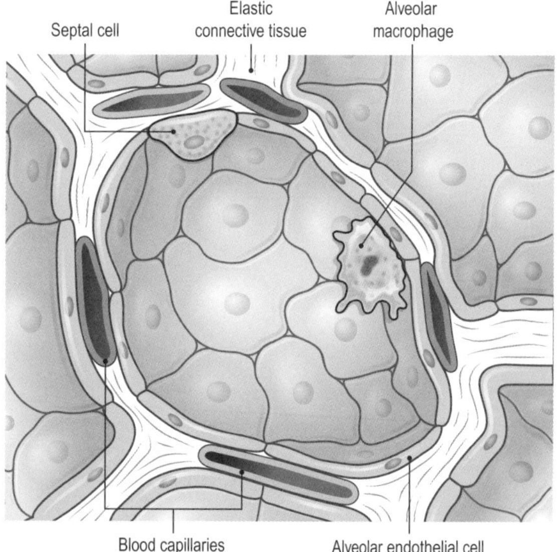

Figure 10.5

11. Cell A: septal; surfactant; surface tension. Cell B: phagocytosis; macrophage.

12. a. Goblet cell; b. larynx; c. anterior nares; d. epiglottis; e. sinus; f. nasopharyngeal tonsil; g. auditory tube.

13. a. Mucus is produced in the upper respiratory tract because this is an efficient way of removing dust and dirt from inhaled air. b. Cilia are present in the upper respiratory tract because mucus needs to be swept away from the lungs. c. Cartilage is present in the upper respiratory tract because the airways have to be kept open at all times. d. Tracheal cartilages are C-shaped because the oesophagus needs to expand during swallowing.

14. The right and left nasal cavities are separated by a plate of bone called the **septum**, which is formed mainly from two facial bones, the **ethmoid** and the **vomer.** The anterior portion of this plate is made of **hyaline cartilage.** The floor of the nasal cavities forms the **roof** of the mouth. Anteriorly, it is made from the **maxillary** bone, also called the **hard palate.** Posteriorly, it is made from **smooth** muscle, is called the **soft palate**, and may be seen through the widely open mouth hanging down in the throat; this section is called the **uvula.** The lateral walls of the nasal cavities are formed partly from the ethmoid bone, which is folded into intricate scroll-like shapes called **conchae**, and are covered in a very vascular **mucous** membrane. The main function of the upper respiratory tract is to **warm, moisten** and **clean** inspired air.

15. The lungs are **nonidentical** in shape and size and their **medial** surfaces face each other across the space between them. Major structures enter and leave the lung through the **medial** surfaces at the area called the **hilum/root.** The broad outer surface of the lungs that lies against the ribs is called the **costal** surface; the surface lying against the diaphragm is the **base**, and the lung tip, also called the **apex**, rises above the clavicles. The space between the lungs is called the **mediastinum.**

16. d; 17. a; 18. c; 19. d; 20. c; 21. a; 22. b; 23. a; 24. a

25. It is very thin and has a large surface area.

26. There are very many capillaries, and the blood cells move through them in single file.

27. a. CO_2; b. CO_2; c. O_2; d. CO_2; e. O_2; f. Both; g. O_2; h. O_2; i. CO_2.

28. External respiration

29., 30. and 31.

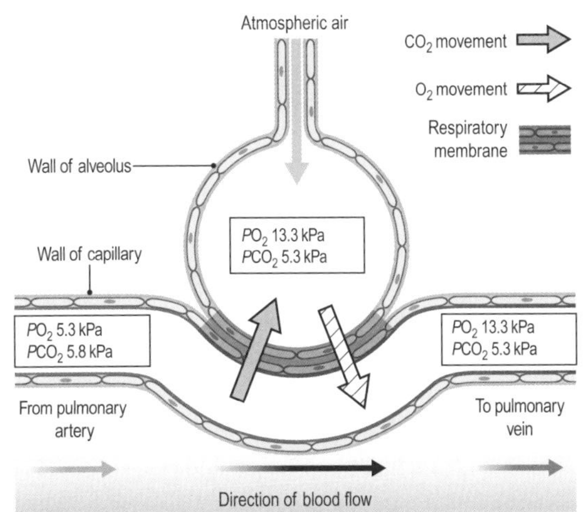

Figure 10.6

32. Internal respiration

33. and 34.

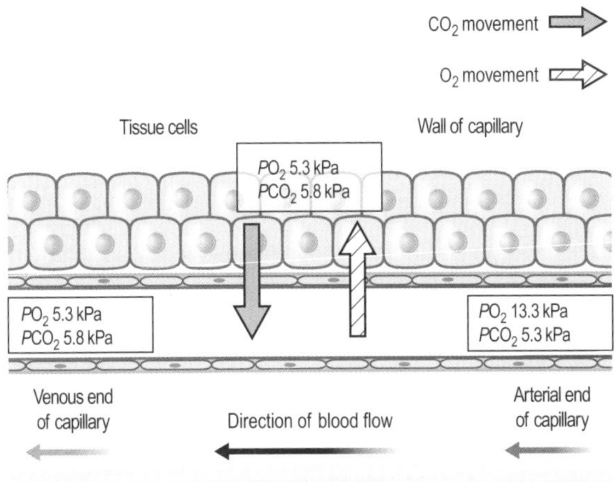

Figure 10.7

35. a. Both; b. IR; c. ER; d. Both; e. IR; f. IR.

36. a. Carbon dioxide diffuses from the body cells into the bloodstream because PCO_2 is lower in the capillary than in the tissues. b. Tissue levels of oxygen are lower than blood levels because body cells are continuously using oxygen. c. Oxygen diffuses out of the capillary because PO_2 is lower in the tissues than in the bloodstream. d. The arterial end of the capillary is higher in oxygen than the venous end because as the blood flows through the tissues it releases oxygen into the cells.

37. Just before inspiration commences, the diaphragm is **relaxed**; this occurs in the pause between breaths in normal quiet breathing. Inspiration commences. The rib cage moves **upwards** and **outwards** owing to contraction of the **intercostal muscles.** The diaphragm **contracts** and moves **downwards.** This **increases** the volume of the thoracic cavity, and **decreases** the pressure. Because of these changes, air moves **into** the lungs, and the lungs **inflate.** Inspiration has taken place.
Unlike inspiration, expiration is usually a **passive** process because it requires no **muscular effort.** So, following the end of inspiration, the diaphragm **relaxes** and moves back into its resting position. The rib cage moves **downwards** and **inwards**, because the **intercostal muscles** have relaxed. This **decreases** the volume of the thoracic cavity and so **increases** the pressure within it. Air therefore now moves **out of** the lungs and they **deflate.** There is now a rest period before the next cycle begins.

38. Increases respiratory effort: fever, pain, acidification of the CSF, exercise, high blood [H+], hypoxaemia, hypercapnia, stimulation of the respiratory centre, decreased CO_2 excretion. Decreases respiratory effort: sedative drugs, sleep, increased alkalinity of the blood, increased pH of the CSF

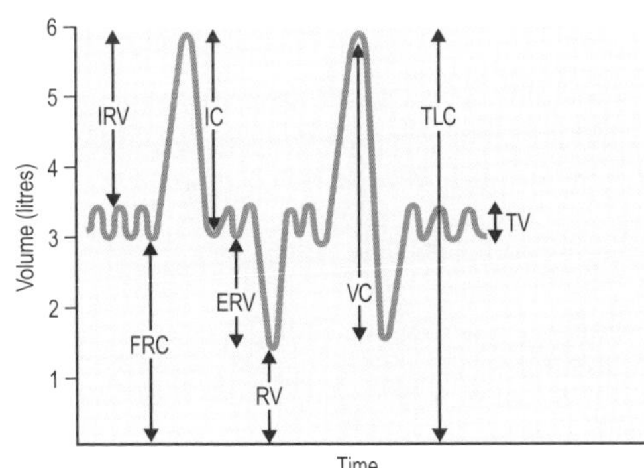

Figure 10.8

39. a. tidal volume; b. vital capacity; c. inspiratory capacity; d. residual volume; e. inspiratory reserve volume; f. expiratory reserve volume; g. total lung capacity; h. functional residual capacity.

40. a. RV; b. VC; c. IRV; d. IRV+ERV; e. TV+IRV; f. RV+IRV+ERV

41. IC is 3000 mL; IRV is 2500 mL.

42. 4800 mL.

43. 3.77 L/min.

44. Residual volume and vital capacity are fixed measures, determined by individual anatomical and physiological constraints, and in health are unaffected by exercise.

45. b; 46. b, c, d; 47. c; 48. a; 49. b, c;
50. d; 51. c; 52. d; 53. a, c; 54. d; 55. a

11 Introduction to nutrition

Answers

1. Carbohydrates, proteins, fats, vitamins, minerals.
2. a. 16.6, underweight; b. 27, overweight; c. 19.5, normal; d. 31.1, obese.
3. Growth and repair of body tissues; an alternative energy source when sufficient dietary carbohydrates and fats are not available; when broken down into their constituent amino acids, building blocks for synthesis of new proteins, e.g. enzymes, plasma proteins, antibodies, some hormones.
4. One that must be eaten in the diet because it cannot be synthesised by the body.
5. Provide energy and heat through the breakdown of monosaccharides, preferred fuel molecule is glucose and in the presence of oxygen; 'protein-sparing' – meaning that when there is sufficient dietary carbohydrate, protein can be used for its main purposes (see above) rather than as an energy source; maintaining energy stores – either as glycogen, an easily broken down short-term storage form found in the liver and skeletal muscles or as fat – long-term storage form found in adipose tissue.
6. Nonstarch polysaccharide (fibre).
7. Bulking diet and satisfying appetite; stimulating peristalsis of the intestines; attracting water that softens faeces; increasing frequency of defaecation and preventing constipation; reducing incidence of certain gastrointestinal disorders.
8. Fruit, vegetables, whole grain cereals.
9. Fats are usually divided into two groups; **saturated** fats are found in foods from animal sources, such as **meat**, **fish** and **eggs.** The second group, the **unsaturated** fats, is found in vegetable oils. Certain hormones, such as **steroids** (e.g. cortisone), are synthesised from the fatty precursor **cholesterol**, also found in the cell membrane. The same precursor substance is transported in the **blood** combined with proteins, forming lipoproteins, such as **low-density lipoprotein** (LDL). This carries **cholesterol** from the **liver** to the body cells. Excessive blood LDL levels have a **harmful** effect on health; LDL is sometimes known as '**bad cholesterol.**' Fats in a meal have the direct effect of **slowing** gastric emptying and **delaying** the return of a feeling of hunger.

   The main use of fat is as a **concentrated** source of **heat** and **energy**. It is stored in **adipose** tissue in cells called **adipocytes**. Fats enable absorption, transport and storage of the **fat**-soluble vitamins **A, D, E** and **K**. Fats are essential constituents of **myelin sheaths**, the outer covering of some nerve fibres that enables rapid transmission of impulses and **sebum**, the oily substance secreted by sebaceous glands in the skin.
10. a. Vitamins C and E; b. Vitamin C; c. Vitamin A; d. Vitamin B_6; e. Vitamin A; f. Vitamins B_1, B_2 and biotin; g. Vitamin K; h. Vitamins B_6, B_{12}, folate (folic acid); i. Pantothenic acid, Vitamin B_6; j. Vitamin B_{12}.

11.

Table 11.1 Functions of minerals

Function	Calcium	Phosphate	Sodium	Potassium	Iron	Iodine
Needed for haemoglobin synthesis					✓	
Used in thyroxine manufacture						✓
Most abundant cation outside cells			✓			
99% of body stock is found in bones	✓					
Most abundant cation inside cells				✓		
May be added to table salt						✓
Vitamin D needed for use	✓	✓				
Involved in muscle contraction	✓		✓	✓		
Used to make high-energy ATP		✓				

12. b.
13. d.
14. a.
15. c.
16. b.
17. a, b, d.
18. a, c, d.
19. a.
20. a, b, c, d.

12 The digestive system
Answers

1., 2. and 3.

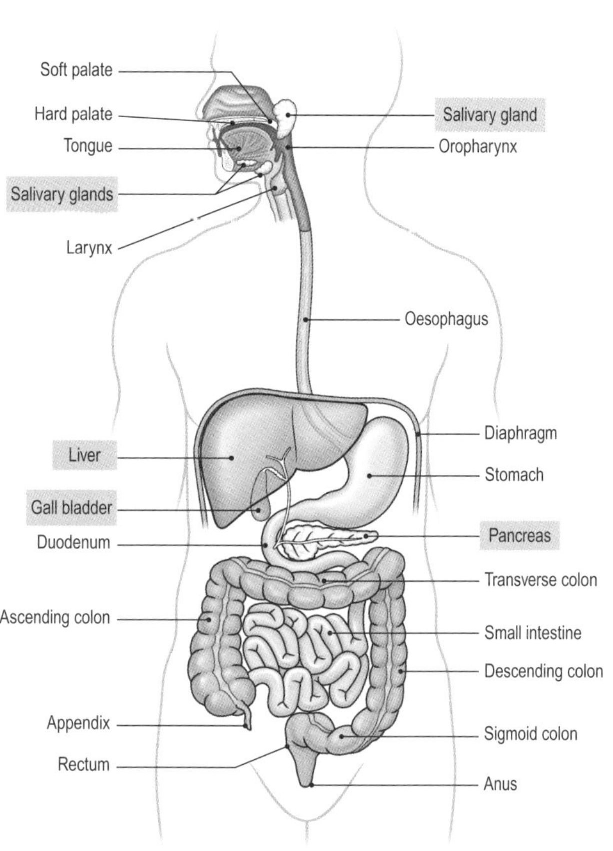

Figure 12.1

4. and 5.

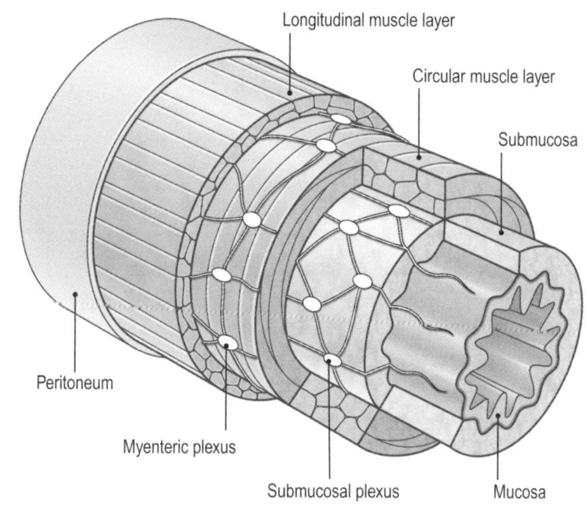

Figure 12.2

6. Columnar epithelium

7.

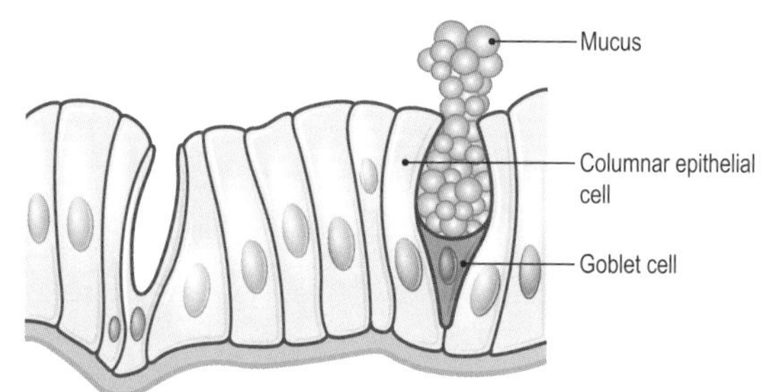

Figure 12.3

8. Mucus lubricates the foodstuffs in the gastrointestinal tract and protects the lining of the gastrointestinal tract.
9. In areas where secretion and absorption occur, such as the stomach and small and large intestine.
10. Ingestion, propulsion, digestion, absorption and elimination.
11. Mechanical digestion is the physical squeezing, chopping or cutting of food in the gastrointestinal system, such as chewing by the teeth and churning in the stomach. Chemical digestion involves the breaking down of the molecules that make up the food into smaller ones that can be absorbed; this is accomplished by the gastrointestinal enzymes.
12. a. Rhythmical contraction of smooth muscle in the walls of hollow organs and tubes, such as the alimentary canal. b. Circle of muscle surrounding an internal passageway or orifice that regulates passage of contents through the opening, such as the pyloric sphincter of the stomach.

13. a. 14. d 15. a. 16 c.

17.

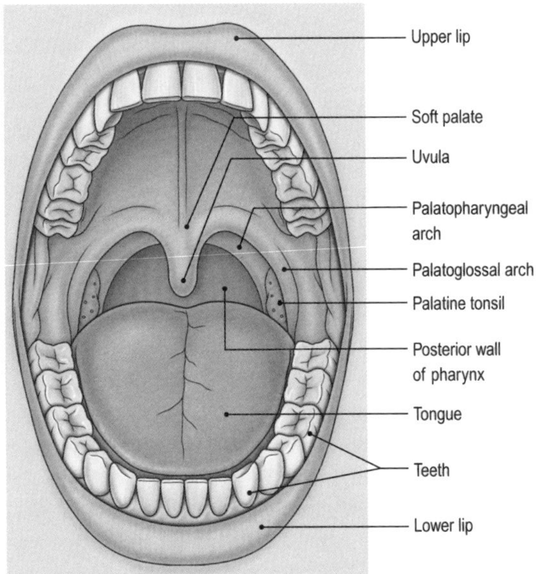

Figure 12.4

18. and 19.

- Cementum – a bonelike substance that secures the tooth in its socket.
- Dentine – layer of the tooth lying below the enamel and surrounding the pulp cavity.
- Enamel – very hard outer layer that forms the crown.

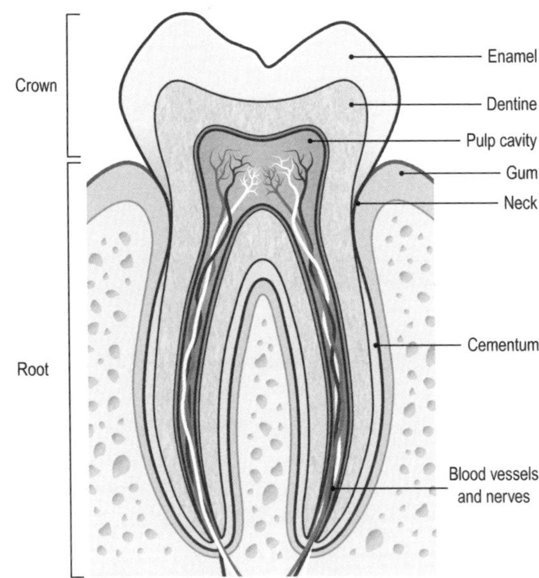

Figure 12.5

20. See Figure 12.6A

21. and 22. See Figure 12.6B

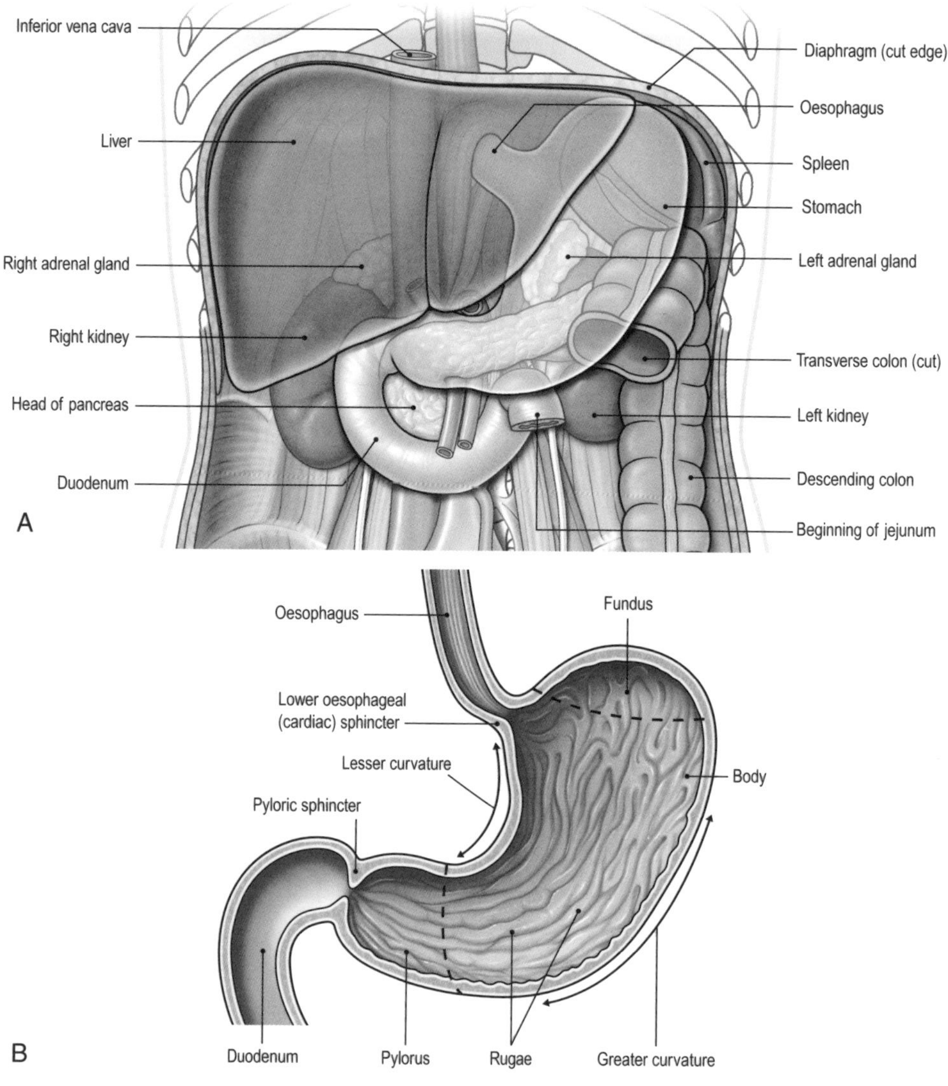

Figure 12.6

23. 3

24. Peristalsis of the three smooth muscle layers enable the stomach to act as an effective churn, mixing and breaking down its contents.

25.

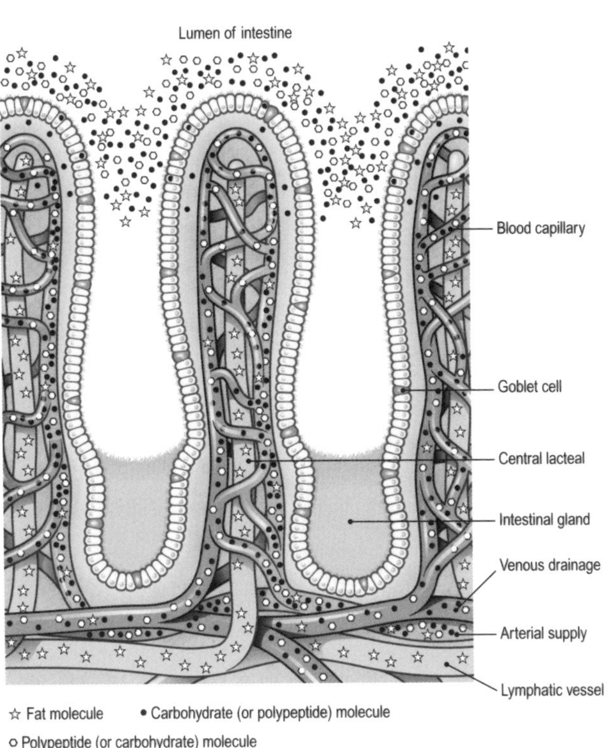

Figure 12.7

29. and 30.

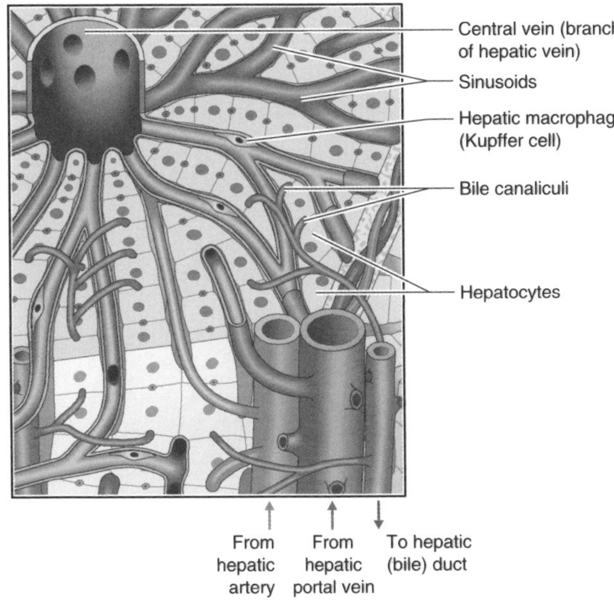

Figure 12.9

26., 27. and 28.

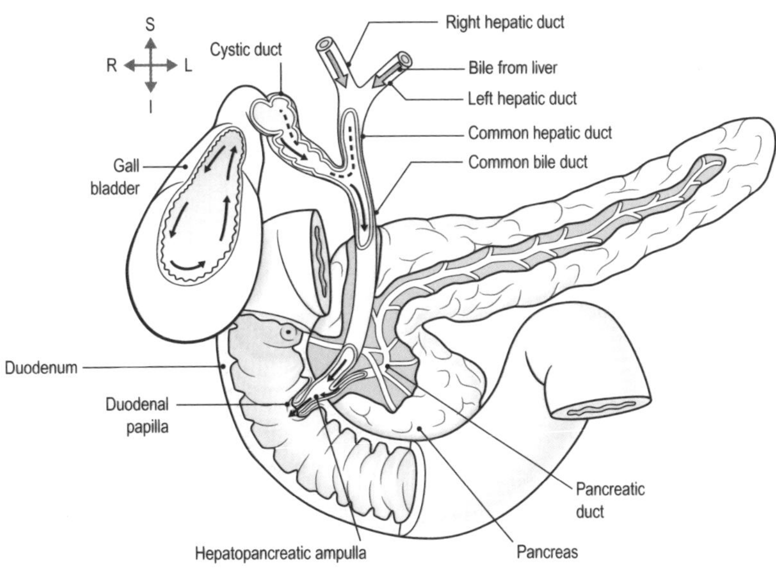

Figure 12.8

31. The arterial supply is from the hepatic artery and nourishes the liver tissues; the venous supply is from the hepatic portal vein, which brings nutrient-rich blood from the intestines for purification before being returned to the venous circulation.

32. and 33.

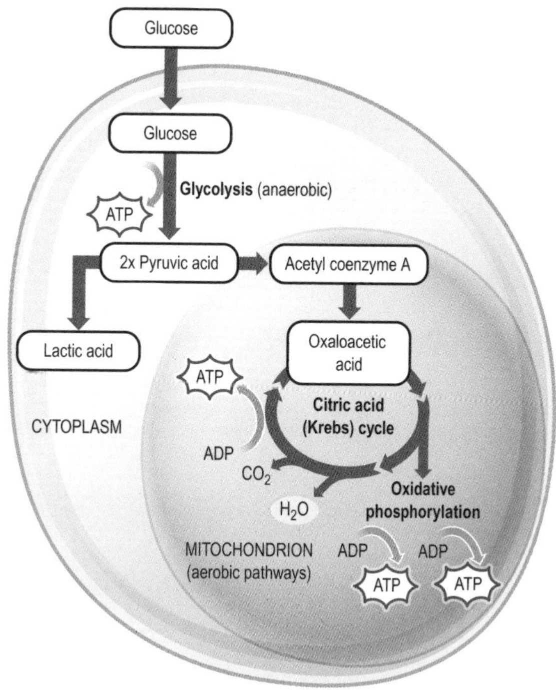

Figure 12.10

34. and 35.

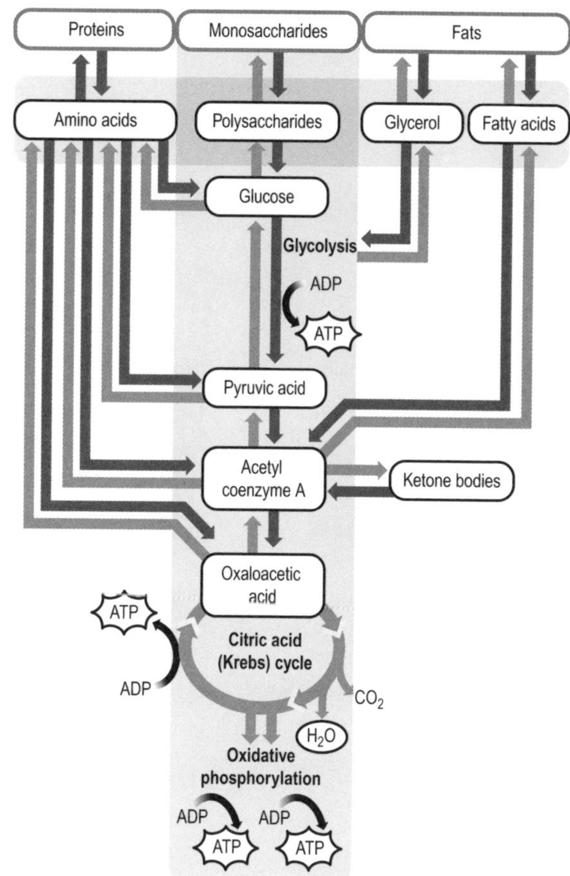

Figure 12.11

36. Oxygen.

37. Oral, pharyngeal and oesophageal.

38. a. Hydrochloric acid, intrinsic factor; b. hydrochloric acid; c. mucus; d. hydrochloric acid; e. pepsinogens; f. pepsinogens; g. pepsinogens; h. intrinsic factor; i. hydrochloric acid; j. mucus; k. pepsinogens; l. hydrochloric acid.

39. Bolus.

40. a. Catabolism is the breaking down of large molecules into smaller ones, often to release stored energy.
b. Anabolism is the synthesis of large molecules from smaller ones, usually requiring energy.

41. On a daily basis, the intestine secretes about **1500 mL** of intestinal juices, and its contents are usually acidic because the pH of the contents coming from the stomach is **acidic.** In the small intestine, chemical digestion is completed and the end products are absorbed. The main enzyme secreted by the enterocytes is enterokinase, which **activates enzymes from the pancreas.** However, other enzymes from accessory structures are passed into the **duodenum** as well.

The pancreas secretes **amylase**, which is important in reducing large sugar molecules to **disaccharides.** In addition, pancreatic lipase breaks down fats into **fatty acids and glycerol**, which can be absorbed in the intestine. The third major nutrient group, the proteins, are broken down to **dipeptides** by pancreatic **trypsin and chymotrypsin.** Pancreatic juice is also rich in **bicarbonate** ions, important in neutralising the acid chyme from the stomach.

Even after the multiple digestive actions of these enzymes, the digested proteins and carbohydrates are still not in a readily absorbable form, and digestion is completed by enzymes made by the **enterocytes.** Thus, the final stage of protein digestion produces **amino acids,** and the final stage of carbohydrate digestion produces **monosaccharides.**

42. The liver is involved in the metabolism of carbohydrates; it converts glucose to **glycogen** for storage; the hormone that is important for this is **insulin.** In the opposite reaction, glucose is released to meet the body's energy needs, and the important hormone for this is **glucagon.** This action of the liver maintains the blood sugar levels within close limits. Other metabolic processes include the formation of waste, including **urea**, from the breakdown of protein, and **uric acid**, from the breakdown of nucleic acids. Transamination is the process whereby new **amino acids** are made from **carbohydrates.** Proteins are also made here; two important groups of plasma proteins are the **clotting proteins** and the **plasma proteins.**

    The liver detoxifies many ingested chemicals, including **alcohol** and **drugs.** It also breaks down some of the body's own products, such as **hormones.** Red blood cells and other cellular material such as microbes are broken down in the **Kupffer** cells. It synthesises vitamin **A** from **carotene**, a provitamin found in plants such as carrots, and stores it, along with other vitamins. The liver is also the main storage site of **iron** (essential for haemoglobin synthesis).

    The liver makes **bile**, which is stored in the gall bladder and facilitates the digestion of **fats.** Bile salts are important for **emulsifying** fats in the small intestine and are themselves reabsorbed from the gut and returned to the liver in the **blood.** This is called the **enterohepatic** circulation, and helps to conserve the body's store of bile salts. Bilirubin is released when **red blood cells/erythrocytes** are broken down (this occurs mainly in the **spleen** and the **liver**). On its passage through the intestine, it is converted by bacteria to **stercobilin**, which is excreted in the faeces; some, however, is reabsorbed and excreted in the urine as **urobilinogen.** If levels of bilirubin in the blood are high, its yellow colour is seen in the tissues as **jaundice.**

43.

44. d.

45. b.

46. b.

47. a.

48. b.

49. d.

50. c.

51. d.

52. b.

53. a. and d.

54. b.

55. b. and d.

56. a. and c.

57. d.

58. c.

59. d.

60. b.

61. c.

62. c.

63. a.

64. c.

65. b.

66. b., c. and d.

67. c.

68. a.

Table 12.1 Functions of the pancreas

Exocrine functions	Endocrine functions
Secretion of enzymes	Secretion of insulin
Passes secretions into duodenum	Control of blood sugar levels
Secretions leave via the pancreatic duct	Secretion of hormones
Role is in digestion	Substances are passed directly into blood
Synthesis takes place in pancreatic alveoli	Secretion of glucagon
Secretions include amylase, lipase and proteases	Synthesis takes place in pancreatic islets

13 The urinary system

Answers

1., 2. and 3.

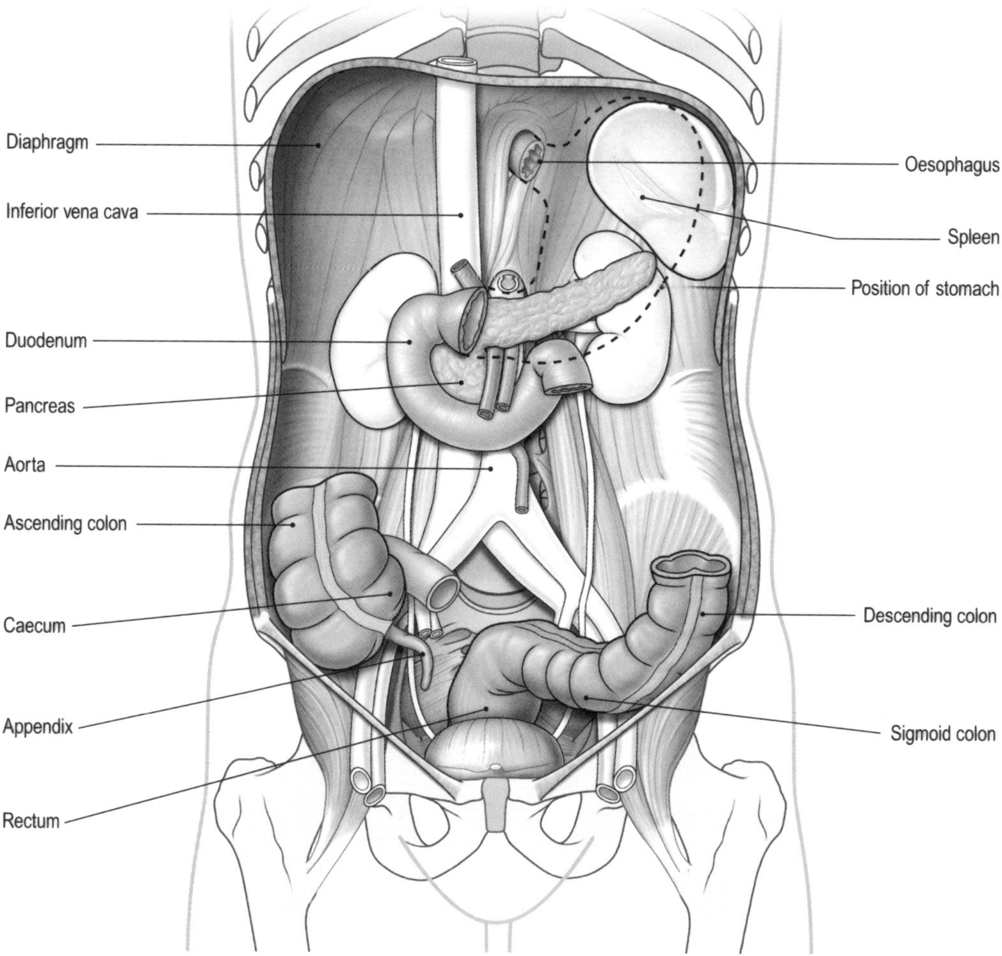

Figure 13.1

4.

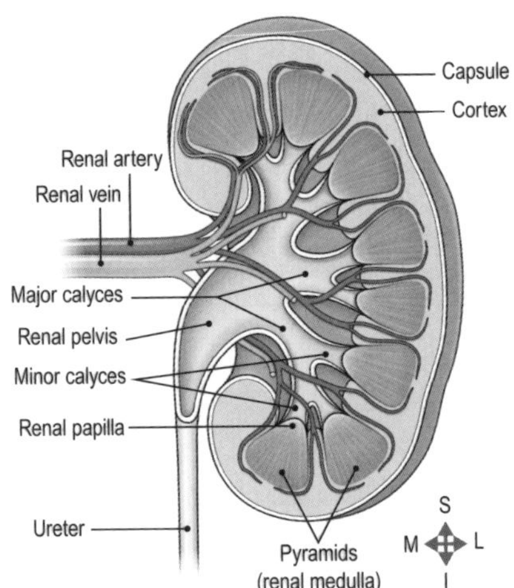

Figure 13.2

5., 6. and 7.

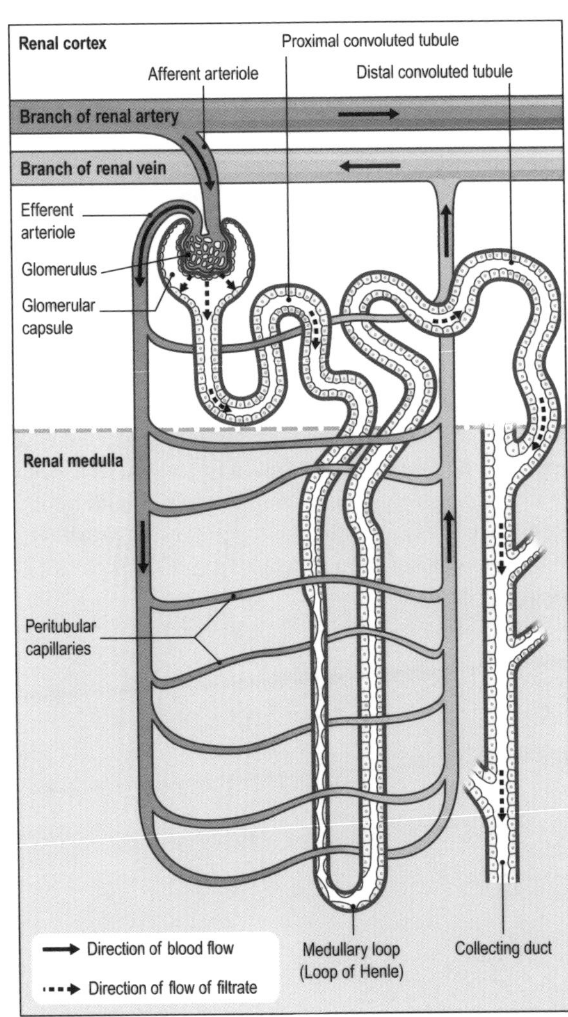

Figure 13.3

8., 9. and 10.

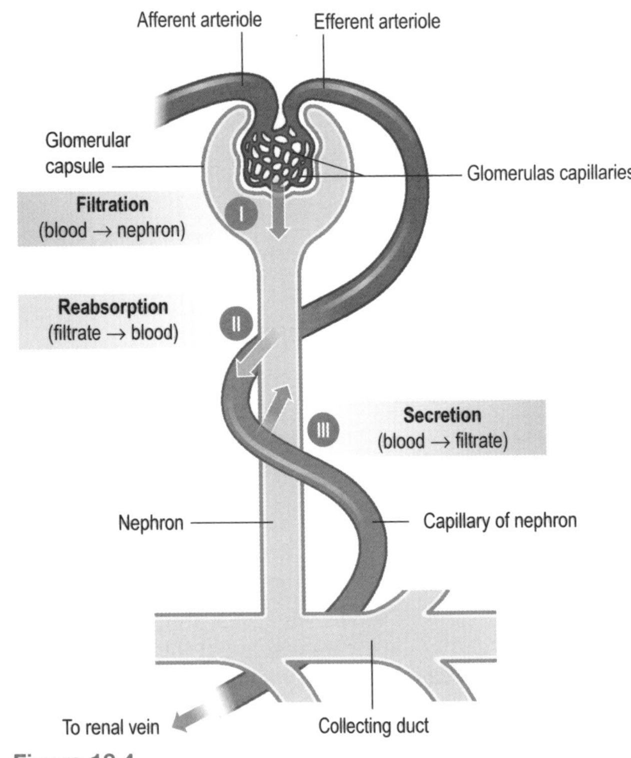

Figure 13.4

11.

Table 13.1 Normal constituents of glomerular filtrate and urine

Constituent of blood	Presence in glomerular filtrate	Presence in urine
Water	Normal	Normal
Sodium	Normal	Normal
Potassium	Normal	Normal
Glucose	Normal	Abnormal
Urea	Normal	Normal
Creatinine	Normal	Normal
Proteins	Abnormal	Abnormal
Uric acid	Normal	Normal
Red blood cells	Abnormal	Abnormal
White blood cells	Abnormal	Abnormal
Platelets	Abnormal	Abnormal

12. Water is excreted through the lungs in **saturated expired air**, through the skin as **sweat** and via the kidneys as the main constituent of **urine.** Of these three organs, the most important in controlling fluid balance are the **kidneys.** The minimum urinary output required to excrete the body's waste products is about **500 mL** per day. The volume in excess of this is controlled mainly by the hormone **ADH (antidiuretic hormone).** Sensory nerve cells, called **osmoreceptors**, detect changes in blood osmotic pressure. When the osmotic pressure increases, the secretion of ADH is **increased,** and **water** is reabsorbed by the distal collecting tubules and collecting ducts. These actions result in the osmotic pressure of the blood being **decreased.** This is an example of a **negative feedback** control system.

13. The ureters propel urine from the **kidneys** to the bladder by the process of **peristalsis.** Each ureter is about **25–30 cm** long and **3 mm** in diameter; they are lined with **transitional epithelium.** They enter the bladder at an **oblique** angle that prevents **reflux/backflow** of urine into the ureter as the bladder fills and during **micturition.**

    The bladder acts as a **reservoir** for urine. When empty, its shape resembles a **pear**, and it becomes more **oval** as it fills. The posterior surface is the **base**, and the bladder opens into the urethra at its lowest point, the **neck**. The bladder wall consists of three layers. The outer layer is composed of **connective** tissue and contains **blood** and **lymphatic** vessels. The muscular layer is formed by **smooth** muscle arranged in **three** layers. Collectively, this is called the **detrusor** and, when it **contracts,** the bladder empties. The inner layer is known as the **mucosa**. Three orifices on the posterior bladder wall form the **trigone**. The two upper openings are formed when each **ureter** enters the bladder; the lower one is the opening of the **urethra**.

14. a. True. b. The kidneys secrete renin, an important **enzyme** in the control of blood pressure. c. True. d. Atrial natriuretic peptide is a hormone secreted by the heart that **decreases** reabsorption of sodium and water by the proximal convoluted tubules. e. Antidiuretic hormone (ADH), secreted by the **posterior pituitary**, stimulates reabsorption of water from the distal convoluted tubules.

15. and 16.

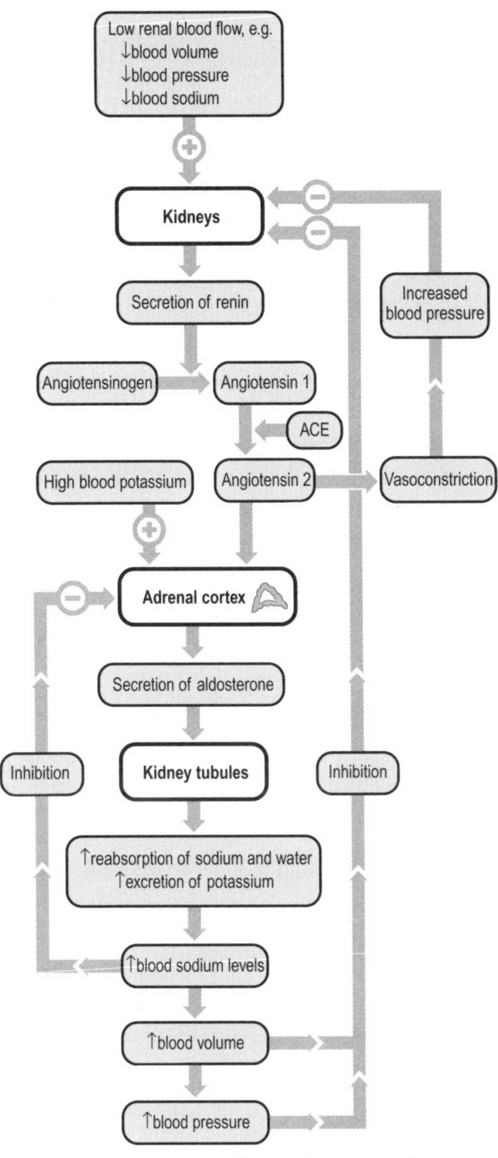

Figure 13.5

17. As the bladder fills and becomes distended, receptors in the wall are stimulated by **stretching.** In infants, this initiates a **spinal reflex,** and micturition occurs as nerve impulses to the bladder cause **contraction** of the **detrusor** muscle and **relaxation** of the **internal** urethral sphincter. When the nervous system is fully developed, the micturition reflex is stimulated, but sensory impulses pass upwards to the **brain.** By conscious effort, the reflex can be **overridden.** In addition to the processes involved in infants, there is **voluntary** relaxation of the **external** urethral sphincter.
18. d.
19. b, c, d.
20. d.
21. c.
22. d.
23. a.
24. b, c.
25. a.
26. d.
27. c.
28. b.
29. c.
30. a, c.
31. Secretion of excessive volumes of urine.
32. Excessive thirst.
33. Presence of ketones in urine.
34. Presence of blood in the urine.
35. Absence of urine.

14 The skin

Answers

1., 2. and 3.

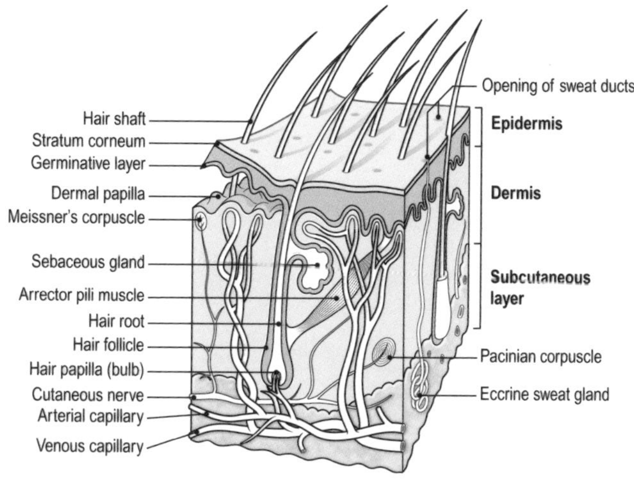

Figure 14.1

4. a. Gain; b. loss; c. loss; d. loss; e. loss; f. gain; g. loss; h. loss.

5. a. Vasoconstriction; b. conduction; c. vasodilation; d. vitamin D; e. dendritic (Langerhans) cell; f. evaporation; g. absorption; h. convection; i. nonspecific defence mechanism.

6. Body temperature is normally maintained around **36.8°C**, although it typically **rises** slightly in the evening. The temperature-regulating centre is situated in the **hypothalamus** and is responsive to the temperature of circulating **blood.** When body temperature rises, sweat glands are stimulated by the **autonomic nervous system.** The **vasomotor** centre in the medulla oblongata controls the diameter of small arteries and **arterioles** and therefore the amount of **blood** circulating in the dermis. When body temperature rises, the skin capillaries **dilate**, and extra blood near the surface increases heat loss by **radiation**, **convection** and **conduction.** The skin is warm and pale skin is **pink** in colour. When body temperature falls, arteriolar vasoconstriction conserves heat and the skin becomes **paler** and feels cool.

   Fever is often the result of **infection.** During this process, there is the release of chemicals, also called **pyrogens**, from damaged tissue. These chemicals act on the **hypothalamus/temperature-regulating centre,** which releases prostaglandins that reset the temperature thermostat to a **higher** temperature. The body responds by activating heat-generating mechanisms, such as **shivering** and **vasoconstriction**, until the new temperature is reached. When the thermostat is reset to the normal level, heat loss mechanisms are activated. There is vasodilatation and profuse **sweating** until the body temperature returns to the normal range again.

7. c.

8. c.

9. a, b, d.

10. a, b, c.

11. a, d.

12. b.

13. and 14.

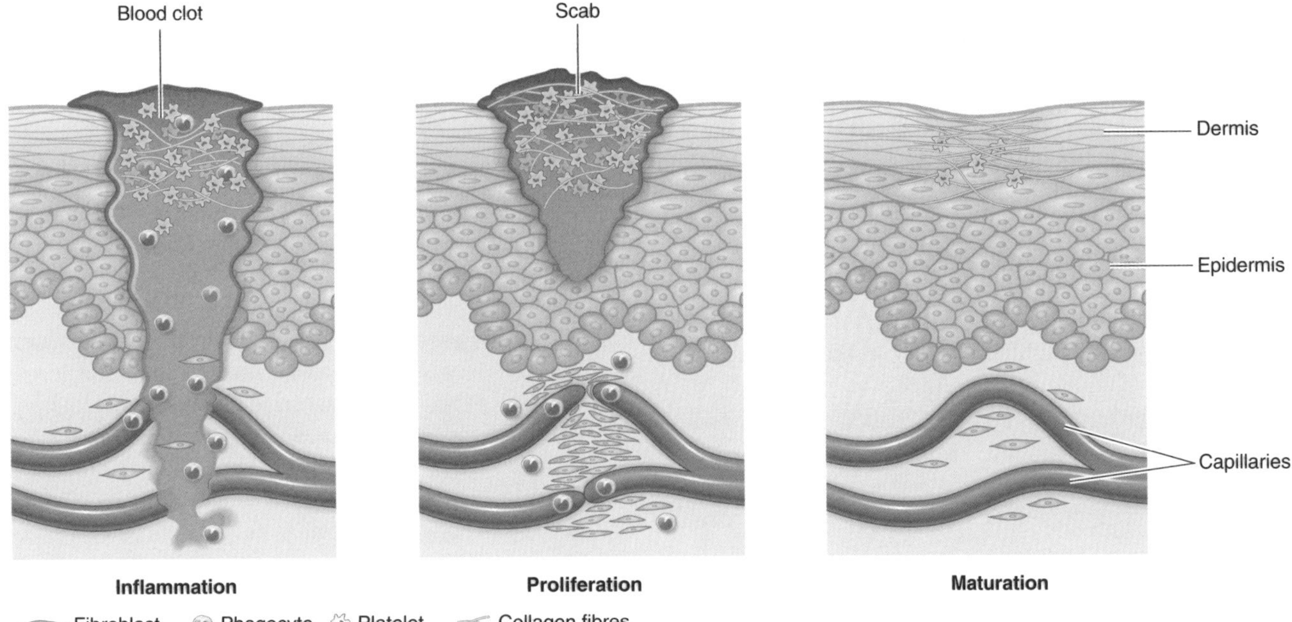

Figure 14.2

15. a. Phagocytes; b. fibroblasts; c. granulation tissue; d. granulation tissue; e. slough; f. scar tissue; g. phagocytes.

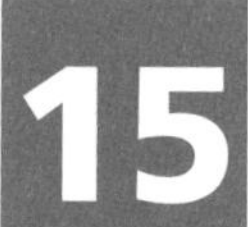

Resistance and immunity

Answers

1. a. NS; b. S; c. S; d. S; e. S/NS; f. S/NS; g. NS; h. S; i. NS; j. NS
2. a. IgE; b. IgM; c. IgA; d. IgA/IgE/IgD/IgG/IgM; e. IgA/IgC/IgM; f. IgM; g. IgE; h. IgD; i. IgA; j. IgG; k. IgM; l. IgA; m. IgG; n. IgA/IgD/IgG/IgM; o. IgG
3. and 4. See Fig. 15.1.

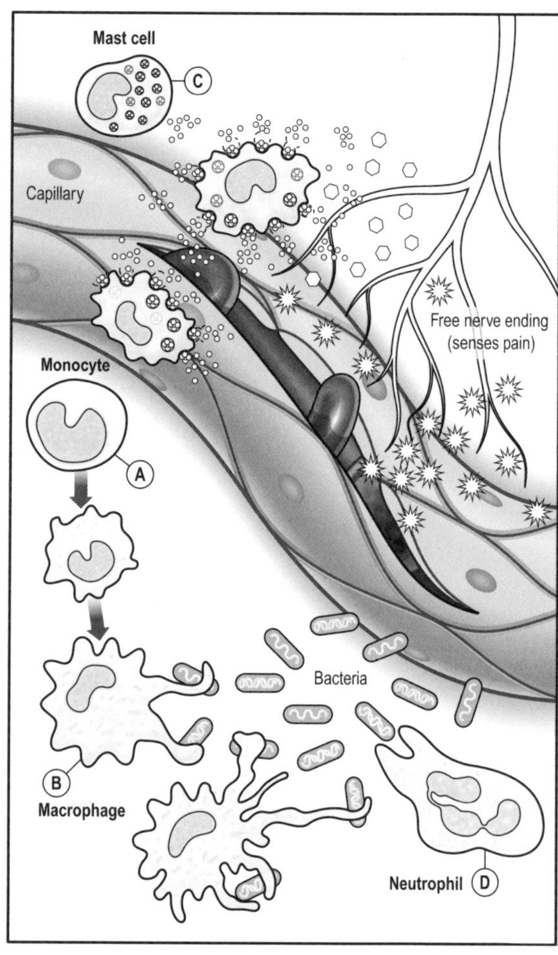

Figure 15.1

5. Cell A, a **monocyte**, travels in the bloodstream and migrates into inflamed tissues. In the tissues, it transforms into cell B, a **macrophage**, which is an active **phagocyte** that engulfs and destroys **microbes** and **cell debris.** Cell D is **smaller** and more **motile** than cell B and is also an active **phagocyte.** It usually travels in the bloodstream and migrates into inflamed tissues by the process called **diapedesis.** It is the first inflammatory cell to appear in damaged tissues. Cell C is fixed in body tissues but, in response to cell damage, releases **histamine**, an important inflammatory mediator associated particularly with **allergic** inflammation. Capillaries respond to this mediator by becoming more **permeable** and widening in diameter, also called **vasodilation.**
6. See Fig. 15.1.
7. 8. and 9. See also Fig. 15.2. Macrophages are nonspecific phagocytes which present antigen to unstimulated T-cells to stimulate an immune response. An unspecialised T-cell has receptors specific for only one antigen but has not yet encountered it; it is activated when presented with this antigen by a macrophage or other antigen presenting cell.A cytotoxic T-cell is one type of differentiated T-cell responsible for direct cell–cell killing – it identifies, attacks and destroys any cell carrying the T-cell's target antigen.A helper T-cell synthesises chemicals called cytokines to promote survival and activity of other immune cells, and is also needed to interact with B-cells to stimulate antibody production. A memory T-cell is long-lived and survives after infection is resolved; it stimulates a faster and stronger response next time, which is the basis of immunity. Regulatory T-cells turn off the immune response once the threat has been dealt with.

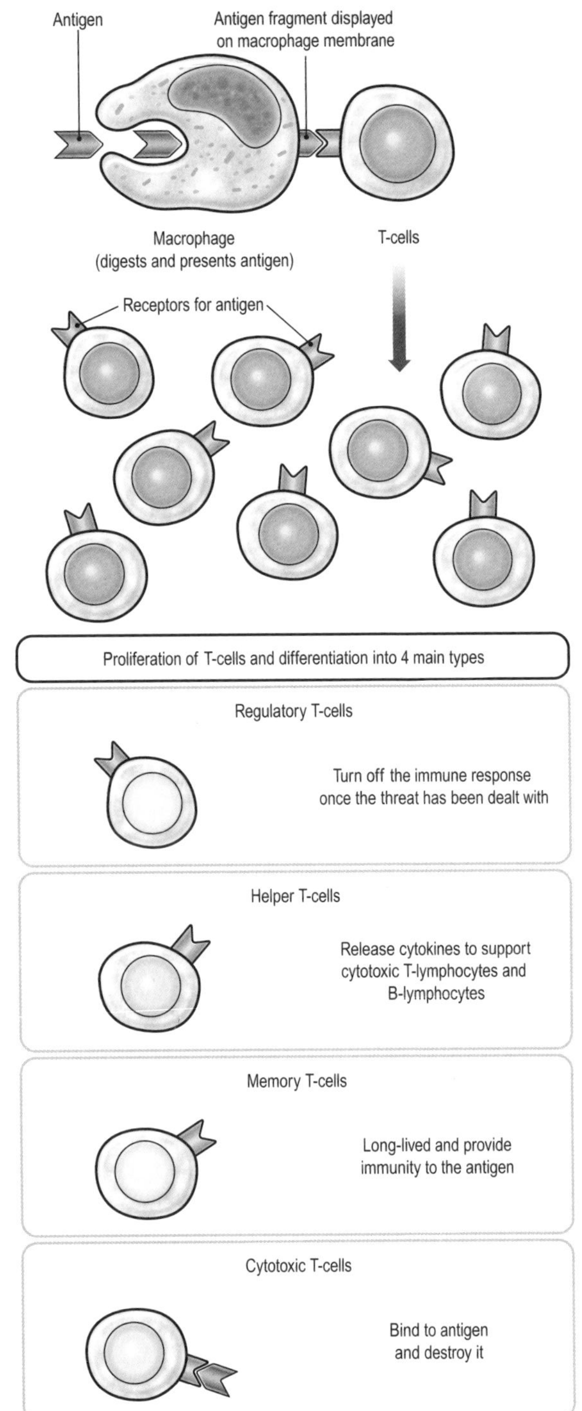
Antigen
Antigen fragment displayed on macrophage membrane
Macrophage (digests and presents antigen)
T-cells
Receptors for antigen
Proliferation of T-cells and differentiation into 4 main types
Regulatory T-cells
Turn off the immune response once the threat has been dealt with
Helper T-cells
Release cytokines to support cytotoxic T-lymphocytes and B-lymphocytes
Memory T-cells
Long-lived and provide immunity to the antigen
Cytotoxic T-cells
Bind to antigen and destroy it

Figure 15.2

9. They are all identical – clonal expansion produces different populations of T-cells which are all specific to the original antigen.
10. Clonal expansion.
11. Redness, heat, swelling, pain, loss of function
12.

Table 15.1 Summary of some important inflammatory mediators

Substance	Made by	Trigger for release	Main actions
Histamine	Mast cells in tissues and basophils in blood	Binding of antibody to mast cell or basophil plasma membrane	Vasodilation, itch, ↑ vascular permeability, degranulation, smooth muscle contraction (e.g. bronchoconstriction)
Serotonin	Platelets, mast cells and basophils; neurotransmitter in central nervous system	When platelets are activated and when mast cells/basophils degranulate	Vasoconstriction, ↑ vascular permeability
Prostaglandins	Synthesised as required from cell membranes	Many triggers, such as drugs, toxins, other mediators, trauma, hormones	Diverse, sometimes opposing, such as fever, pain, vasodilation or vasoconstriction, ↑ vascular permeability
Heparin	Liver, mast cells, basophils	When cells degranulate	Anticoagulant, maintaining blood supply to an inflamed area
Bradykinin	Tissues and blood	Blood clotting, trauma, inflammation	Pain, vasodilation

13.

Table 15.2 Lymphocyte characteristics

Characteristic	T-cell	B-cell
Shape of nucleus	Large, single	Large, single
Site of manufacture	Bone marrow	Bone marrow
Site of post-manufacture processing	Thymus gland	Bone marrow
Nature of immunity involved	Cell-mediated	Antibody-mediated
Specific or nonspecific defence	Specific	Specific
Production of antibodies	No	Yes (as plasma cells)
Processing regulated by thymosin	Yes	No

14. When the body is exposed to an antigen for the first time, the immune response can be measured as blood antibody levels after about **7 days**; this is the **primary** response. The main antibody type here is **IgM.** Antibody levels fall thereafter and do not rise again unless there is a further exposure to the same antigen, which stimulates a **secondary** response. This is different to the first in that it is **faster** and is characterised by high levels of **IgG.** Immunity to an antigen depends on the production of a population of **memory** cells.

    Immunity is not constant throughout life. Unborn babies are vulnerable to infections because **they do not make their own antibodies.** In older age, the immune system can become less efficient. One significant difference in the ageing immune system is **higher levels of autoantibodies.** Additionally, cancer, more common in later years of life, is usually associated with **less efficient immunological surveillance.**

15.

Table 15.3 The four types of acquired immunity

Characteristic	Active natural	Active artificial	Passive natural	Passive artificial
An example is a baby's consumption of antibodies in its mother's milk			✓	
Long-lived protection	✓	✓		
Involves production of memory cells	✓	✓		
An example is vaccination		✓		
Short-lived protection			✓	✓
An example is infusion of antibodies				✓
Involves production of antibodies by the individual	✓	✓		
An example is a child catching chickenpox at school	✓			
Specific	✓	✓	✓	✓

16. b, c; 17. c; 18. a; 19. d; 20. a; 21. b; 22. c;
23. d; 24. b; 25. a, b, c, d; 26. a, c; 27. b;
28. a; 29. a; 30. d; 31. d; 32. a; 33. d; 34. c

16 The musculoskeletal system

Answers

1. and 2.

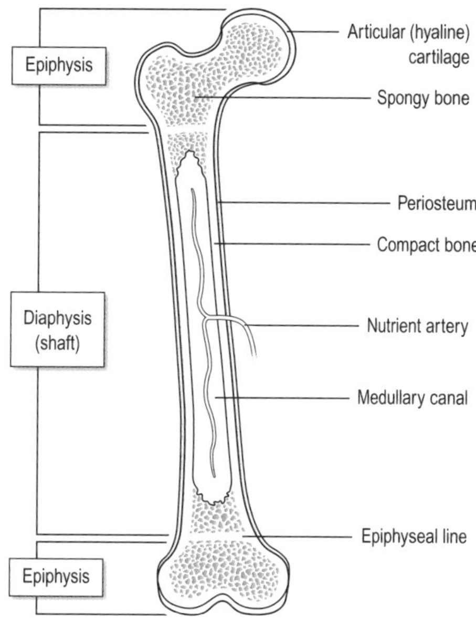

Figure 16.1

3. The spongy bone in the bone ends
4. and 5.

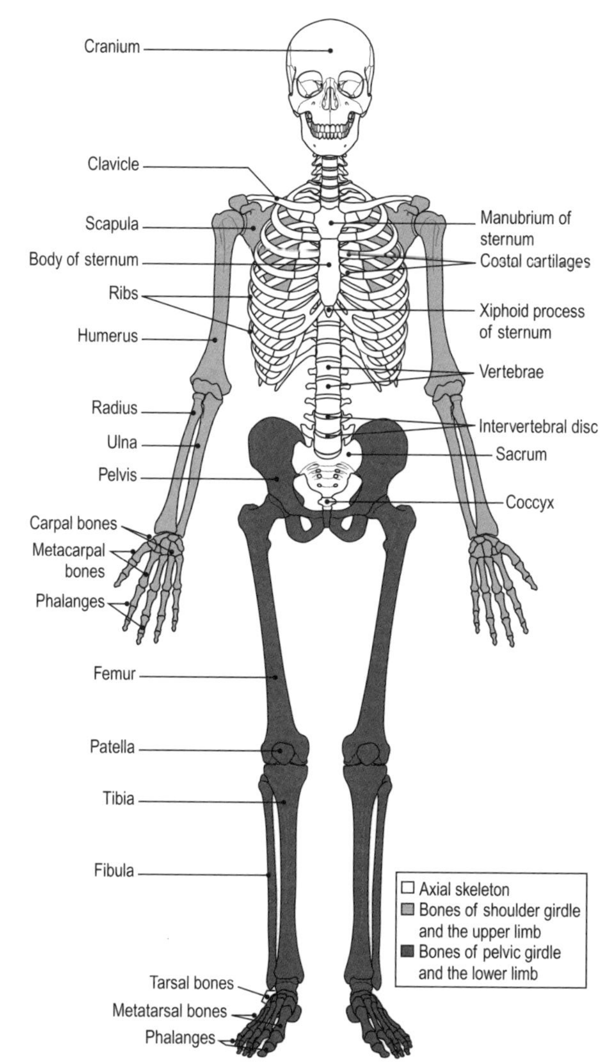

Figure 16.2

6. and 7.

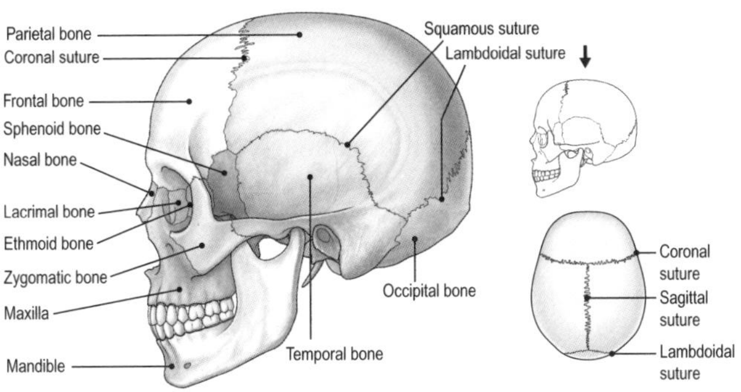

Figure 16.3

8. A. vertebral body; B. Vertebral arch; C. Vertebral foramen; D. Pedicle; E. Transverse process; F. Lamina; G. Spinous process; H. Superior articular process
9. The spinal cord
10. and 11.

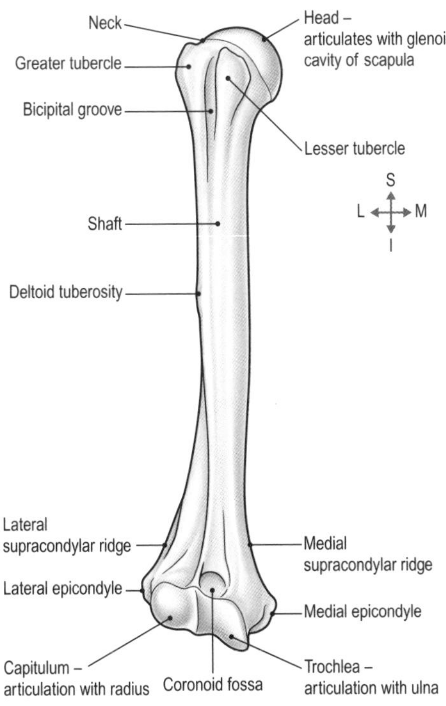

Figure 16.5

12., 13. and 14.

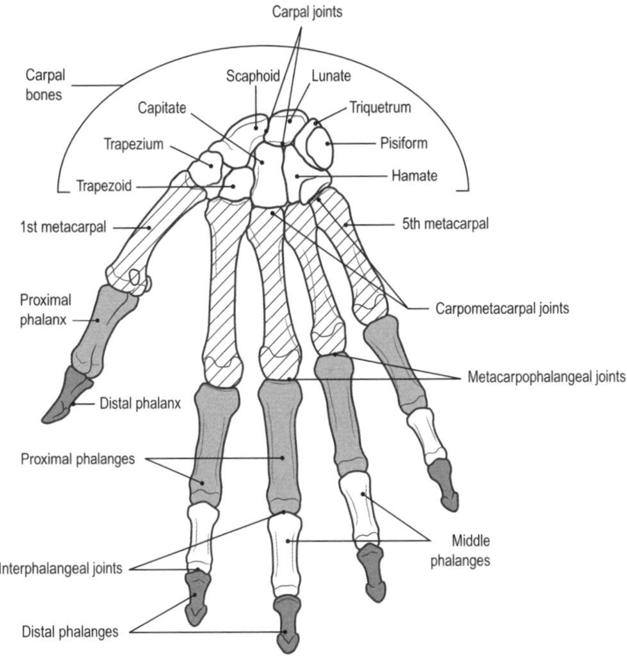

Figure 16.6

15. and 16.

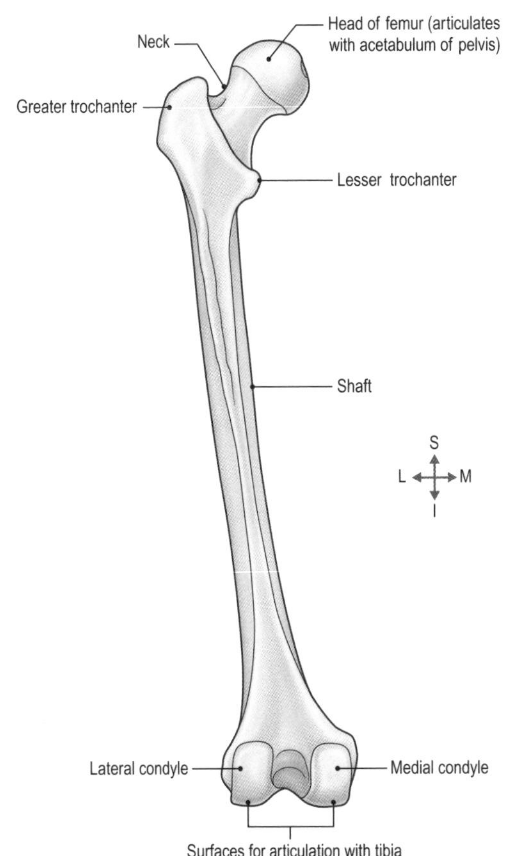

Figure 16.7

17. and 18.

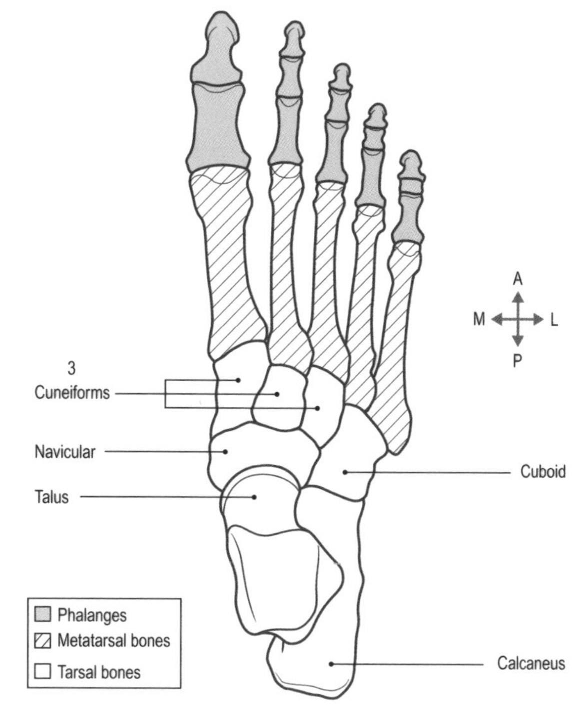

Figure 16.8

19. Long bones: e.g. humerus, radius, ulna, femur, tibia, fibula, metacarpals, metatarsals, phalanges. Short bones: e.g. carpal and tarsal bones. Irregular bones: e.g. vertebrae. Flat bones: e.g. sternum, ribs, cranial bones. Sesamoid bones: e.g. patella, sutural bones.

20. Sinuses contain **air** and are found in the **sphenoid**, **ethmoid**, **maxillary** and **frontal** bones. They all communicate with the **nasal cavity** and are lined with **ciliated epithelium.** Their functions are to give **resonance** to the voice and **lighten** the bones of the face and cranium. Fontanelles are distinct **membranous** areas of the skull in infants and are present until **ossification** is complete and the skull bones fuse. The largest are the **anterior** fontanelle, present until **12–18** months, and the **posterior** fontanelle, which usually closes over by **2–3** months of age. Their presence allows for moulding of the baby's **head** during childbirth.

21.

Table 16.1 Types of fractures

Type of fracture	Characteristics
Simple	Bone ends do not protrude through the skin
Compound	Bone ends protrude through the skin
Pathological	Fracture of a bone weakened by disease

22. Presence of tissue fragments between the bone ends; poor blood supply; poor alignment of bone ends; mobility of bone ends.

23. a. False; there is no cartilage in osteoid. b. True. c. False; bone is broken down by osteoclasts. d. False; osteoclasts are enormous, with up to 50 nuclei. e. False; iron is not an important constituent of bone. f. True.

24. a. Fossa; b. border; c. trochanter; d. foramen; e. condyle; f. meatus; g. suture; h. fissure; i. crest, spine; j. facet; k. sinus.

25.

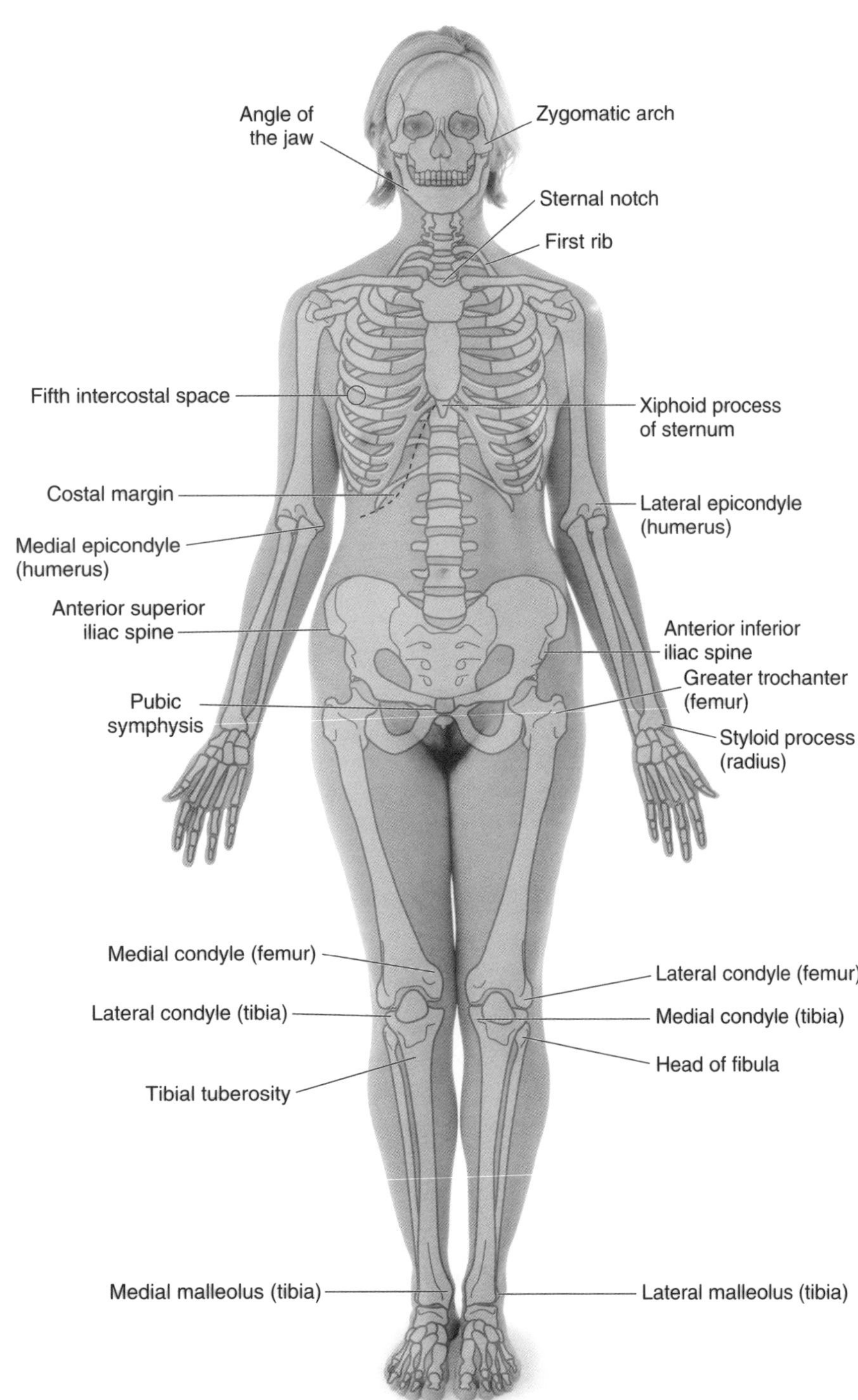

Figure 16.9 Modified from Patton K, et al: Brief Atlas of the Human Body Adapted International Edition, 2019, Elsevier.

26.

Table 16.2 Characteristics of bone

Structure	Characteristic
Spongy bone	Looks like a honeycomb to the naked eye
Osteon	Haversian system
Spongy bone	Cancellous bone
Cortical bone	Compact bone
Trabeculae	Form the framework of spongy bone
Interstitial lamellae	Remains of old osteons
Lacunae	Tiny cavities between lamellae containing osteocytes
Red bone marrow	Found mainly in spaces within spongy bone
Flat bones	Develop from membrane models
Sesamoid bones	Develop from tendon models
Long bones	Develop from cartilage models

27. Oestrogen: a, f; Testosterone: a, f; Parathyroid hormone: d, i; Calcitonin: c; Growth hormone: b, e, g, h; Thyroxine/triiodothyronine: e, g

28. a. Coccyx; b. Transverse foramen; c. Thoracic vertebrae; d. Atlas; e. Axis; f. Sacrum; g. Odontoid process; h. Body; i. Intervertebral disc; j. Annulus fibrosus; k. Nucleus pulposus; l. Spinous process.

29.

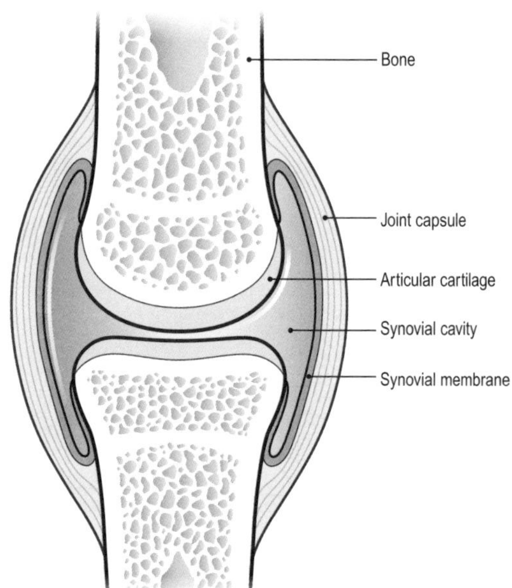

Figure 16.10

30. Epithelial tissue.

31. To cushion the joint and prevent damaging bone-bone contact.

32. and 33.

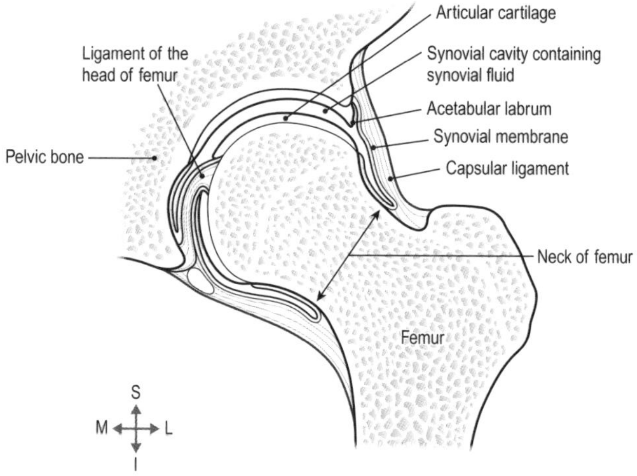

Figure 16.11

34. Neck of femur: see Fig. 16.10

35. Ball and socket

36.

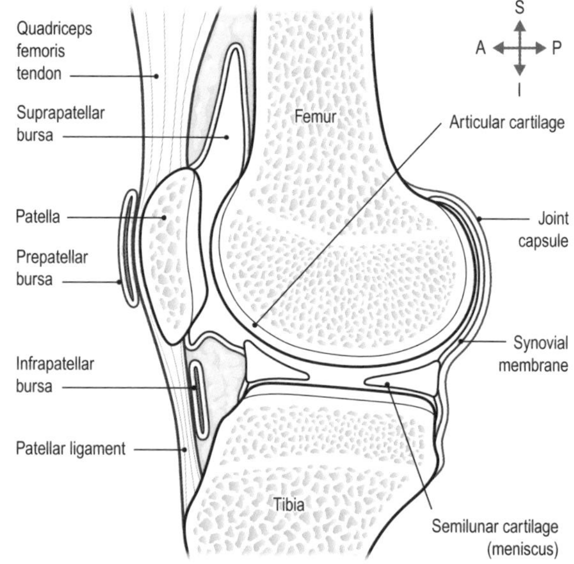

Figure 16.12

37. a. Flexion; b. Extension; c. Abduction; d. Adduction; e. Circumduction; f. Rotation; g. Pronation; h. Supination; i. Inversion; j. Eversion.

38.

Table 16.3 Joints and movements

Joint	Type (S, F or C)	Movement (I, SI, Fr)
Suture	F	I
Tooth in jaw	C	I
Shoulder joint	S	Fr
Symphysis pubis	C	SI
Knee joint	S	Fr
Interosseous membrane	F	SI
Hip joint	S	Fr
Joint between phalanges	S	Fr
Intervertebral discs	C	SI

C, Cartilaginous; *F*, fibrous; *Fr*, freely movable; *I*, immovable; *S*, synovial; *SI*, slightly movable.

39. Nourishes the structures within the joint cavity; protects as phagocytes remove microbes and cellular debris; lubricates and maintains joint stability; keeps the ends of the bones together.

40. a. Bands of tough connective tissue which attach the bones of a joint to each other and stabilise the joint.
b. Tendons fasten muscles to bone; they provide stability and transmit the force of a contracting muscle to the bone to allow movement at a joint.

41. Bursae are fluid-filled sacs which pad, cushion and stabilise joints.

42. a; 43. b; 44. d; 45. a; 46. c; 47. b; 48. d;
49. b; 50. d; 51. a; 52. a, b, c; 53. d

54. Cardiac, smooth and skeletal

55.

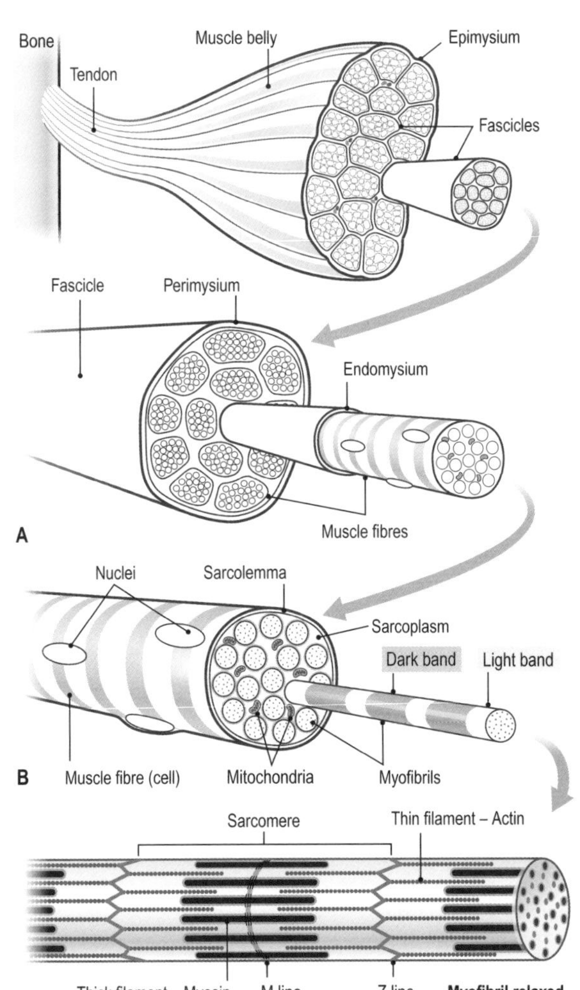

Figure 16.13

56.

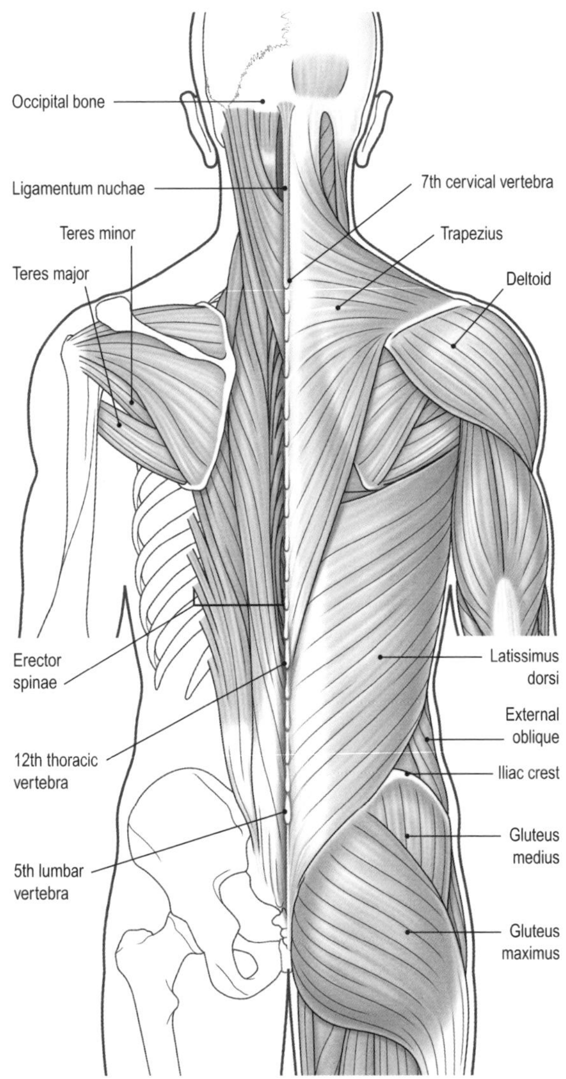

Figure 16.14

57.

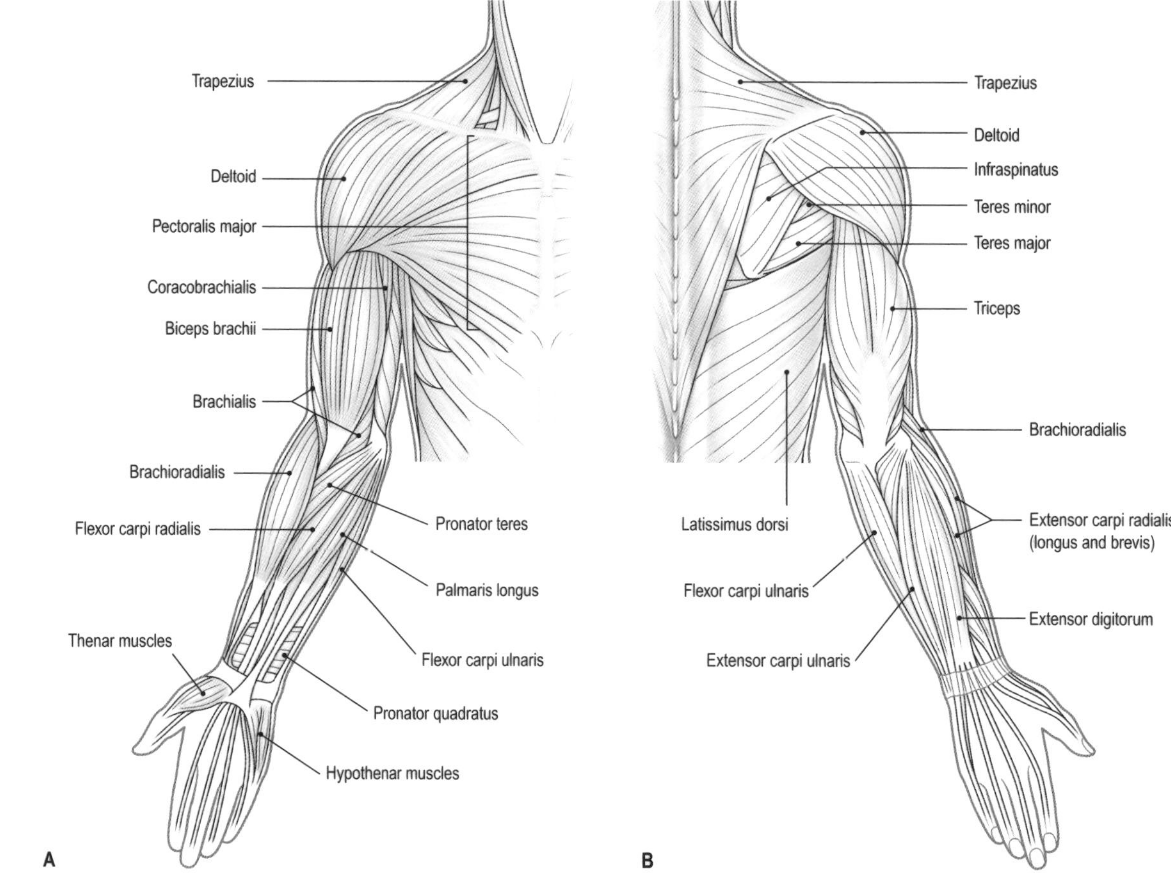

Figure 16.15

58.

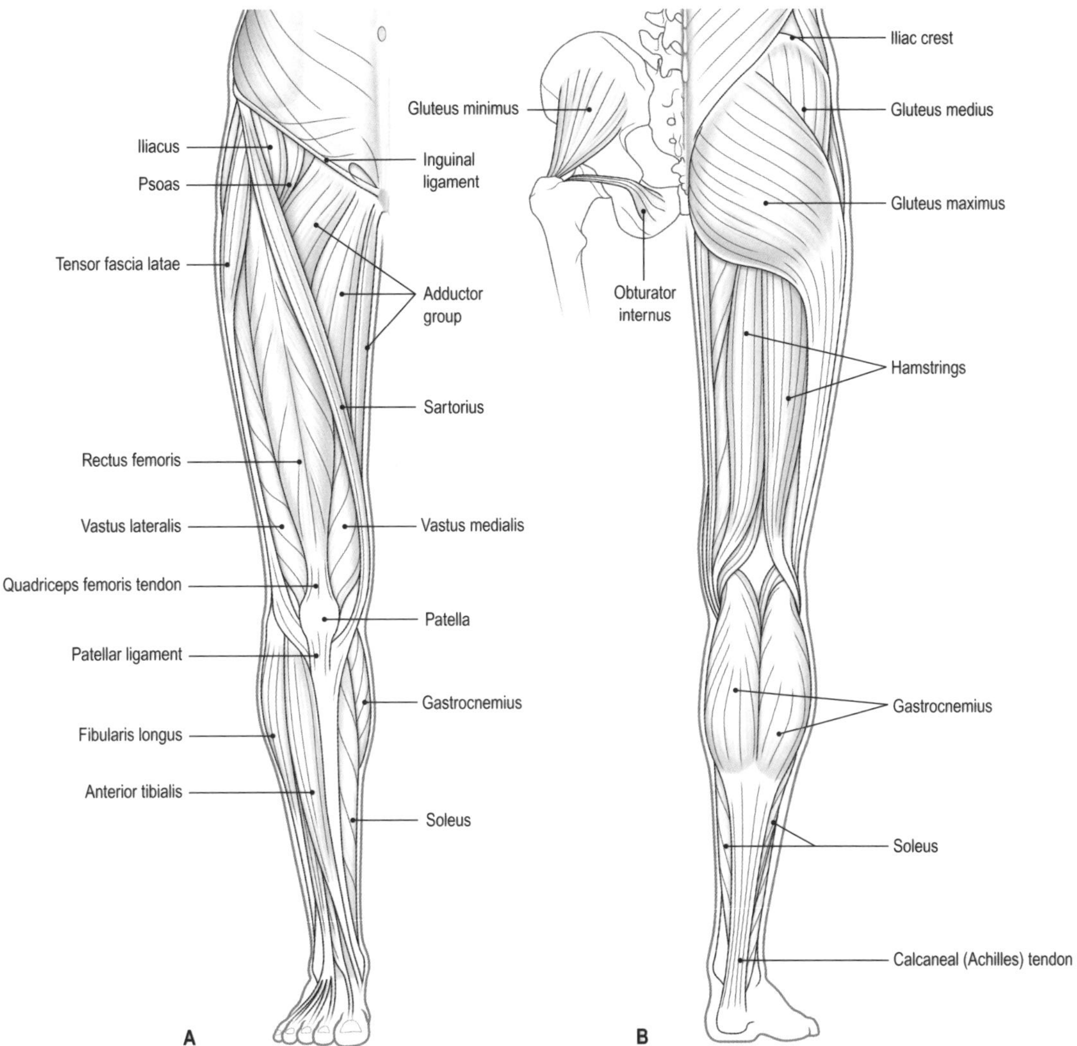

Figure 16.16

59.

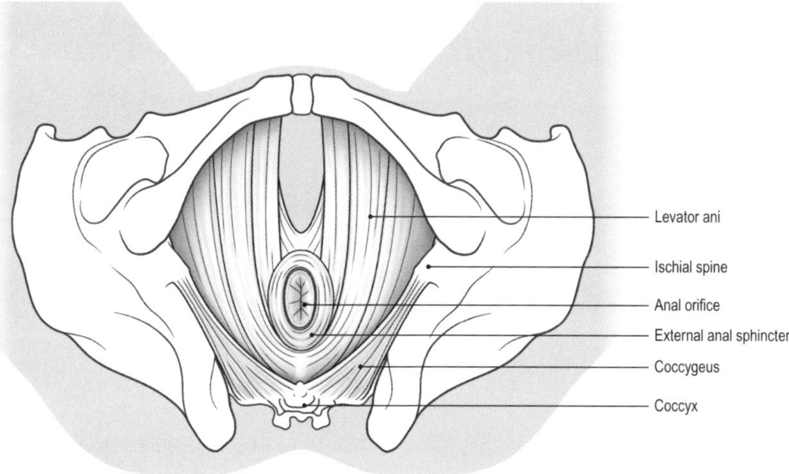

Figure 16.17

60. The functional unit of a skeletal muscle cell is the **sarcomere.** At each end of this unit are lines called **Z**-lines. Within the unit are two types of filament, thick filaments (made of **myosin**), and thin ones, made of **actin.** When the muscle cell is relaxed, these two filaments are not connected to each other. Contraction is initiated when an electrical impulse, called an **action potential**, passes along the cell membrane (also called the **sarcolemma**) of the muscle cell and penetrates deep into the sarcoplasm via the network of **channels** that run through the cell. This electrical stimulation causes **calcium** ions to be released from the **calcium stores** within the cell; these ions cause links, called **cross bridges,** to form between the thick and thin filaments. The filaments pull on each other, which causes the functional unit to **shorten** in length, pulling the **Z-lines** at either end towards one another. If enough units are stimulated to contract at the same time, the entire **muscle** will also **shorten (contract).**

61.

Table 16.4 Functions of muscles of the face and neck

Muscle	Paired/unpaired	Function
Occipitofrontalis	Unpaired	Raises the eyebrows
Levator palpebrae superioris	Paired	Raise the eyelids
Orbicularis oculi	Paired	Close the eyes and screws them up
Buccinator	Paired	Draw in the cheeks and expel air forcibly
Orbicularis oris	Unpaired	Closes the lips; involved in whistling
Masseter	Paired	Draw the mandible up to the maxilla for chewing
Temporalis	Paired	Close the mouth and involved in chewing
Pterygoid	Paired	Close the mouth and pull the lower jaw forwards
Sternocleidomastoid	Paired	Contraction of one – draws the head towards the shoulder; contraction of both – flexion of the cervical vertebrae drawing the sternum and clavicles upwards
Trapezius	Paired	Pull the head backwards, square the shoulders and control movements of the scapula when the shoulder is in use

62. Muscle work that allows the muscle to shorten, as when lifting a manageable load.

63. Muscle work when the muscle is trying to lift an immoveable load, so it cannot shorten but it develops increased tension.

64. The (usually proximal) attachment point of a muscle, which usually remains steady when the muscle contracts.

65. Two muscles that work in opposition to each other across one or more joints.

66. c, d; 67. b; 68. d; 69. c; 70. a; 71. d; 72. c

17 Introduction to genetics

Answers

1. The nucleus contains the body's **genetic** material, in the form of DNA, which is built from nucleotides, each made up of three components: a **phosphate** group, the sugar **deoxyribose** and one of four **bases.** DNA is a double strand of nucleotides that resembles a **helix**, or twisted ladder. DNA and associated proteins called **histones** are coiled together, forming a substance called **chromatin.** In preparation for cell division, the DNA becomes very tightly coiled and can be seen as **chromosomes** under the microscope. There are 23 pairs of them in most human cells. Each consists of many functional subunits called **genes.** Any given type of cell uses only part of the whole genetic code, also called the **genome**, to carry out its specific activities. Each **gene** contains the genetic code, or instructions, for the synthesis of one **protein**, that could, for example, be an **enzyme** needed to catalyse a particular chemical **reaction**, a hormone, or it may form part of the structure of a cell. The coded instructions have to be transferred to the **cytoplasm** of the cell, because that is where the organelles that make protein, the **ribosomes**, are found. DNA itself does not transfer, but a copy of the genetic code is made in the form of **mRNA**, which leaves the **nucleus.** When its instructions have been read and the new protein synthesised, the copy is destroyed.

2. All nucleated body cells, with the exception of spermatozoa and ova, contain **46** chromosomes, arranged in pairs. One chromosome of each pair is inherited from the mother and one from the father, so there are **two** copies of each gene in the cell. Two chromosomes of the same pair are called **homologues**, and the genes are present in paired sites called **alleles.**

   When the paired genes are identical, they are called **homozygous**, but if they are different forms they are called **heterozygous.** Dominant genes are always **expressed over recessive genes.** Individuals homozygous for a dominant gene **cannot** pass the recessive form on to their children, and individuals heterozygous for a gene **can** pass on either form of the gene to theirs.

3. and 4.

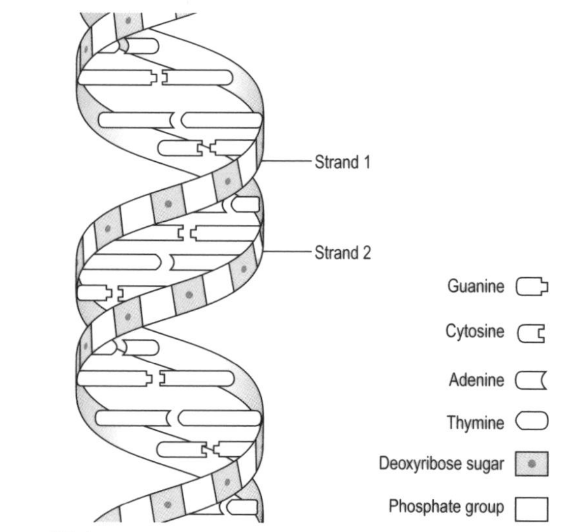

Figure 17.1

5.

Table 17.1 The DNA code

DNA Strand 1	C	C	G	T	A	A	C	T	C	A	A	T	G	T
DNA Strand 2	G	G	C	A	T	T	G	A	G	T	T	A	C	A
mRNA	G	G	C	A	U	U	G	A	G	U	U	A	C	A

6. b, d, g and h are true.
   a. Translation takes place on the ribosomes in the cytoplasm.
   c. A codon is a piece of RNA carrying information.
   e. Some new proteins are made for export, e.g. insulin.
   f. Red blood cells have no nucleus, and gametes carry only half.

7.

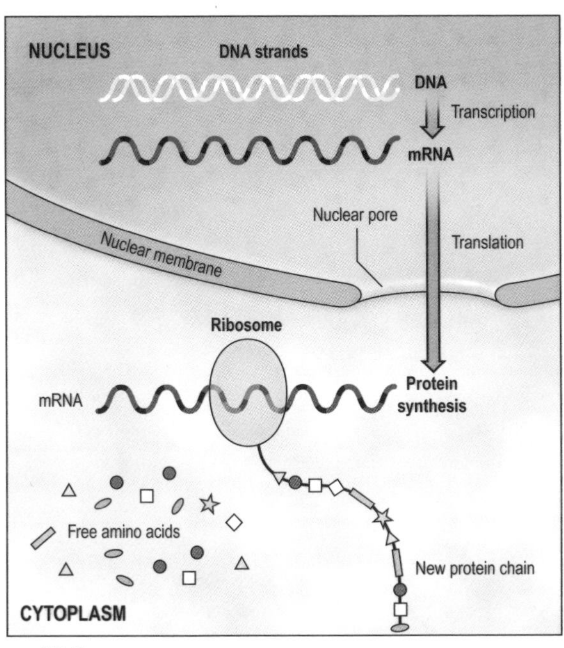

Figure 17.2

8.

Box 17.1

	T	t
T	TT	Tt
t	Tt	tt

9. TT and Tt, because they both have the dominant tongue rolling gene T.

10. TT and tt: the two copies of their genes are the same.

11.

Box 17.2

	B	B
b	Bb	Bb
b	Bb	Bb

12. None; a blue-eyed child needs two recessive b genes, one from each parent, but the father has two copies of the dominant B gene and so does not have a recessive gene to pass to his children.

13.

Box 17.3

	X^B	Y
X^b	X^BX^b	X^bY
X^b	X^BX^b	X^bY

14. 50:50.

15. 100% (both of them).

16. Carriers: they are heterozygous for the gene with one dominant, healthy gene and one recessive gene for colour blindness. Although they have normal colour vision, they can pass the recessive gene to their children.

17. c; 18. c; 19. d; 20. a; 21. b; 22. a; 23. d;
24. b; 25. d.

18 The reproductive systems

Answers

1.

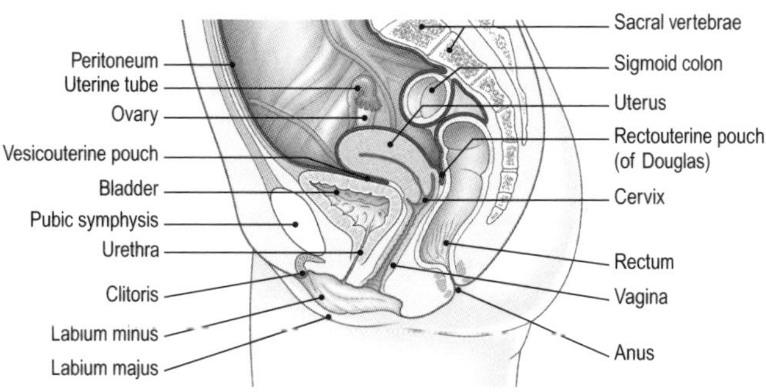

Figure 18.1

2.

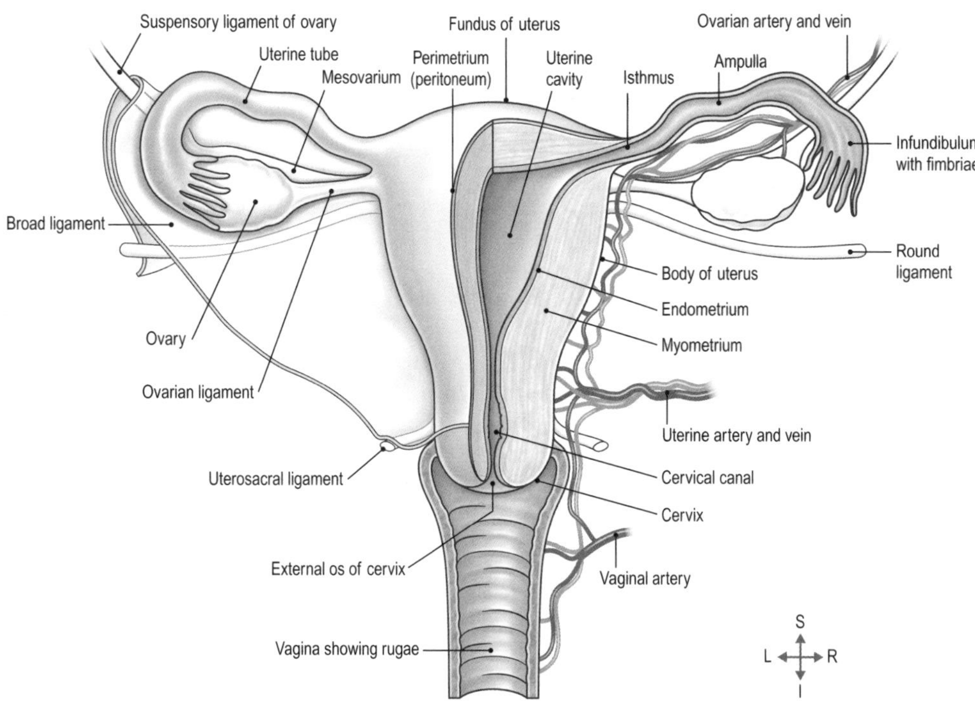

Figure 18.2

3., 4. and 5.

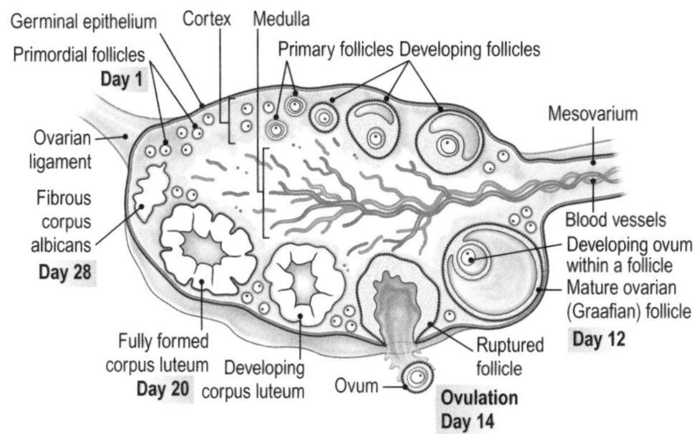

Figure 18.3

6. Oestrogen
7. See Fig. 18.3
8. Maturation of the uterus, uterine tubes and ovaries; beginning of the menstrual cycle; development of the breasts; growth of pubic and axillary hair; increase in body height and pelvic width; deposition of subcutaneous fat, especially at hips and breasts.

9. and 10.

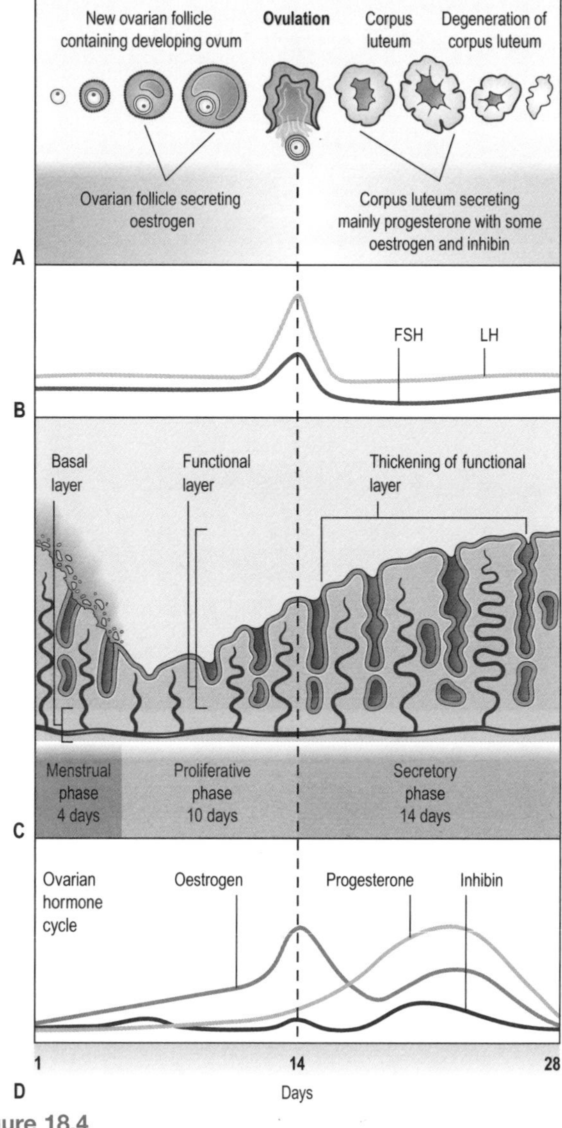

Figure 18.4

11. Anterior pituitary
12. Ovulation (event E) is triggered by the mid-cycle surge in LH, which in turn is triggered by rising oestrogen levels.
13. and 14. See Fig. 18.4
15. Inhibin, with oestrogen and progesterone, suppresses the hypothalamus and pituitary in the second half of the cycle to prevent maturation and release of another ovum.
16. Oestrogen and progesterone are synthesised by the corpus luteum in the second half of the cycle. If pregnancy does not occur, this structure begins to degenerate and so levels of these hormones fall.
17. If pregnancy occurs, the developing embryo secretes human chorionic gonadotrophin (hCG) which maintains the corpus luteum for the first 3–4 months of pregnancy, during which time the oestrogen and progesterone it secretes supports the pregnancy. After this time, the placenta is developed enough to be secreting adequate levels of these hormones and takes over this role from the corpus luteum.
18. Blastocyst: f, i, m; Embryo: n; Trophoblast: c; Gestation: l; Fetus: g, j, k; Zygote: h, i.

19.

Table 18.1 The effect of hormones on the breast

Statement	Hormone(s)
Stimulates body growth and development in puberty	Oestrogen and progesterone
Initiates release of milk	Oxytocin
Stimulates production of milk	Prolactin
Stimulates growth and development in pregnancy	Oestrogen and progesterone

20. c; 21. c, d; 22. a; 23. c; 24. c; 25. b;

26. d; 27. d

28.

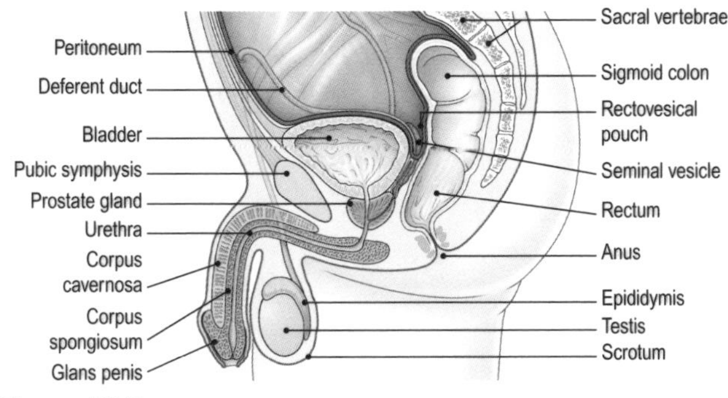

Figure 18.5

29.

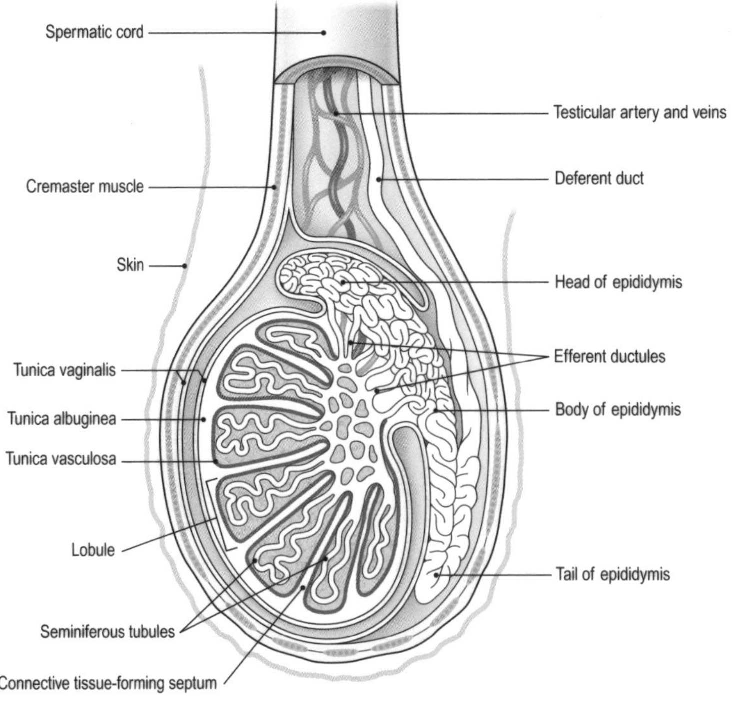

Figure 18.6

30. b; 31. d; 32. c; 33. a